Canceling Appointment with Death:

COVID-19 PANDEMIC

Using Divine Missile Defense System against
Invisible Global Weapon of Mass Destruction

How COVID-19 Changed the World
What to do During Future Pandemics
True Life Stories of COVID-19 Survivors

AKINTAYO EMMANUEL

ISBN 978-1-63874-421-4 (paperback)
ISBN 978-1-63903-912-8 (hardcover)
ISBN 978-1-63874-422-1 (digital)

Christian Faith Publishing, Inc.
832 Park Avenue
Meadville, PA 16335
www.christianfaithpublishing.com

Printed in the United States of America

To my Redeemer and the Redeemer of my family,
our Savior, Lord, and King whom we know
intimately as "the Resurrection and the Life."

CONTENTS

ACKNOWLEDGMENTS

In all aspects of life, the beauty and breadth of God's wisdom have made it impossible for man to do justice to the burgeoning theological discourse that surrounds God's Resurrection life that terminates all appointments with death. This makes me express my appreciation to my biological parents, Honorable Claudius and Mrs. Elizabeth Brown, for their words of encouragement. They reminded me of the critical events that occurred in my childhood. Their words of encouragement and love have been a blessing and source of inspiration to me. My dad and mom testified that the divine mandate of God upon life is my paternal grandmother's answered prayers.

I am exceptionally and eternally grateful for the life of my father in the Lord, Pastor Enoch Adeboye, whose walk with and for the Lord has been a source of inspiration to me. I also want to bless the Lord for Daddy (Bishop) David Oyedepo who has imparted unto me the spirit of faith from a spiritual father-son platform that enables the recipient to believe God for the impossible and to experience the incredible. The proofs of a vital and real father-son relationship are intrinsically evident.

My children have sacrificed the time that was rightfully theirs for the sake of this research and in conjunction with my very busy workload and tasking schedule without complaint. I am exceptionally thankful to God for their precious lives, and I owe everything to God for the perfect and good gifts that my bright and morning star children are to me and this world.

I cannot adequately express my gratitude to my sweetest sweetheart, the bone of my bone, and flesh of my flesh. She is my best friend, editor (a difficult and often thankless task), helper, and the only one that knows and understands me without explanation. She is the glorious mother of our children. We have all flourished together like a palm tree in the courts of our God as lovers. My children and I bless the Lord for her tenacity and passion for the Lord. Our family exists to become like Jesus Christ and to fulfill "*missio dei.*"

Finally, I am humbled to be loved and saved by our merciful and gracious God, our High Priest after the order of Melchizedek. I am highly honored that He chose me among many to proclaim His Word and to advance His kingdom in and through me. He has whispered to other true apostles and prophets and to me confirming that I am one of His beloved sons in whom He is well pleased.

I pray for all those who have confessed Jesus Christ as their Savior, Lord, and King and that we will all allow the Holy Spirit to complete the work He has started in our lives. I pray that God's perfect will, plan, and purpose will be fulfilled in our lives as we keep His commandments of love without spots and remain unrebukable until the appearing of our Lord Jesus Christ who is the only blessed Potentate, King of kings, and Lord of lords; the only one who hath immortality, dwelling in the light which no man can approach unto whom no man hath seen, nor can see, and to Him alone be honor and power everlasting. Amen (1 Tim. 6:14–16).

Bene est anima nostra (It is well with our soul)*!*

PREFACE

Writing this book, *Cancelling Appointment with Death*, in an unprecedented time when the world is under siege by the COVID-19 global pandemic is thought-provoking. During this time, some have discovered much about Jesus Christ. He is the resurrection and life, while many are questioning the perfect nature of the Almighty God and His glorious character. What is God saying during this pandemic? And who is truly at fault?

The COVID-19 global pandemic stunned the year 2020, revealing how unprepared, fragile, and incapable we are as individuals and as a global community. This pandemic has enacted a global shift, impacting our approach to life and death. However, the immutability of God's eternal life, His resurrection, and transfiguration power remain eternally steadfast and sure.

I have been humbled by the challenges of putting together these helpful insights into words, not only for this time but for the years to come. Some of the issues addressed in this book require sober musings and result-oriented actions. I launch into significant areas that are yet to be fully explored. It was only the mercy and grace of God that enabled me to dive into uncharted and unpopular topics in this book, despite limitations caused by this global crisis.

There is no new revelation in much of what I wrote in this book since there is no new thing under the earth. I am only standing on the shoulders of people who genuinely love the Lord, men of great faith, skill, and passion who have covered much on overcoming the fear of death. No one book can cover all issues surrounding cancelling appointments with death or spiritual weapons of mass destruction because the subject is broad, but the all-knowing and the only wise God has all the answers. Even though all of your theological questions might not be answered in this book, I am glad that others have done extensive work on some of the topics in this book, and my knowledge has been broadened through their research.

There are additional components that could have been integrated but were intentionally left out. Sometimes it is much easier to leave some things unsaid and only highlight the most needful areas. I have attempted to provide balanced information in the book, taking into consideration both the theological aspect as well as what the scientists, contemporaries, and market people are rationalizing. I have intentionally embraced other people's perspectives and discoveries and contextualized theologically through the present neo-generational lenses to restore hope to the hopeless. I have cited those who might not be on the same theological plane or beliefs as Christians because I believe they will also find answers in Jesus Christ who is the only solution to all difficult life situations.

I am trusting that this book will assist you in fulfilling your life goals in joy and peace and provide assistance in your spiritual journey. You are called to live and not die and to be satisfied with long life as you declare the works of God in the land of the living. I desire to be practical yet give you the basics of what it takes to cancel every appointment with death from God's Word.

In times like this, we all need to stop, reflect, repent, and ponder upon the love and mercy of God. The storms of life and the toughest of times have been designed for us to humble ourselves before God, the Most High, turn from our wicked ways, and seek His divine assistance. The Good News Translation of Psalms 119:71 declares, "My punishment was good for me because it made me, learn your commands."

The New Living Translations says, "My suffering was good for me, for it taught me to pay attention to your decrees."

We must learn so much through COVID-19 lockdowns and be humbled while going through its desert phase more than when we have the comfort of the greener pastures of ease and freedom. Many who have previously given up on praying have started to pray again. Those going through spiritual lethargy have been awakened out of slumber into a closer relationship with the Lord Jesus Christ. Those that have drifted away have come back to God during this crisis.

This is the time for us to begin to live the crucified life by the faith of the Son of the living God. Storms do come to everyone, but only those who have ears to hear and are committed to doing the Word of God will remain in faith. The Lord will not prevent us from being thrown into the lion's den, but He will send His angels ahead to shut the mouth of the lions; neither will He keep us from being thrown into the fiery furnace of life, but He will ensure that not even a single hair on our head is burned. We are to pass through waters as in Noah's flood, the Red Sea, and the River Jordan but never to be drowned by them (Isa. 43:2).

It is time to live by the faith of the son of God who loves us and gave Himself for us. We must progress from faith to faith during any trying times, and in the end, we will come out greater, stronger, more powerful, and impactful. Remember, death and life are in the power of our tongues. Death and life have been set before us, and we are admonished by God to choose life so that we and our children can live (Deut. 30:19; Prov. 18:21).

In this book, I have endeavored to help all the readers embrace a different methodology of how we perceive the love of God during and post-COVID-19 pandemic from a biblical context, how we are to conduct ourselves in any future pandemic, how we can recover from this present pandemic, and the primary mission of the church who is the salt and light of the world.

My prayer is that you will find encouragement, hope, love, strength, and practical help during this global pandemic and in a post-COVID-19 world.

INTRODUCTION

The year 2020 was marked by a coronavirus pandemic that spread to every corner of the globe, forcing border closures, stay-at-home orders, and triggering a global economic downturn. This deadly coronavirus (COVID-19) pandemic is one of many things the Lord Jesus Christ instructed Christians to look out for before His second return. Jesus Christ declares in Matthew 24:7, "For nation shall rise against nation, and kingdom against kingdom: and there shall be famines, and pestilences, and earthquakes, in divers' places."[1]

Nearly four billion people, which is more than half the world's population, are on some form of stay at home governmental orders. We have become the subjects in this grand experiment of global quarantine. None have experienced the specific details of the challenges ahead—nations' battles with disruption of work, lockdowns, flattening the curve, first and second wave, etc.

The advent of coronavirus has brought into our space new normal, now normal, and new vocabulary. From social distancing to regular use of protective face masks, mass temperature checks, monitoring of cellphone locations, and other personal information, new happenings with new adjustments can best be called the new normal. There are floor plans that make distancing conducive. The educational environment has become very different from what it used to be. Measures are being put in place to increase sanitization, deep cleaning, adjust school assemblies, physical education, and recess should the schools be allowed to open at the beginning of the 2020/2021 school year.

---

[1] Unless otherwise noted, all biblical passages referenced are in the King James Version (Nashville, TN Broadman & Holman, 1996).

Our national leaders have urged everyone to practice social distancing, which could have seriously led to social isolation from families and friends, if not for technology. Social distancing increases the physical space between people to avoid the spread of the illness. It means staying at least six feet away from other people, which lessens the chance of catching COVID-19.

Jeff Green connotes that COVID-19 will be remembered as the disease that divided and split us. He observed that the pandemic affects some groups more than others, stirring up a toxic mix of fear, resentment, and schadenfreude. Additionally, he cited Jason Beckfield who narrated that the dividing is a function of what people are choosing to do with the virus since people can shift blame away from themselves or shift blame onto people they dislike.[2]

Fear, stress, and worry are already combating many people. COVID-19 has made the world's inhabitants search for answers, true light, and hope for the hopeless. Many are searching for the light at the end of the tunnel and are finding that their usual heroes cannot get them out of this mess. Technology, Hollywood, actors and actresses, world governments, and scientists have failed to deliver the prompt answer, and many are finally beginning to realize we need God, the Father of our Lord Jesus Christ, more than ever.

Robert Redfield restated that global health officials have repeatedly warned of the rise of bacteria and other microbes resistant to most available drugs, raising the specter of untreatable infectious diseases that could spread rapidly.[3]

Antibiotic-resistant bacterial infection and viruses are just among many agents of the last enemy that shall be destroyed, ushering us into a future when we will never need antibiotics or vaccines again. There will indeed be a post-antibiotic and vaccine era

---

[2] Jeff Green, "COVID-19 Is Becoming the Disease That Divides Us: By Race, Class and Age." Bloomberg Business, 2020, Accessed April 29, 2020, https://www.bloomberg.com/news/articles/2020-03-21/covid-19-divides-u-s-society-by-race-class-and-age.

[3] Whitcomb 11/14, KHN Morning Briefing, 2019, Accessed April 14, 2020, https://khn.org/morning-breakout/the-post-antibiotic-era-isnt-coming-its-already-here-startling-report-reveals-scope-of-superbug-crisis/.

made available to us through faith in Christ Jesus. Paul elucidated in 1 Corinthian 15:26, "The last enemy that will be destroyed is death," and obedience to the command of our Creator is the only thing that triggers heaven's release of God's divine missile defense systems that will destroy every invisible pandemic global weapons of mass destruction.

While most nations have been traumatized by COVID-19, including those who are not infected, many have experienced overwhelming fear, emotional heaviness, hyper-vigilance trauma, and a general worldwide state of trauma because of the pandemic and its negative impact on their lives and the world's economy. On the other side of the coin, it has brought togetherness, a reassuring touch, effective communication, and an anxious need to talk to someone. Some can integrate mental health steps that deal with trauma and take the lead in prayer that heals and makes men rise above the traumas it brings.

Sanya Penili indicated that touch heals, and an increasing amount of evidence suggests that touch has more power than we could ever imagine. She suggested some benefits of healing by touch therapy, including pain and stress relief, faster recovery and mobility after surgery, a strengthened immune system, a more profound spiritual connection, and reduced trauma and chronic pain.[4] She added that there is now evidence that touch may affect the brain as well and that it has been discovered through long-standing evidence that touch is so deeply a part of being human that does affect our physical, social, and psychological well-being and that it has been found to help in kids' physiological and neurological development to decrease anxiety and deepen bonding.[5]

Children who need at least a hundred touches every day are being deprived of touch because they live in the new climate of "no touching." We are starving our innate God-designed need for touch

---

[4] Sanya Penili, "Science & Wellness: How the Power of Touch Helps Kids Thrive," Parent Co., 2017, Accessed April 30, 2020, https://www.parent.com/how-the-power-of-touch-helps-kids-thrive/.

[5] Ibid.

that our heavenly Father has provided for healing and refreshing the wounded, fatigued, and heartbroken. The result of the touch of Jesus Christ to humanity can be seen in Matthew 8:3, 15, 9:20, 29, 14:36, 17:7, and 20:34. He is always touched with the feelings of our infirmities (Hebrews 4:15).

With the onset of COVID-19, some have turned from false gods to the God of heaven and earth. Stadiums have been closed down, civic centers shut down, and all major concerts have been canceled. Theaters have been shuttered with no new films forthcoming, and lovers of money already are experiencing a downward spiral movement of the stock market. This single virus attack has exposed man's arrogance against God and futile attempts to claim authority over the earth. This is another confirmation that the enormous resources spent on manufacturing weapons of mass destruction that could not deliver humankind in the day of trouble might have been directed toward providing global resources to solve the devastating problem of poverty, underdevelopment, and hunger worldwide.

The United States, China, Russia, Great Britain, Italy, Spain, France, and many other nations have not deployed any weapon against COVID-19. None have been able to go out and confront the virus head-on at any battlefield. Instead, they shut down their borders, markets, schools, and sports arenas in dread of this invisible world destroyer, and the so-called mighty nations, G7, G20, NATO, EU, UN Security Council, and WHO have not developed solutions that will protect the people against this virus. However, they are relentlessly working to produce a vaccine against this pandemic.

Richard Burns highlighted that the development of ballistic missiles by Nazi Germany launched the United States on a quest to defeat the then new weaponry. He cited American's first Secretary of Defense, James Forrestal, who maintained that history has shown that all new weapons always develop a countermeasure, beginning with what the Romans developed to counter Hannibal's use of elephants. Burns rationalized that President George Bush's decision to proceed with the deployment of antiballistic missile defensive systems in 2002 was the culmination of a series of increasingly partisan political controversies that reached back to the1950s.[6]

Similarly, the Almighty God has numerous and invisible spiritual missile defense systems that can be activated through fasting, prayer, and doing God's Word to counterattack any invisible lethal bacteria and viruses in forms of missiles sent to destabilize the world.

Paul stated in 2 Corinthians 10:4–6:

> For the weapons of our warfare are not carnal, but mighty through God to the pulling down of strongholds. Casting down imaginations, and every high thing that exalteth itself against the knowledge of God and bringing into captivity every thought to the obedience of Christ; And having in a readiness to revenge all disobedience, when your obedience is fulfilled.

Has this pandemic made you doubt God's Word, love, and care? Are you wondering how the story will end? Have you lost every hope? I want to remind you that the *Lord* sees everything, and *He* has it all in control. He hears our prayers and the cries of our hearts. He understands how big this situation is, and He is touched with the feeling of our infirmities and has provided a way out of this pandemic. We are never alone. God who is our refuge and strength is bigger than this COVID-19 and all other future pandemics.

Are you brokenhearted? Remember that God uses broken things beautifully. He uses broken clouds to pour out rain. He uses broken sets of soil as fields. He uses broken fruit crops to produce seeds. God uses broken seeds to give life to new plants, and so when you feel broken by COVID-19, rest assured that God will use it to produce something beautiful and worth praising Him in our lives. We must be ever ready and alert for a new heaven and earth that Isaiah prophesied in Isaiah 65:17, "For, behold, create new heavens

---

6   Richard D. Burns, *The Missile Defense Systems of George W. Bush: A Critical Assessment* (Santa Barbara, CA: ABC-CLIO, 2010), 1–2.

and a new earth: and the former shall not be remembered, nor come into mind."

Apostle John caught a glimpse of this new heaven and earth on the Island of Patmos as recorded in Revelation 21:1, 4:

> And I saw a new heaven and a new earth: for the first heaven and the first earth were passed away; and there was no more sea
>
> [A]nd God shall wipe away all tears from their eyes; and there shall be no more death, neither sorrow, nor crying, neither shall there be any more pain: for the former things are passed away.

It is the raw will of God that we destroy by the power of the Holy Spirit this last enemy called "death" by putting it under the feet of the body of Christ before the Lord Jesus returns at the close of this age. David declares in Psalms 110:1–2, "The LORD said unto my Lord, sit thou at my right hand until I make thine enemies thy footstool. The LORD shall send the rod of thy strength out of Zion: rule thou in the midst of thine enemies."

The Church of Jesus Christ must walk out of every harassment and intimidation of death into eternal life in an abundant measure. Those who have been appointed to death must cancel all such appointments right now by the power of the Holy Spirit in the precious name of Jesus Christ. It is time to not only walk in the light but become the light of the world. Nothing shatters darkness like the light. The Word of God declares in Hosea 4:6, "My people are destroyed for lack of knowledge," but the light of God shines in darkness even over death, and the darkness can never comprehend it (John 1:5).

CHAPTER 1

Death Is a Personality

Death and hell are spirit personalities (Rev. 6:8, 20:13) that will be cast into the lake of fire. The Bible declares, "And death and hell were cast into the lake of fire. This is the second death. And whosoever was not found written in the book of life was cast into the lake of fire" (Rev. 20:14–15). Death is both spiritual and physical. Physical death is the exit of the human spirit from the physical body. The book of James 2:26 states, "For as the body without the spirit is dead, so faith without works is dead also." Spiritual death is separation from God and so from the power of His eternal life.

When Adam sinned in the Garden of Eden, he died first spiritually and later died physically (Gen. 2:17, 5:5). When he died spiritually and was separated from God's life, faith became distorted to fear; light (wisdom, understanding, and revelation of God's Word) became distorted to darkness (foolishness and ignorance); righteousness became distorted to sin; health to sickness; prosperity to poverty because the force of eternal life that God placed inside man to maintain what God had created to be good was no longer in force because of man's separation from God.

Immediately after the sin of Adam, life was absent, which is death, just as the absence of light is darkness, absence of righteousness is sin, absence of knowledge is foolishness, absence of healing is sickness, absence of peace is conflict, and the absence of prosperity is poverty. Ultimately, the distortion in the physical body caused it gradually to grow older and weaker to the point where it could no longer be suitable for the human spirit to inhabit. Then the man died physically when the human spirit departs from the human body.

There is no experience in life so generally dreaded as death. No one wants to confront death; everyone wants to avoid it. However, the fact remains that death is very real, and being caught to meet the Lord in the air (known as rapture) is also very real. The birth of man is celebrated as is marriage, and finally, death or being caught up to meet Jesus Christ in the air. The epitaph of all generations is: "He was born; he lived; he died, or it shall be said one day about the overcomer that he was caught up to meet the Lord in the air."

All the efforts of science to increase human life spans, the consummation of civilizations, the endeavors to build a better world, and all the joys and sorrows of billions of individuals that eternity alone possesses can be summarized inside these following three scriptural accounts.

Genesis 2:17 states, "In the day that thou eatest thereof thou shalt surely die."

Also, 1 Thessalonians 4:16–18 connotes Christians that are alive and remain at the Second Coming of our Lord Jesus Christ as being caught up to meet Him in the air when He descends for the saint:

> For the Lord, himself shall descend from heaven with a shout, with the voice of the archangel, and with the trump of God: and the dead in Christ shall rise first: Then we which are alive and remain shall be caught up together with them in the clouds, to meet the Lord in the air: and so shall we ever be with the Lord. Wherefore comfort one another with these words.

The book of Revelation 21:4 states, "There shall be no more death." Actually, that which men call "death," God calls it "birth."

Paul elucidated in 1 Corinthians 5:6 and Philippians 1:21–24:

> Therefore we are always confident, knowing that, whilst we are at home in the body, we are absent from the Lord.
>
> For to me to live is Christ, and to die is gain. But if I live in the flesh, this is the fruit of my labor, yet what I shall choose I wot not. For I am in a strait betwixt two, having a desire to depart, and to be with Christ; which is far better: Nevertheless, to abide in the flesh is more needful for you.

Paul, speaking by the revelation of God, substantiated this truth by explaining that to be absent in the body as a child of God (known as death to man) is to be present with the Lord (ultimate birth in God's presence). There is a movement from one world to the other. The baby begins life and existence in the matrix of the womb. However, after nine months, the baby dies to everything in the womb and is born into another world, and later on, when the baby, "now ninety years old or a hundred and twenty years old," depending on the lifetime of the baby, now a matured individual after being redeemed by the blood of Jesus Christ, will also die to this world to be born (birth) or enter into an eternal world in God's presence. As God's people, even though we have been birthed physically, we are still birth spiritually, emotionally, and experientially going from strength to strength, faith to faith, and glory to glory. Therefore, we must never give up on ourselves or our God-given dreams, even though there could be some stretch marks, pain, nausea, or sickness along the way.

As of December 23, 2020, the Institute for Health Metrics and Evaluation estimated 561,669 COVID-19 deaths in America by April 2021 based on current projection scenario. Testing supplies have been inadequate around the world, and the US Centers for Disease Control and Prevention says about 25 percent of people infected with the virus may exhibit no symptoms at all. The practice of social distancing by avoiding nonessential travel, telecommuting, homeschooling, and staying at least six feet away from other people outside the home has become the new normal.

According to the Centers for Disease Control and Prevention (CDC), the novel coronavirus is a new coronavirus that has not been previously identified. In the 2019 (COVID-19), the virus causing coronavirus disease was not the same as the coronaviruses that commonly circulate among humans and cause mild illnesses, like the common cold. The CDC stated that the diagnosis of coronavirus 229E, NL63, OC43, or HKU1 is not the same as a COVID-19 diagnosis. Patients with COVID-19 are being evaluated and cared for differently than patients with common coronavirus diagnoses.

CDC documented that on February 11, 2020, the World Health Organization (WHO) announced an official name for this disease that has caused the 2019 novel coronavirus outbreak first identified in Wuhan, China. The new name for this disease was coronavirus 2019, abbreviated as COVID-19. In analyzing the word *COVID-19*, "CO" stands for "corona," "VI" for "virus," and "D" for disease. Formerly, this disease was referred to as the "2019 novel coronavirus" or "2019-nCoV." The CDC elucidated that there are many types of human coronaviruses, including some that commonly cause mild upper-respiratory tract illnesses, but COVID-19 is a new disease caused by a novel (or new) coronavirus that has never been seen in humans. The name of this disease was selected following the World Health Organization (WHO) best practice for new human infectious diseases.[7]

The Spanish flu 1918 pandemic (H1N1 virus) with the avian origin gene was the most severe in recent history. Jeffrey Taubenberger and David Morenst stated that the Spanish flu infected and caused symptoms in as much as five hundred million people worldwide and spread over two years. They explained that the Spanish flu sickened almost one-third of the entire world's population, and the total death

---

[7] Center for Disease Control and Prevention, 2020, Accessed April 14, 2020, https://www.cdc.gov/coronavirus/2019-ncov/faq.html#Coronavirus-Disease-2019-Basics.

from this flu (without one single gunshot) was estimated to be fifty to a hundred million, rivaling the total death toll of World War II.[8]

Taubenberger and Morenst state:

> Even with modern antiviral and antibacterial drugs, vaccines, and prevention knowledge, the return of a pandemic virus equivalent in pathogenicity to the virus of 1918 would likely kill more than 100 million people worldwide. A pandemic virus with the (alleged) pathogenic potential of some recent H5N1 outbreaks could cause substantially more deaths.[9]

They ascertained while answering the question of whether the 1918 pandemic could appear again, and if so, what could be done about it? They explained that until we can determine the factors that gave rise to the 1918 pandemic mortality patterns and learn about its formation, all predictions are only educated guesses. They stated that we could only conclude that analogous conditions could lead to an equally devastating pandemic since it happened once.[10]

This substantiated the likelihoods that the conditions of the world right now are ripe for an even worse outbreak than the Spanish flu because of an increasing and unprecedented world population that is approaching about eight billion according to the pew research center, with overcrowding in urban areas in countries such as China and India and largely throughout the world.[11] This situation cou-

---

[8] Jeffrey K. Taubenberger and David M. Morenst, "1918 Influenza: The Mother of All Pandemics, Emerging Infectious Diseases," www.cdc.gov/edi 12:1, 2006, Accessed April 14, 2020, https://www.researchgate.net/publication/31591640_1918_Influenza_The_mother_of_all_pandemics.

[9] Ibid., 21.

[10] Ibid., 20.

[11] Anthony Cilluffo and Neil Ruiz, "World's Population Is Projected to Nearly Stop Growing by the End of the Century," Pew Research Center. Fact Tank: News in Numbers, 2019, Accessed, April 15, 2020, https://www.pewresearch.org/fact-tank/2019/06/17/worlds-population-is-projected-to-nearly-stop-growing-by-the-end-of-the-century/.

pled with poor sanitation conditions in many countries is resulting a global village characterized by ease and air travel prevalence. The stage is now set for the world to continuously accommodate highly contagious diseases that can spread faster than ever before in human history. But how battle-ready are the nations prepared to quickly produce a miracle vaccine that can stop or minimize a plague of such magnitude?

Kevin Brown enumerated on the first modern antibiotic, penicillin, that was discovered in 1928 by Sir Alexander Fleming, a Scottish bacteriologist who was put into medical use from 1942. This was hailed as a modern miracle, and its effectiveness against bacterial infections was seen as an unprecedented triumph of science. Fleming was recognized for that achievement in 1945 when he received the Nobel Prize for Physiology or Medicine along with Australian pathologist, Howard Walter Florey, and German-born British biochemist, Ernst Boris Chain, who isolated and purified penicillin.[12] However, the world has entered an era where some miracle vaccine cannot be quickly developed or will no longer prevent a new strain of viruses, thereby enabling invisible enemies to rip families and individuals apart by death.

While antibiotics are used to treat or prevent some types of bacterial infections, they cannot treat viral infections because they are not lethal to viruses just because viruses insert their genetic material into human cells' DNA to reproduce, and because of this, antibiotics have no target to attack in a virus. Robert Redfield, an American virologist and the director of CDC and administrator of the Agency for Toxic Substances and Disease Registry, states:

> I don't think anybody would disagree that, for decades, collectively, our nations underinvested in public health. Now I think people understand that can have significant conse-

---

[12] Kevin Brown, "Sir Alexander Fleming, Scottish Bacteriologist," *Encyclopedia Britannica*, 2020, Accessed April 14, 2020, https://www.britannica.com/biography/Alexander-Fleming.

quences. Furthermore, now is the time for us to overinvest, overprepare in public health. This virus is going to be with us.[13]

We are in an era where there is little hope in future vision where the world will experience a zero fight for survival against devastating, merciless, and invisible enemies. However, there is a way of escape for humanity, and that is faith in the Lord Jesus Christ and in His Word. The Bible supports this in Hosea 13:14, "I will ransom them from the power of the grave; I will redeem them from death: O death, I will be thy plagues; O grave, I will be thy destruction: repentance shall be hid from mine eyes."

The Lord Jesus Christ suffered and died to bring an end to all of humankind sufferings, including disease, contrary to the CDC dreary projection about COVID-19 that this pandemic will never stop. It is clearly stated in Isaiah 53:4–5:

> Surely he hath borne our griefs, and carried our sorrows: yet we did esteem him stricken, smitten of God, and afflicted, and He was wounded for our transgressions, He was bruised for our iniquities: the chastisement of our peace was upon Him, and with His stripes, we are healed.

The surging aimless mass of lost humanity has been impelled by fear of the dark, fear of disease, fear of the unknown, and the fear of death, but the fear of death is but the acme of all fears. Men avoid it, hate it, and fight against it. However, death will continue until that day when through the glorious power of Christ who was triumphant over death, the scroll of heaven will be rolled back, the saints of God

---

[13] Robert Redfield, "US Readiness and Latest Guidance for Coronavirus," Speech with Sam Whitehead of member station WABE, 2020, Accessed April 14, 2020, https://www.npr.org/2020/03/30/824021895/cdc-director-redfield-speaks-on-u-s-readiness-and-latest-guidance-for-coronavirus.

shall enjoy the blissful ages of eternity, and "there shall be no more death."

The COVID-19 pandemic has mandated us to admit that the classes, levels, and tiers that we spent so much effort perfecting have blinded us to the reality of who we are. It takes a virus to open our eyes that we are not as different from each other as we have always thought. For the wealthy traveling to a smaller community to escape coronavirus to avoid the pandemic, how far can we travel? And how far can we run away from the present reality?

Hillary Hoffower documented that the wealthy had left their urban dwellings behind, escaping to smaller communities that offer them the luxury of more space and access to nature as they ride out the pandemic. She narrated that some have taken refuge in their second homes, a part-time residence in the summer, while others have rented vacation homes. Furthermore, while they tend to favor some of the most traditionally popular hot spots for the rich and famous, these locales spread far and wide.

However, no matter the location, the problem remains the same as residents are disgusted about the influx of people because they are concerned that their more rural communities will not manage a coronavirus outbreak with medical supply shortages, less access to food groceries, and stretched hospitals.[14]

The good news is that Jesus had swallowed up death in victory, so it is not a matter of fleeing from death or going to a more secure destination. Death and hell are spirit personalities (Rev. 6:8, 20:13–14) that are present in one form or the other everywhere on earth. Jesus Christ has the keys of death and hell (Rev. 1:18). Moreover, when you have these keys, you have the authority and dominion. You can open and close, and you can close and open. You determine those who go in and go out, and Jesus has given us these keys so we

---

[14] Hillary Hoffower, "Rich Urbanites Are Fleeing Big Cities and Draining Resources in Smaller, More Remote Vacation Spots. Here's Where They're Going," *Business Insider*, 2020, Accessed May 2, 2020, https://www.businessinsider.com/wealthy-fled-big-cities-vacation-homes-during-coronavirus-pandemic-2020-4.

can walk in His authority and dominion. You can cancel all appointments with death with the revelation knowledge of God, which is the key. As the book of Luke 11:52 states, "Woe unto you, lawyers! for ye have taken away the key of knowledge: ye entered not in yourselves and them that were entering in ye hindered."

Now, by the power of the resurrection of the Lord Jesus, man's connection with God is restored when we turn our lives over to God and are born again and thereby make man experience the inflow of the divine life into man's spirits, souls (wills, minds, and emotions), and bodies, which will enable him to reverse the distortions that have been caused by spiritual death; that is, separation from God.

The book of 1 Peter 1:3 states, "Blessed be the God and Father of our Lord Jesus Christ, which according to his abundant mercy hath begotten us again unto a lively hope by the resurrection of Jesus Christ from the dead." This reversal of spiritual death and its debilitating effects is what is called the destruction of death. Paul explains in Romans 8:11, "But if the Spirit of him that raised up Jesus from the dead dwell in you, he that raised up Christ from the dead shall also quicken your mortal bodies by his Spirit that dwelleth in you."

Death is the last enemy that must be conquered by God's last days people. All enemies must be placed under the feet of Jesus Christ before the return of our Lord Jesus, including the last enemy, which is death. Jesus declares in Matthew 22:44, "The Lord said unto my Lord, sit thou on my right hand, till I make thine enemies thy footstool?"

While death is no longer to be feared by the Christian, death itself is an enemy. It is a penalty. It brings grief and misery. However, in a higher sense, since Jesus has "abolished death and hath brought life and immortality to light through the Gospel," then every appointment with death must be canceled by God's people. The spirit of death operated by the law of sin and death (Rom. 8:1) is governed by the enemy through sin to exterminate human life on the earth. Paul described death as "the last enemy" with a horrific sting like that of an adder, and Jesus wept as He stood, sorrowing at the death of Lazarus.

The Bible declares:

> Let the sighing of the prisoner come before thee; according to the greatness of thy power preserve thou those that are appointed to die.
>
> [T]o hear the groaning of the prisoner; to loose those that are appointed to death. (Ps. 79:11, 102:20)

Death is in all ramifications. The physical death or emotional death could shut down the emotion and make the person indifferent and numb to feelings. Relational death, such as divorce, family, or friendship breakups, could bring the relationship to a dead end. Social death could result in loss of influence, reputation, or even life imprisonment. Financial death can be caused by failure to perceive opportunities or plague, such as COVID-19, which can destroy national economies. However, the most severe of all these is spiritual death, which is separation from God in this life and throughout eternity, and it is called eternal death.

There is a tendency for many people to avoid any severe thought or discussion on death, but it is just as natural to die as it is to be born. The Bible says, "What man is he that liveth, and shall not see death" (Psalm 89:48)?

> Man, that is born of a woman is of few days, and full of trouble. He cometh forth like a flower, and is cut down; he fleeth also as a shadow, and continueth not.
>
> His days are determined, the number of his months are with thee, thou have appointed his bounds that he cannot pass.
>
> If a man die, shall he live again all the days of my appointed time will I wait, till my change come. (Job 14:1, 2, 5, 14)

Death and the future state are by their very nature mysteries that cannot be solved apart from the revelation that has been given in the Bible. At death, your body will be placed in a grave, and it will decay back to the dust of the earth and await the resurrection morning. At death, the soul of the Christian will immediately pass into glory. The body returns to the dust of the earth.

The angels will carry the soul of one who is a Christian into God's heaven above. According to the Holy Scriptures, the soul of one who has never been born anew by faith in Jesus Christ will suffer torment in hell. There is undoubtedly the death of the righteous, and John Wesley was once asked, "If you knew you would die at midnight tomorrow, how would you spend the intervening time?"

He responded, "Why, I would spend it just as I intend to spend it. I would preach tonight at Gloucester and again tomorrow evening. I would then repair to my friend's house as he expects me. I would converse and pray with the family, retire to my room about 10 o'clock, commend myself to my heavenly Father, lie down to sleep, and wake up in glory."[15]

The Entrance of Death into the World

Death has never been part of God's creation. He never even wanted any of His children to die. His plan was for them to live in His goodness and blessings forever. He wanted everything to be well with them. He wanted them to enjoy a life without stress or strain in an environment full of everything good and excellence. His plan was and still is to make a man walk in the fullness of God's blessings.

The first time that death was mentioned in the Bible was when God warned Adam and Eve about the consequence of disobeying His command, and through their disobedience, death was introduced into the world. However, before then, Adam was enjoying blissful communion with God. He was a stranger to the subject of

---

[15] Loraine Boettner, *Immortality* (Phillipsburg, NJ: Presbyterian and Reformed Publishing Company, 1956), 36.

death until he heard about the consequence of sin, which was death from God. Adam knew that to obey God would mean continuous and unending life, and to disobey him would bring the sentence of death. The power of choice and the right to decide was now left with man.

> And the LORD God commanded the man, saying, of every tree of the garden thou mayest freely eat: but of the tree of the knowledge of good and evil, thou shalt not eat of it: for in the day that thou eatest thereof thou shalt surely die. (Gen. 2:16–17)

However, Satan would not allow the situation to go unchallenged. Though he provoked and tempted Eve, he could not force her to eat the fruit. Both she and her husband partook of it by their own choice, and in so doing, they experienced the displeasure of God, and God, holy and righteous in all His judgments, passed the sentence of death to them as he has earlier instructed. The Bible stressed that the wages of sin is death, and the gift of God is eternal life through Jesus Christ our Lord (Rom. 6:23).

Immediately, Adam and Eve ate the forbidden fruit, and God's verdict was passed upon them; their bodies commenced the process of death and decay. Death opened the door for all sicknesses and diseases, including COVID-19. "And all the days that Adam lived were nine hundred and thirty years: and he died" (Genesis 5:5). Therefore, death entered the world by sin through Adam's choice to disobey God when he fell into the temptation of Satan through the serpent. Paul affirms in Romans 5:12, 19, 21:

> Wherefore, as by one man sin entered into the world, and death by sin; and so death passed upon all men, for that all have sinned.
>
> For as by one man's disobedience many were made sinners, so by the obedience of one shall many be made righteous.

> [T]hat as sin hath reigned unto death, even
> so might grace reign through righteousness unto
> eternal life by Jesus Christ our Lord.

That is why until we align ourselves to obeying God by the help of the Holy Spirit through God's mercy and grace, which contrarywise Adam disobeyed, we cannot experience the eternal life that God promised us. This will be the only condition that will usher in eradicating death and healing all those who are diseased, fulfilling the promises spoken to God's people. The Lord promised his people when it comes to all sickness and diseases, including COVID-19:

> And said, If thou wilt diligently hearken to
> the voice of the Lord thy God, and wilt do that
> which is right in his sight, and wilt give ear to
> his commandments and keep all his statutes, I
> will put none of these diseases upon thee, which
> I have brought upon the Egyptians: for I am the
> Lord that healeth thee. (Ex. 15:26)

Jesus questioned the Pharisees:

> For whether is easier, to say, Thy sins be for-
> given thee; or to say, Arise, and walk? But that ye
> may know that the Son of man hath power on
> earth to forgive sins (then saith he to the sick of
> the palsy,) Arise, take up thy bed, and go unto
> thine house. And he arose and departed to his
> house. But when the multitudes saw it, they mar-
> veled, and glorified God, which had given such
> power unto men. Matt. 9:5–8

Whenever sin, which is the root of all sicknesses and diseases, is out of anyone's life, its product or fruit will automatically and ultimately wither. The end of sin in any man's life will always be death, except it is terminated by the eternal life of God through the precious blood of Jesus, for the life of the flesh is in the blood (Lev. 17:11). That is why Jesus has come to become our sin-bearer so we can become His righteousness (2 Cor. 5:21). He paid the ultimate penalty for our sin.

We read Paul's very words in Ephesians 1:7 that we have redemption through his blood, even the forgiveness of sins, according to the riches of his grace; and James 1:13–15 explains what happens when the heart is pregnant of sin:

> Let no man say when he is tempted, I am tempted of God: for God cannot be tempted with evil, neither tempteth he any man. However, every man is tempted when drawn away from his lust and enticed. Then when lust hath conceived, it bringeth forth sin: and sin, when it is finished, bringeth forth death.

To Adam and Eve, God said, "In the sweat of thy face shalt thou eat bread, till thou return unto the ground; for out of it wast thou taken: for dust thou art, and unto dust shalt thou return" (Gen. 3:19). God reiterated that the soul that sinneth, it shall die (Eze. 18:4), and that the wages of sin is death (Rom. 6:23) and interestingly, all have sinned (in Adam) and come short of the glory of God (Rom. 3:23).

Sin will allow you to enjoy its pleasures for a season (Heb. 11:25). It will allow you to pursue happiness, worldly pleasure, and power, but the game of life is brief. In the end, sin will track down each of its players with death. We endlessly search in vain in our efforts to discover the secret of victory over death, for "what man is he that liveth, and shall not see death" (Ps. 89:48)?

Because our nature is sinful and our hearts are desperately wicked (Jer. 17:9), death continues to prick human life and drives them to the grave as the goad drives an ox to slaughter. However, shortly before the return of Jesus Christ the second time, the Church of Jesus Christ would have destroyed the last enemy, which is death. "The last enemy that shall be destroyed is death" (1 Cor. 15:26).

The Church of Jesus Christ would have perfected how to operate the law of the Spirit of life in Christ Jesus, which is the law of keeping the commandment of love and keeping oneself in love, "For the law of the Spirit of life in Christ Jesus hath made me free from the law of sin and death" (Rom. 8:2).

> "We know that whosoever is born of God sinneth not; but he that is begotten of God keepeth himself, and that wicked one toucheth him not" (1 John 5:18).

Solomon, the preacher of old, said, "For the living know that they shall die" (Eccles. 9:5), but death does not end it all. The Bible declares in Hebrews 9:27, "It is appointed unto men once to die, but after this the judgment." Out in the great beyond, the soul will live forever.

The epistle to the Hebrews speaks of men "who through fear of death were all their lifetime subject to bondage… These all died in faith, not having received the promises, but having seen them afar off and were persuaded of them and embraced them and confessed that they were strangers and pilgrims on the earth" (Heb. 2:15, 11:13).

Life insurance companies become rich by merely pointing out that all men must die. The insurance agents have little difficulty selling a policy by merely saying that death may come suddenly and unexpectedly. Even architects and builders take death into account whenever they embark on building a structure in the transportation or aviation industry.

However, there are some conditions you must fulfill if you want to die the death of the righteous. You must believe that Jesus Christ is the Son of God and that He brought from heaven the Gospel of eternal redemption to save humankind (Acts 16:31–33). You must repent of your sins and renounce Satan with all his pernicious ways and all the sinful pleasures of this world. This is possible, and you can do it right now as you read this book by confessing that Jesus Christ is now Savior, Lord, and King of your life (Acts 2:38, 3:19, 17:30, 26:20; 1 John 2:15–17).

You also need to covenant with God by experiencing Christian water baptism, letting God's Word have the only say in your life and in the choices you make and begin to live as His disciple (Mark 16:16). Then the precious blood Jesus Christ shed for us on the cross of Calvary will become your shield and preserve you from the wrath of God (Rom. 3:25; 1 John 2:2, 4:10).

Whenever a sinner surrenders his life to the Lord, He is drawn nearer and nearer to God by the blood of Jesus Christ. Ephesians 2:12–14 declares:

> That at that time ye were without Christ, being aliens from the commonwealth of Israel, and strangers from the covenants of promise, having no hope, and without God in the world: But now in Christ Jesus ye who sometimes were far off are made nigh by the blood of Christ. For he is our peace, who hath made both one, and hath broken down the middle wall of partition between us.

There are two people in the Bible who never tasted death here on earth, which is a foreshadow of God's remnant overcomers that will put death under their feet. With regard to Enoch's translation, Hebrews 11:5 declares, "By faith Enoch was translated that he should not see death; and was not found, because God had translated him: for before his translation he had this testimony, that he pleased God."

However, Hebrews 11:13, affirms that, "These all died in faith, not having received the promises, but having seen them afar off, and were persuaded of them, and embraced them, and confessed that they were strangers and pilgrims on the earth."

We do know that Abraham faced the grim reality of death when he offered Isaac as a sacrifice to the Lord. Though Isaac was spared, a ram died in his stead. Then we read, "And Sarah died" (Gen. 23:2).

"And the Lord said unto Moses, Behold, thy days approach that thou must die" (Deut. 31:14).

The patriarchs, prophets, and apostles did not hesitate to declare that death is certain. Noah preached righteousness and the judgment of God. He warned men that if they would not repent, the Lord would destroy them from the face of the earth (Gen. 6:7). Men only mocked this preacher of righteousness, and then God struck the whole earth with death and destruction. God's Word accounted that the waters prevailed for forty days on the earth until every hill was covered. Additionally, Isaiah said to Hezekiah, "Set thine house in order; for thou shalt die, and not live" (2 Kings 20:1). Jeremiah declared unto Hananiah, "This year thou shalt die" (Jer. 28:16). Ezekiel prophesied God's Word by saying, "The soul that sinneth, it shall die" (Eze. 18:4); and "that wicked man shall die in his iniquity" (Eze. 33:8).

When Jesus told the story of the rich man and Lazarus, He said, "The beggar died... The rich man also died" (Luke 16:22). Luke documented the initial death event of Dorcas, "[S]he was sick and died" (Acts 9:37). The book of Proverbs 30:15–16 declares:

> The horseleach hath two daughters, crying,
> Give, give. There are three things that are never
> satisfied, yea, four things say not, It is enough:
> The grave; and the barren womb; the earth that is
> not filled with water; and the fire that saith not,
> It is enough.

The good news is that whenever a true believer dies, he is said to fall asleep (1 Thess. 4:13, 15; 1 Cor. 15:6), and immediately. his soul takes the upward course to be with the Lord. Ecclesiastes 3:21 clarifies this thought, "Who knoweth the spirit of man that goeth upward, and the spirit of the beast that goeth downward to the earth?"

We can better understand this when we know the true purpose of the death of Jesus Christ. The wisdom of God here is Jesus went to the cross as man and died to receive the punishment for sin. He offered Himself to pay the price for us because the sin of man must be punished by death. Peter declares that "Christ also hath once suffered for sins, the just for the unjust, that He might bring us to God, being put to death in the flesh" (1 Pet. 3:18).

Stewart Salmond explained that people like the Egyptians, Babylonians, Assyrians, Persians, and Phoenicians had associations with the Hebrews, which at times were both intimate and influential, and it is natural to conclude with strong verification that they left a stamp of their minds and words upon Hebrew thought and Hebrew language. He stated that the practical universality of the belief in some sort of a life after death does not exclude belief in an absolute cessation of being for some, and not all who have believed in a continuance of life have allowed all and sundry to be heirs of it.

He asked several questions with regard to various ethnic preparation of the subject of immortality. How did the idea of a future life originate? Was it a divine gift bestowed upon primitive man by his Creator which, as it travelled down the ages, became broken up, perverted, or lost in some races? While in others it was retained in comparative purity and with all the capacities of growth? Or did it only emerge in course of time as was the case with the ideas of art and science? Did it appear first in a rudimentary form and then gradually unfold and take shape and gather precision? Was it the product of man's gifts of reflection and imagination? Did it rise in the incapacity of primitive man to think of one who had been living as having utterly ceased to live? Or in his thoughts on the mystery of sleep? Or in what is its genesis to be sought?

How did man come to think of a soul and to ascribe to it a continuance, which failed the body? Did he begin by a ghost tenanting his body, yet distinct from it, making itself visible at times? Or by fancying the forms which he saw in dream at times? Or by fancying the forms which he saw in dream or vision to be the dead themselves in surviving shadow figures?

Furthermore, he asked why the idea of a retributive future always appears anytime the idea of an afterlife is discovered. Or is it rather the case that the conception of rewards for virtue and penalties for vices in the other world was a later development of the belief?[16]

---

[16] Stewart D. Salmond, *The Christian Doctrine of Immortality* (Edinburg: Morrison & Gibb Limited, 1907), 7–9.

Laungani, et al., elucidated that science may delay death, but it can neither prevent it nor can it explain anything about what, if anything, lies beyond death or what can be done to prepare for that transition. They noted that this understanding does not prevent people from behaving as if, even now, scientific medicine could provide a solution to the problem of death. They added that doctors and nurses tend to collude with this, and most Westerners still go to a hospital to die, many of them in the naïve belief that scientific medicine will prevail over death.[17]

Moreover, they explained that most students of comparative religion see each faith as comprehensible in the time and place in which it has arisen. There is a search for meaning in life and death which must take place within a particular historical and geographical context. They inferred that despite current attempts at ecumenicity between the many sects of the Christian church, the rites and beliefs of other people seem alien or, at best, quaint, and we allow license to poets, but no such license is given to the clerics, and those who hold most passionately to the truths of their own religions often deride the beliefs of others.[18]

They concluded that improvements in palliative care for the dying are setting a good example of open communication about prognosis as people approach the end of their lives. They stated that doctors still collude with the family in maintaining the pretense of immortality, and all societies see death as a transition for the person who dies. How people prepare themselves for this transition and how the survivors feel and behave after death has occurred varies a great deal, and the search for meaning in life and death must take place within a particular historical and geographical context with possibilities for fundamental consistencies, themes, and truths that appear and reappear in one culture after another. They stipulated that times of death and bereavement are times when people need people, provided people have sufficient knowledge of and sympathy

---

[17] Laungani, et al…, *Death and Bereavement Across Cultures* (East Sussex: Routledge T&F Group, 2015), 4.
[18] Ibid., 5.

for the other person's culture to be able to understand what they need from us; then we shall have a great deal to offer.[19]

In God's Holy Word, those who fall asleep in the Lord take the upward course to heaven and to God because they die the death of the righteous. The Bible explains, "Who can count the dust of Jacob, and the number of the fourth part of Israel? Let me die the death of the righteous, and let my last end be like his" (Numbers 23:10)!

You have nothing to lose but all to gain by accepting Jesus Christ as your Lord and Savior from sin. In so doing, you will be brought to God by virtue of Jesus's sacrificial and vicarious death. Believers are able to say, "The Lord hath laid on Him the iniquity of us all" (Isaiah 53:6). As Jesus hung dying upon the cross, He was the true sin-offering for His people. We were, by nature, on the downward course, doomed to be separated from God; but Jesus, by virtue of His death, provided a new destiny.

But what course does death pursue in the case of someone that has not accepted Jesus Christ as Lord and Savior? That will take that declining path into eternal death? However, since the death of Christ has paid for the believers, the punishment of sin and death to him is a pleasant ascension into the Father's presence. It follows that the death of the unbeliever is an unpleasant descent away from the presence of God. When the unbeliever takes his last breath, he passes from this world into a spiritual and eternal death. Both are conscious, but death was forced to pursue a different course for each.

God's Word: An Inestimable Asset Against Death

If we will stick with the Lord, our lives will be more packed with faith and power with every passing year. We will develop a history of walking with God that makes us ever more dangerous to the devil. We will accumulate so many victories that instead of panicking when trouble arises, we will be like David when he came up against Goliath or Daniel when he entered the lion's den after praying intensively.

---

[19] Ibid., 8.

They both had confidence because they remembered what the Lord had done for them in the past. If we keep storing the Word in our hearts and developing our relationships with the Lord, the good fight of faith will get easier, not harder, as we age. If we keep abiding in God's Word, the more years we pile up, the more fulfilling our days will be.

Thomas O'Loughin explained that Genesis 5 describes itself as the book of Adam's genealogy, and in each verse, except verse 24, where it presented one of Adam's descendants through Seth, Enoch who disappeared because God took him, and in this chapter which runs from the birth of Seth to the birth of the three sons of Noah along with Genesis 7:6, 11, 8:13, and 9:28 were based all Judeo-Christian efforts at a world chronology down to the middle of the nineteenth century.[20]

God's people continued to enjoy such extended lives that patriarchs born centuries apart lived at the same time. Noah's father (Lamech) must have known Adam. And Noah, who was born 1,056 years after the time of Creation, must have also lived to see Abraham who was born 1,948 years after Creation. Job, too, who is believed to have lived during the same era Abraham did, enjoyed a life span that would shock us today. Although the devil came after him with vengeance and moved through his wife who had cooperated with the devil to advise Job to curse God and die, Job still refused her counsel and stood with God.

Job's friends who were famous for criticizing and accusing him also spoke iniquitous things about their friend, Job, but one thing they said of him came true: "Thou shall come to thy grave in a full age, like season" (Job 5:26). After God had restored Job with a double portion of blessing, He gave him another 140 years to enjoy the blessings. Job 42:16–17 states, "After this lived Job an hundred and

---

[20] Thomas O'Loughlin "The Controversy Over Methuselah's Death: Proto-chronology and the Origins of the Western Concept of Inerrancy." *JSTOR: Recherches De Théologie Ancienne Et Médiévale*, 62, 182–225, 1995, Accessed 12 May, 2020, www.jstor.org/stable/26189089.

forty years, and saw his sons, and his sons' sons, even four genera-tions. So Job died, being old and full of days."

The Bible says one day with the Lord is as a thousand years, and a thousand years is as one day. The day of the Lord in comparison to the life span of man is very brief regardless of color, race, religion, or ethnicity. The world is right now in the day of the Lord, the seven thousand years according to Scriptures, which is the prophetic sab-bath year of the Lord as we count from Adam. It is no more the day of the white man, black man, or brown man. Man has had their days in the six previous days, but this seventh day in the day which the Lord has made, we will rejoice and be glad in it. Our sovereign God will do whatever he chooses to do and however He chooses to do it according to His Word. Psalms 115:3 and 135:6 speaks about the sovereignty of God that "our God is in the heavens: he hath done whatsoever he hath pleased… Whatsoever the Lord pleased, that did he in heaven, and in earth, in the seas, and all deep places."

Human life is so short as compared to one single day of the Lord that it cannot continue to exist on the earth. The brevity is lik-ened to "a tale that is told" (Ps. 90:9), "a pilgrimage" (Gen. 47:9), "a swift post" (Job 9:25), "a swift ship" (Job 9:26), "a handbreadth" (Ps. 39:5), "a shepherd's tent removed" (Isa. 38:12), "a thread cut by the weaver" (Isa. 38:12), "a dream" (Job 20:2–8), "a sleep" (Ps. 90:4–5), "a shadow" (Ps. 144:4; Eccles. 6:12, 8:13), "a flower" (Job 14:1–2), "a weaver's shuttle" (Job 7:6), "a water split on the ground" (2 Sam. 14:14), "grass" (Ps. 90:5–6, 103:15, 92:7, 102:11, 129:6; Isa 37:27, 40:6–8; James 1:10–11; 1 Pet, 1:24; Rev, 8:7, 9:4), "wind" (Job 7:7, 30:15), "a vapor" (James 4:14), and "nothing or vanity" (Ps. 144:4; Job 7:16; Ps 62:9; Eccles. 1:2, 12:8).

God had invested years of training to prepare Moses for His divine mission on earth. For forty years, he was educated in the house of Pharaoh, and for another forty years, he tended his father-in-law's flock on the back side of the desert. God designed these to get Moses ready for the most important assignment of his life. Moses was eighty years old when he received the mandate. He was so invigorated with divine life that his health and strength remained undiminished for the rest of his life. He lived to be 120 years old (Deut. 34:7). Moses' secret for long strong life reverberated throughout the Bible and is intriguing. Moses stayed fresh and fruitful up to a youthful ripe old age of one hundred and twenty tears. He truly experienced a youthful old age despite his rugged life in the wilderness and his potentially high stress job of leading about three million plus belligerent and unbelieving people to the promised land.

He tapped into a fountain of divine youthfulness that kept him young year after year and decade after decade. What kept him going was nothing else but God's Word. This could not have been possible because of a special type of gene or DNA nor because of a certain kind of food, although they were feeding on angels' food; it could not be due to a special kind of exercise program, although they had a wilderness walking program that was exceptional. It was only due to the living Word of the Almighty God that he encountered. It was the Word Moses received on Mount Sinai in the midst of the fire of God's glory, the Word he believed and obeyed that kept him young, vibrant, and strong till that age.

Starting from the time he was eighty years until his mission was finished forty years later, it was God's Word that prolonged his days. The Word from God was his life. God's Word protected him, preserved him, and kept him going from strength to strength, faith to faith, and glory to glory. That is why just before he led Israelites into the edge of the promised land, Moses called them together and pronounced, according to Deuteronomy 32:46–47,

> And he said unto them, Set your hearts unto all the words which I testify among you this day, which ye shall command your children to observe to do, all the words of this law. For it is not a vain thing for you; because it is your life: and through this thing ye shall prolong your days in the land, whither ye go over Jordan to possess it.

Moses died for just one reason because God told him to. Who knows how long Moses might have lived if he had not violated God's commandment in the wilderness? Maybe he would spend another forty years to witness and enjoy the Israelites living in the promised land. He might have been gathered to his people at around 160 years of age instead of 120.

Moses was gathered unto his people. The Lord "gathered" him as He gathered Abraham, Isaac, Jacob, and Aaron unto their people (Gen. 25:8, 35:29; Num. 20:24, 26, 27:13), and this is a biblical proof that no matter how old a child of God is, you do not have to get sick and be feeble before dying or suffering untimely death. We must not allow the devil to evict us from our bodies by inflicting sickness, disease, or injury upon us. We can just finish our divine assignments and then let God gather us to Himself or at best be a part of the generation that will be changed, caught up, and meet the Lord in the air.

No one can do away with the reality and veracity of God's Word and for the fact that it is going to come to pass. But the question is, "Which part of His Word do we choose?" The coming to pass is incontestable; the Word of God is coming to pass, especially regarding cancelling appointments with death. God's Word will surely come to pass just as in the case of the contemporary nation of Israel that was founded and declared her independence on May 14, 1948. God fulfilled what prophet Ezekiel prophesied in Ezekiel chapter 37:1–14 in Israel against all odds. Ezekiel 37:13–14 declares:

> And ye shall know that I am the Lord, when I have opened your graves, O my people, and brought you up out of your graves. And shall put my spirit in you, and ye shall live, and I shall place you in your own land: then shall ye know that I the Lord have spoken it, and performed it, saith the Lord.

In 1947, when the United Nations declared Israel as a nation, all the Arab states such as Iran, Jordan, Iraq did not agree, and over fifty million Arabs immediately declared war against the state of Israel. At that time, the state of Israel was no more than a few hundred thousand. It looked as if it was going to be a total annihilation of Israel because they were just a new nation without weapons and no standing army. They practically had nothing because they had just come out from the Holocaust. They only had a ragtag army. All observers had perceived it was going to be over in a week. But there is a God in heaven who watches over His Word to perform it (Jer.1:12). God had also said in Ezekiel 36:24, "I will bring them back and establish them in the land.'

The Lord used the United States of America to come to their aid, but the summary of their conquest was that it was God who kept His Word on Israel, and it was God alone.

According to the office of historian milestones:

> 1945–1952, after Israel declared its independence on May 14, 1948, the fighting intensified with other Arab forces joining the Palestinian Arabs in attacking territory in the former Palestinian mandate. The milestones specified that on the eve of May 14, the Arabs launched an air attack on Tel Aviv, which the Israelis resisted but this action was followed by the invasion of the former Palestinian mandate by Arab armies from Lebanon, Syria, Iraq, and Egypt. The Milestone detailed that Saudi Arabia sent a formation that fought under the Egyptian command and the British trained forces from Transjordan eventually intervened in the conflict, but only in areas that had been designated as part of the Arab state under the United Nations Partition Plan and the "corpus separatum" of Jerusalem. Finally, after tense early fighting, Israeli forces, now under joint command, were able to gain the offensive.[21]

---

[21] "The Arab-Israeli War of 1948," Office of the Historian, Milestone, 1945–1952, Accessed May 9, 2020, https://history.state.gov/milestones/1945-1952/arab-israeli-war.

If God can do it for the nation of physical Israel, then our own promises are easy because theirs was against all odds! As of today, Israel is an industrial, scientific, and military powerhouse. It is one of the most powerful nations on the earth. As a desert nation, they have perfected the art of irrigation, and they will never allow one drop of water to waste. This is God's Word being fulfilled to a backsliding, rebellious, disobedient people because of their fathers, Abraham, Isaac, and Jacob, who are looking at God's face in heaven every day. The promise was made to their fathers in Romans 11:28, "As concerning the gospel (they are) enemies for your sakes: but as touching the election (they are) beloved for the fathers' sakes."

Caleb and Joshua were young and strong and ready to receive the fulfillment of God's promise. They were confident God would keep His word. At about forty years of age, they declare in Numbers 14:8–9:

> If the Lord delight in us, then he will bring us into this land, and give it us; a land which floweth with milk and honey. Only rebel not ye against the Lord, neither fear ye the people of the land; for they are bread for us: their defence is departed from them, and the Lord is with us: fear them not.

At about forty years after they entered into their inheritance, Caleb took his possession when he was about eighty-five years. He was eighty-five years old when he placed a demand for his inheritance in Joshua 14:10–14:

> And now, behold, the Lord hath kept me alive, as he said, these forty and five years, even since the Lord spake this word unto Moses, while the children of Israel wandered in the wilderness: and now, lo, I am this day fourscore and five years old. As yet I am as strong this day as I was in the day that Moses sent me: as my strength

was then, even so is my strength now, for war, both to go out, and to come in. Now therefore give me this mountain, whereof the Lord spake in that day; for thou heardest in that day how the Anakims were there, and that the cities were great and fenced: if so be the Lord will be with me, then I shall be able to drive them out, as the Lord said. And Joshua blessed him and gave unto Caleb the son of Jephunneh Hebron for an inheritance. Hebron therefore became the inheritance of Caleb the son of Jephunneh the Kenezite unto this day, because that he wholly followed the Lord God of Israel.

We need the Word of God every day. We need to keep reading and meditating on it until it comes alive in us and takes control of our lives. We must thrive to be an obedient doer of God's Word. We must receive, believe, and profess the promises of God as we grow literarily younger. It was the Word of God that Caleb held on to for years and that kept him young and strong enough to whip a hillside full of giants at eighty-five. The Word did for him (and will do for us) just what Isaiah 40:28–31 says.

As God's children, when we celebrate our birthdays, we are actually going back to the days of our youth. The scripture enumerated in the book of Job 33:23–25:

> If there be a messenger with him, an interpreter, one among a thousand, to shew unto man his uprightness: Then he is gracious unto him, and saith, Deliver him from going down to the pit: I have found a ransom. His flesh shall be fresher than a child's: he shall return to the days of his youth.

Sarah's body went back to her youthful days. Her flesh was fresher than a child's. Abraham also fathered a son at one hundred years old, and after Sarah died, he remarried at about one hundred and thirty-seven years since he was about ten years older than Sarah and also fathered five more sons and lived another forty years. The Bible indicated in Genesis 25:7–8 that he enjoyed those years. When Abraham was still just a youngster of eighty or ninety years, the Lord had spoken to him and said, "Thou shall go to thy fathers in peace, thou shalt be buried in a good old age" (Gen. 15:15). And God's Word was fulfilled in his life. Surely, the counsel of the Lord stands forever (Ps. 33:11).

God's Word Cancels Every Appointment with Death

It is the raw will of God that we destroy spiritual and physical death in our souls and bodies by the power of the Holy Spirit so as to manifest the reality of the resurrection of the Lord Jesus Christ to men in the earth. Second Corinthians 4:10–11 declares:

> Always bearing about in the body the dying of the Lord Jesus, that the life also of Jesus might be made manifest in our body. For we which live are always delivered unto death for Jesus' sake, that the life also of Jesus might be made manifest in our mortal flesh.

The book of 2 Corinthians 5:4 speaks further, "For we that are in this tabernacle do groan, being burdened: not for that we would be unclothed, but clothed upon, that mortality might be swallowed up of life."

Now, this does not mean that Christians will not die physically, but it means that those who die in Christ Jesus will determine when, where, and how they die and will not have to die from sickness. Other Christians who will be around at the Second Coming of our Lord Jesus Christ shall be caught up to meet the Lord in the air with a glorified body. This is a mystery that Paul shows us in 1 Corinthians 15:51–52:

> Behold, I shew you a mystery; we shall not all sleep, but we shall all be changed, in a moment, in the twinkling of an eye, at the last trump: for the trumpet shall sound, and the dead shall be raised incorruptible, and we shall be changed.

The Bible is God's authentic Word. It is honest, reliable, consistent, and eternally true.

Our God has magnified His Word above His name which means God Himself is subject to His own Word (Ps. 138:2). God cannot break His Word (Num. 23:17), and it is impossible for God to lie or not to fulfill His Word or promises (Heb. 6:17–19). The book of Titus states, "In hope of eternal life, which God, that cannot lie, promised before the world began."

God is constantly paying attention to watching over His Word to perform it so that when you speak or pray according to His Word, you have His attention to see to it that His Word is fulfilled in your situation. God's Word is honest because God is righteous. God's Word is reliable because God is omnipotent and omniscient. God's Word is eternally consistent because God is omnipresent.

Did you know God has a schedule? He has time all mapped out. He knows the exact moment of your entrance to the world and has packaged a perfect and smooth exit for you. He knows when the glorious church is going to be caught up to meet Jesus Christ in the air, and He has known it from the beginning. In Job 9:8, God treads upon the waves of the sea, and in chapter 24 and verse 14, He walks in the circuit of heaven, while in Psalms 104:3, He walks upon the wings of the wind. However, in Psalms 89:3, He has a mighty arm, a strong hand, and high is His right hand. Paul declares in Colossians 2:2–3, "In whom are hid all the treasures of wisdom and knowledge."

CHAPTER 2

Origin of COVID-19: Socioeconomic and Theological View

In God's Word, we are warned not to eat animals, like bats (Lev. 11:13–19), but men decided to eat them because of their special taste, and the result is coronavirus.

Jane Qiu mentioned that the Wuhan-based virologist, Shi Zhengli, identified dozens of deadly SARS-like viruses in bat caves. She explained that the Wuhan Center for Disease Control and Prevention had detected a novel coronavirus in two hospital patients with a typical pneumonia, and it wanted Zhengli's renowned laboratory to investigate the same. The mysterious patient samples arrived at the Wuhan Institute of Virology at 7:00 p.m. on December 30, 2019.

Subject to the confirmation of their discovery, the new pathogen would pose to be a serious public health threat because it belonged to the same family of viruses that caused severe acute respiratory syndrome (SARS), a disease that plagued 8,100 people and killed nearly eight hundred people between 2002 and 2003. Zhengli, often called China's "bat woman" by her colleagues because of her virus-hunting expeditions in bat caves over the past sixteen years, was hoping this would not be the case in Wuhan, central China. Her previous studies had shown that the southern subtropical provinces of Guangdong, Guangxi, and Yunnan had the greatest risk of coronaviruses jumping to humans from animals, particularly bats, which was a known reservoir.

This China's bat woman felt she was fighting a battle in her worst nightmare, even though it was one she had been preparing for over the past sixteen years by using a technique called polymerase chain reaction, which can detect a virus when its genetic material is amplified. The research team found that samples from five of seven patients had genetic sequences present in all coronaviruses.

By January 7, the Wuhan team had determined that the new virus had indeed caused the disease those patients suffered, a conclusion based on results from analyses using polymerase chain reaction, full genome sequencing, antibody tests of blood samples, and the virus's ability to infect human lung cells in a petri dish. The genomic sequence of the virus, eventually named SARS-CoV-2, was 96 percent identical to that of a coronavirus the researchers had identified in horseshoe bats in Yunnan. The data also points to a single introduction into humans followed by sustained human-to-human transmission,

In Wuhan, the region's burgeoning wildlife markets sells a wide range of animals such as bats, civets, pangolins, badgers, and crocodiles, and they all are perfect viral melting pots. Although humans could have caught the deadly virus from bats directly, independent teams have suggested that pangolins may have been an intermediate host. Zhengli's research teams had reportedly uncovered SARS-CoV-2-like coronaviruses in pangolins that were seized in anti-smuggling operations in southern China.

Back in Wuhan, where the lockdown was finally lifted on April 8, China's bat woman was not in a celebratory mood. She was distressed because stories from the media had repeated a tenuous suggestion that SARS-CoV-2 accidentally leaked from her lab despite the fact that its genetic sequence did not match any that her lab had previously studied.[22]

---

[22] Jane Qui, "Public Health: How China's 'Bat Woman' Hunted Down Viruses from SARS to the New Coronavirus," *Scientific American*, 2020, Accessed April 30, 2020, https://www.scientificamerican.com/article/how-chinas-bat-woman-hunted-down-viruses-from-sars-to-the-new-coronavirus1/.

In retrospect, the Lord warned us about the danger of eating mice (Lev. 11:1–47; Isa. 66:17; 1 Cor. 8:1–13), but men chose to make young uncooked mice their delicacy.

According to Christopher Intagliata, mice trapped in New York City apartment buildings harbored disease-causing bacteria and anti-biotic-resistant genes. He cited the battery of genetic tests of swabs of mice's rear ends and their feces from traps performed by Simon Williams and his colleagues where the mice harbored an array of disease-causing bacteria, like shigella, *Clostridium difficile*, salmonella. This also carried a suite of antibiotic-resistance genes and viruses associated with insects, dogs, chickens, and pigs. They observed that mice from a Chelsea apartment building had the most pig viruses because they lived near the meatpacking district, which used to have pork-processing facilities before fashionable nightclubs took over.[23]

Jordan Rubin explained that statistics show that the United States is not the world's healthiest nation. Although the United States does enjoy one of the highest standards of living in the world with extraordinary emergency, medical technology, trauma care, and first-class access to emergency health care—still, all these do not make Americans healthy. He added that most Americans eat great quantities of food frequently based on convenience, which has made the entire fast-food and TV dinner industries to flourish due to the fast-paced lifestyles that demand eating convenient foods.

Rubin observed that under primitive conditions, food was vital for survival because primitive people "ate to live," but many people have allowed food to become their idol and "eat to live" has become "live to eat." He substantiated that most modern men and women have strayed from the Creator's foods which are the same foods that traditionally nourished the world's healthiest people, and because this is a promiscuous society where many say yes to virtually every whim and desire of the palate, it has resulted into a national dilemma

---

[23] Christopher Intagliata, "Biology 60-SECOND SCIENCE: NYC Mice Are Packed with Pathogens," *Scientific American*, 2020, accessed April 30, 2020, https://www.scientificamerican.com/podcast/episode/nyc-mice-are-packed-with-pathogens/.

of becoming overweight, sedentary, and has created an increasingly sick population.[24]

The Lord instructed us to desist from eating animal fat and blood which can increase the risk of breast cancer and raise human "bad" cholesterol subsequently subjecting one to heart disease (Lev. 3:17). The origin of the Human Immunodeficiency Virus (HIV) has been a subject of scientific research and debate since the virus was identified in the 1980s.[25] Just as HIV crossed from chimps to humans, the 2019 coronavirus outbreak was due to contact between people and wild animals. Beatrice Hahn and Paul Sharp states:

> Acquired immunodeficiency syndrome (AIDS) of humans is caused by two lentiviruses, human immunodeficiency viruses types 1 and 2 (HIV-1 and HIV-2). Both HIVs are the result of multiple cross-species transmissions of simian immunodeficiency viruses (SIVs) naturally infecting African primates.[26]

They concluded that most of these transfers resulted in viruses that spread in humans to only a limited extent. In their findings, one transmission event, involving SIVcpz from chimpanzees in southeastern Cameroon gave rise to HIV-1 group M—the principal cause of the AIDS pandemic. They proved that AIDS had likely afflicted chimpanzees long before the emergence of HIV. They cited CDC and Greene that acquired Immune Deficiency Syndrome (AIDS) was first recognized as a new disease in 1981 when increasing num-

---

[24] Jordan S. Rubin, *The Maker's Diet—The 40-Day Health Experience that Will Change Your Life Forever* (Florida: Siloam, 2005), 31–32.

[25] "Origin of HIV AIDS, Avert Global Information and Education on HIV and AIDS," Accessed April 29, 2020, https://www.avert.org/professionals/history-hiv-aids/origin.

[26] Beatrice Hahn and Paul Sharp, "Cold Spring Harbor Perspective in Medicine: Origins of HIV and the AIDS Pandemic," 1:1, 2011, Accessed April 30, 2020, https://www.ncbi.nlm.nih.gov/pmc/articles/PMC3234451/.

bers of young homosexual men succumbed to unusual opportunistic infections and rare malignancies.

Additionally, they cited Barre-Sinoussi, et al., Gallo, et al. and Popovic, et al., that a retrovirus now termed human immunodeficiency virus type 1 (HIV-1) was subsequently identified as the causative agent of what has since become one of the most devastating infectious diseases to have emerged in recent history.[27] In their words, they rationalized, "Tracing the genetic changes that occurred as SIVs crossed from monkeys to apes and from apes to humans provides a new framework to examine the requirements of successful host switches and to gauge future zoonotic risk."[28]

Are you surprised that you are required to wash your hands frequently during this COVID-19 pandemic? The Lord has commanded this hygienic practice in His Word before now (Ex. 30:17–21). God is really serious about cleanliness. Our Lord Jesus Christ was all out to clean the unclean (Mark 1:23–27) because only clean people will inherit the kingdom of God (Rev. 19:8–14). Those who will live a long and healthy life must go back to God's Word, the Bible.

Don Colbert buttressed this notion by clarifying that we live in a toxic world and a toxic planet that is taking a heavy toll upon our bodies every day due to our technological advances since the industrial revolution. He observed that we have continued to pour dangerous chemicals and pollutants into our streams, soil, and air. He maintained that if our earth is sick and toxic, then there is a very good chance that most people will be sick and toxic. Colbert supported his claim by the mysterious deaths in 1976 of 182 Legionnaires that were staying at a Philadelphia hotel while attending a conference whose deaths were caused by contracting pneumonia from legionella bacteria that had contaminated the hotel's air conditioning system. He attested that eating right can keep us healthy as conventional medicine with its prescriptions might not help many times. He suggested that medical science will have to address the root of this problem. He cited Thomas Edison who said, "The doctor of the future

---

[27] Ibid.
[28] Ibid.

will give no medicine but will interest his patients in the care of the human frame, in diet and in the cause and prevention of disease." Colbert corroborated that what we need is better prevention.[29]

The Lord has desired that we quarantine a long time ago as found in the book of Leviticus, chapter 15. According to Johanna Mayer, the word *quarantine* was first used in the fourteenth century, and it is from the Latin *quadraginta* and the Italian *quaranta*, both meaning "forty." She expounded historically by looking back to the mid-fourteenth century in Europe. At the time, the bubonic plague, infamously known as the Black Death, was ripping through the continent starting from 1343. The disease wiped out an estimated one-third of Europe's population during a particularly nasty period of three years between 1347–1350. She stated that this sweep of the plague resulted in one of the biggest die-offs in human history and was an impetus to take action.

Mayer added that within a century, cities extended the isolation period from thirty to forty days, and the term changed from *trentino* to *quarantine*, the root of the English word *quarantine* that we use today, and that there is a lot of cultural meaning packed into the number "forty" with plenty of biblical events drawn upon the number, such as Jesus's fast in the desert, Moses' time on Mount Sinai, and the Christian observation of Lent. She clarified that although we can trace the word *quarantine* to the time of the black death, the practice of isolating the sick stretches back much further and references to isolating people with leprosy that can be found in the Bible and hospitals, called lazarettos, which were intentionally constructed outside the city center, existed by the first half of the fourteenth century in Venice. She mentioned that the name lazaretto itself is named after the beggar Lazarus, the patron saint of lepers in Catholicism.[30]

Joe Schwarcz elucidated that the cause of the Black Death disease was unknown, but it was clear that it was contagious, and once

---

[29] Don Colbert, *Toxic Relief* (Florida: Siloam, 2003), 6–34.
[30] Johanna Mayer, "Where Does the Word 'Quarantine' Come From?", *Science Friday Massive Science*, 2020, Accessed May 7, 2020, https://massivesci.com/articles/quarantine-coronavirus-COVID-19-etymology-science-friday/.

it took hold, it always spread like wildfire. As of that time in Milan, Italian doctors had advised that victims should be walled up in their homes along with healthy family members, which literarily worked. Schwarcz expounded that it would not be until 1894 that Alexandre Yersin of France's Pasteur Institute identified a bacterium as the causative agent of black death while investigating an outbreak of the plague in Hong Kong. The bacterium, eventually named *Yersinia pestis* in his honor, is thought to have originated in Asia where it found a hospitable environment in fleas, which would readily transmit it through their bites. Since fleas infected rats and mice, rodents that were regular passengers on ships, the disease spread throughout the Mediterranean and Europe.

Schwarcz explicated that infection with the bacterium could take several forms with "bubonic plague" being the most notorious, adding that this term originates from the Greek for "groin" due to the characteristic swellings of the lymph glands, particularly in the groin, an area close to the legs where flea bites are most likely to occur. He stated that in "septicemic" and "pneumonic plague," bacteria enter the bloodstream and can be transmitted from person to person, especially though the coughing associated with pneumonic plague. He stressed that whenever science fails to find an explanation for a phenomenon, superstition and quackery rush in to fill the void. And there certainly was no scientific explanation for the plague in the fourteenth century.

The Church decreed that the Black Death was punishment for human sin. Lepers, because of their outward signs that resembled the plague, were blamed as were astrological alignments and volcanic eruptions.

He buttressed that "Flagellants"[31] believed God's punishment could be avoided by stripping to the waist and whipping themselves as they marched from town to town. Jews were also targeted, accused of poisoning wells. Many Jewish communities in Europe were exter-

---

[31] Editors, "Flagellants are medieval religious sects that included public beatings with whips as part of their discipline and devotional practice. They arose in northern Italy and had become large and widespread by about 1260," *Encyclopedia Britannica*, Accessed May 7, 2020, https://www.britannica.com/topic/flagellants.

minated in hopes of bringing an end to the plague, and also in Cologne, thousands of Jews were burned alive after being accused of starting the plague.

Black cats also became victims. They were thought to be witches in an animal form, casting their spells on the population. Since cats were a natural enemy of the disease-carrying rats, hunting them actually increased the spread of the plague.

Schwarcz emphasized that as far as treatments went during those days, there were none, and since the plague was often accompanied by a terrible smell, people walked around with flowers under their noses, hoping to ward off the stench and the disease, which did not produce any reasonable results. The belief that pleasant smells were of some help persisted through the seventeenth century when the great plague once again terrified Londoners. He stated that holding garlic in the mouth, swishing vinegar, or burning Sulphur to get rid of the "bad air" did no good. Smoking was also thought to be protective, and even children were forced to smoke tobacco with threats of being whipped if they refused. He underlined that the first effective treatment appeared in 1932 with the advent of the sulfonamide drugs, but today, the standard treatment is in the form of such antibiotics as streptomycin, chloramphenicol, tetracycline, and the fluoroquinolones.[32]

The development of a national quarantine policy in the United States took a bit of a process to develop. In 1793, when yellow fever hit Philadelphia, sailors were quarantined in a hospital outside the city. Also, when typhus landed in New York City in 1892, at least seventy people were quarantined on a nearby island. Additionally, when an outbreak of SARS (severe acute respiratory syndrome) moved through Canada in 2003, about 30,000 people in Toronto were quarantined. And during the 2014 Ebola outbreak in West Africa, health workers returning to the United States from affected areas were quarantined.[33]

---

[32] Joe Schwarcz, "The Word 'Quarantine' Comes from the Italian Word 'Forty Days.'" McGill Office for Science and Society, 2020, Accessed May 7, 2020, https://www.mcgill.ca/oss/article/did-you-know-health/word-quarantine-comes-italian-word-forty-days.

[33] Ibid.

COVID-19 Hazards to First Responders and Special Tribute

There have been tributes for COVID-19 health workers from around the globe since the coronavirus pandemic. These frontline health care workers have been on the forefront as they save the lives of others in overstretched hospitals. They have worked around the clock at the risk of their own lives and their loved ones. There are also people that served alongside health workers on the frontlines of COVID-19 in essential services. From nurses, technicians, transporters, truckers, EMTs, pharmacists, pulmonologists, epidemiologists, virologists, cardiologists, neurosurgeons, infectiology personnel, immunologists, first responders, grocery store clerks, gas station attendants, postal employees, delivery drivers, auto mechanics, and many more who are rising to the occasion and caring for the most vulnerable populations.

The gratitude and respect from the public to these heroes of the nations are immeasurable, but that hasn't stopped many from around the world trying to express it. These essential workers placed themselves in the path of the coronavirus just to help others to survive. Their dedication, selflessness, sacrifices, commitment, and courage deserve profound and deepest gratitude and admiration. Their service to patients has saved countless lives and made a millionfold difference, and their sacrifices are appreciated to the utmost. Our brave doctors, nurses, and first responders fought to save lives; medical workers race to develop critical medical supplies. Scientists are working around the clock to develop life-saving therapeutics. Everyone is making selfless sacrifices to put an end to this pandemic.

Health care workers comfort, care, and cure patients and put the nations at ease. They place others before themselves. They do not give up when things seem very hard, stressful, and pressuring. They focus on the patients, even at the expense of little or no lunch break, and are not available to their own loved ones. Not only do they ensure that people have essential care, supplies, and services, but they often do it while interacting with members of the public who can potentially make them ill. They are indeed an inspiration, and we do honor and pray for their own safety too.

CHAPTER 3

Fight COVID-19 from the Throne of Grace

Richard Bartlett's and Alexandria Watkin's understanding is that there is more than one way to treat SARS-CoV-2. According to them, other related studies in addition to their own case studies has led to the discoveries of arsenals of powerful therapies that can be used to treat SARS-CoV-2. They buttressed that when the call to arms was sounded on January 20, 2020, after the first case of SARS-CoV-2 was first identified in the United States by the month of March 2020, a successful empirical treatment plan was already put into place (budesonide 0.5mg nebulizer, twice daily, clarithromycin (Biaxin) 500mg tab, twice daily for ten days, Zinc 50mg tab, twice daily, and aspirin 81mg tab, daily).[34]

What then is the Christian theological response to COVID-19 pandemic? This is the time for us to cry to the Lord for mercy and for the speedy discovery of medication and vaccination from this lethal effect of this pandemic. We must humble ourselves, turn from our sins and wicked ways, and pray to the Lord for His mercy for the nations of the world. We must now come to the throne of grace to obtain mercy and find grace to help us in our time of need,

---

[34] Richard Bartlett and Alexandria Watkins, "The COVID Silver Bullet. SARS-C0V-2 and the Case for Empirical Treatment," Case Study Report, 2020, Assessed August 3, 2020, http://covidsilverbullet.com/wpcontent/uploads/2020/07/Bartlett_COVID_Case_Study.pdf.

and as we do so, millions of souls will come to Jesus Christ, families will become more prayer devoted, the church will be united, and the COVID-19-plagued year will go down in history not as the year where the nations collapsed but as the year of historical advance of prayer, worldwide evangelism, soul winning, and discipleship.

COVID-19 cannot bring the death of globalization because several countries will still depend on goods and services from one another, just as it has been from centuries past. They will still need to trade with one another. Indeed, COVID-19 has brought to revival a healthy fear of God which is a factor for the foundation of the wisdom of God into the world.

Alissa Rubin, et al., narrated that experts are trying to figure out why the coronavirus is so capricious, and the answers could determine how best to protect ourselves and for how long we have to. They observed that the coronavirus has killed so many people in Iran that the country has resorted to mass burials, but in neighboring Iraq, the body count is one-fourth of Iran's number of fatalities.

As of December 23, 2020, Dominican Republic has reported nearly 161,930 cases of the virus, but just across the border, Haiti has recorded about 9771 cases. They observed that in Indonesia, thousands are believed to have died of the coronavirus, but a strict lockdown has kept fatalities to about four hundred and thirty-nine in nearby Malaysia as of December 23, 2020.

They also considered global metropolises like New York, Paris, and London that have been devastated while teeming cities like Bangkok, Baghdad, New Delhi, and Lagos have been largely spared. This has raised the question of why the virus has overwhelmed some places and left others relatively untouched, although there are already hundreds of studies underway around the world that are looking into how demographics, preexisting conditions, and genetics might affect the wide variation in impact. They reflected on doctors in Saudi Arabia that are studying whether genetic differences may help explain varying levels of severity in COVID-19 cases among Saudi Arabs and just as scientists in Brazil are looking into the relationship between genetics and COVID-19 complications.

Alissa Rubin, et al., also observed that many developing nations with hot climates and young populations have escaped the worst of coronavirus, suggesting that temperature and demographics could be factors, but they resolved that countries like Peru, Indonesia, and Brazil, tropical countries in the throes of growing epidemics, throw cold water on that idea. However, according to an unproven theory but impossible to refute, the virus may just have to reach those countries yet, and doctors who studied infectious diseases around the world have confessed that they do not have enough data to get a full epidemiological picture and that gaps in information in many countries make it dangerous to draw conclusions.

The woeful testing in many places has led to vast underestimates of the virus's progress, and deaths are almost certainly undercounted. Still, the broad patterns are clear. Even in places with abysmal record-keeping and broken health systems, mass burials, or hospitals turning away sick people by the thousands would be hard to miss, and a number of places are just not seeing them.

Furthermore, Alissa, et al., explained that the power of youth has made many countries with younger populations escape this mass pandemic. Africa is the world's youngest continent with more than 60 percent of its population under the age twenty-five. Contrarily, in Thailand and Najaf in Iraq, local health officials found that the twenty to twenty-nine age group had the highest rate of infection but often showed few symptoms.

Additionally, along with youth, relatively good health can lessen the impact of the virus among those who are infected while certain preexisting conditions, notably hypertension, diabetes and obesity, can worsen the severity according to researchers in the United States. They cited epidemiologists who observed cultural factors, like the social distancing that has been built into certain societies which has given some countries more protection. Anne Soy cited Moeti, who established that one of the big drivers of the spread of COVID-19 in Western countries is that the elderly people were living in specialized nursing homes and these became places where the transmission was very intense. Alternatively, these homes are rare in most African countries where older people are more likely to be living in rural areas. It is the norm in many African countries for people to return to their rural homes when they retire from employment in urban areas. Additionally, the population density in rural areas is lower; therefore maintaining social distance is much easier. Furthermore, an under-developed transport system within and between countries appears to have been a blessing in disguise. This has resulted in many Africans not traveling as much as people do in more developed economies, thereby minimizing contact.[35] However, there are notable exceptions to the cultural distancing theory. In many parts of the Middle East, such as Iraq and the Persian Gulf countries, men often embrace or shake hands on meeting, yet most are not getting sick.

What might be called "national distancing" has also proven advantageous. Countries that are relatively isolated have reaped health benefits from their seclusion. Far-flung nations, such as some in the South Pacific and parts of sub-Saharan Africa, have not been as inundated with visitors bringing the virus with them. Health experts in Africa cited limited travel from abroad as perhaps the main rea-son for the continent's relatively low infection rate, and the lack of public transportation in developing countries may have also reduced the spread of the virus there. The geography of the outbreak, which spreads rapidly during the winter in temperate zone countries like Italy and the United States and was virtually unseen in warmer coun-tries such as Chad or Guyana, seems to suggest that the virus does not take well to heat. But researchers say the idea that hot weather alone can repel the virus is wishful thinking because some of the worst outbreaks in the developing world have been in places like the Amazonas region of Brazil as tropical a place as any.

The ultraviolet rays of direct sunlight inhibit this coronavi-rus according to a study by ecological modelers at the University of Connecticut. Thus, the surfaces in sunny places may be less likely to remain contaminated, but transmission usually occurs through contact with an infected person, not by touching a surface. They

---

[35] Anne Soy, "Coronavirus in Africa: Five reasons why Covid-19 has been less deadly than elsewhere," BBC News Africa, (2020), https://www.bbc.com/news/world-africa-54418613 (accessed December 22, 2020).

remarked that early and strict lockdowns in countries like Vietnam and Greece have been able to avoid out-of-control contagions, which is the evidence of the power of strict social distancing and quarantines to contain the virus. Additionally, they indicated that in some African countries with bitter experience with previous killer diseases like HIV, drug-resistant tuberculosis, and Ebola, the initial drill to these diseases was well-triggered, which makes these nations to react quickly.

Counterintuitively, some countries where authorities reacted late and with spotty enforcement of lockdowns appear to have been spared. Cambodia and Laos both had brief spates of infections when few social distancing measures were in place, but neither has recorded a new case in about three weeks. Also, Lebanon, whose Christian and Muslim citizens often go on pilgrimages, places rife with the virus but should have had high numbers of infections but did not. They then concluded that some countries that should have been inundated are not, leaving researchers scratching their heads, especially when countries do all the wrong things and still end up seemingly not as battered by the virus as one would expect.[36]

COVID-19 was expected to sink globalization, but it has actually become an incentive for it to take deeper roots. China had started deglobalizing long ago with its "Made in China 2025" plan, which is a mechanism to deglobalize by reducing the nation's purchases of other countries.

Martin Jacques cited Goldman Sachs projections which suggest the three largest economies in the world will deglobalize by 2050. The first will be China, followed by a closely matched America and India, then Brazil, Mexico, Russia, and Indonesia with only two European countries featuring in the top ten, namely the UK and Germany in the ninth and tenth places respectively. According to Jacques, if

---

[36] Alissa, et al., "The COVID-19 Riddle: Why Does the Virus Wallop Some Places and Spare Others?" *The New York Times*, 2020, Accessed May 3, 2020, https://www.nytimes.com/2020/05/03/world/asia/coronavirus-spread-where-why.html.

these projections are borne out in practice, then during the next four decades, the world will come to look like a very different place.[37]

Jacques citation from the neoconservative think-tank, Project for the New American Century, stated that as the twentieth century draws to a close, the United States does stand as the world's pre-eminent power having led the West to victory in the Cold War that predisposes America with an opportunity with a challenge of whether the United States has the vision to build upon the achievements of past decades and whether it can have the resolve to shame the new century favorable to American principles and interests.[38] He cited the influential neoconservative Charles Krauthammer who documented that the Soviet Union died and something new was born, something utterly new which was a unipolar world that is dominated by a single superpower unchecked by any rival and with decisive reach in every corner of the globe which was a staggering development that has never been seen right from the fall of Rome.[39]

Jacques observed that America's present superpower status has been a product of its rapid economic growth between 1870 and 1930 and that it was the world's largest and often most dynamic economy during the second half of the twentieth century. He added that this economic strength underpinned and made possible its astonishing political, cultural, and military power form 1945 onward.[40]

He elaborated that we were so used to the world being Western, even American, that we have little idea what it would be like if it was not, and the West has a very strong vested interest in the world being cast in its image because this brings multifarious benefits. However, he clarified that hegemonic powers seek to project their values and institutions on to subordinate nations, and the latter, in response, will adapt or genuflect toward their ways depending their circumstances. If they refuse, hegemonic powers will then impose those values and arrangements on them and, in some instances, by

---

[37] Martin Jacques, *When China Rules the World: The Rise of the Middle Kingdom and the End of the Western World* (New York: Penguin Group, 2009), 3.

[38] Ibid., 4.

[39] Ibid., 4.

[40] Ibid., 5–6

the snood-type mask is underway while a 3D design of the handle has been widely circulated.

The BBC stated that Plaid Cymru leader Adam Price, who was part of the impetus to get the ventilator into mass production, said the innovations put Wales "on the front foot" in the battle against the pandemic. Price concludes, "It shows that Wales as a small nation, can get things done quickly as we face the biggest challenge of our generation."

According to BBC, Dr. Rhys Thomas from Glangwili Hospital in Carmarthen in Wales was "desperately concerned" at the lack of intensive care unit (ICU) ventilators to deal with the expected influx of patients.[44]

On the other hand, Andrew Murray stated that along with engineering company CR Clark & Co of Ammanford created a machine that not only helps patients to breathe but cleans the room of viral particles. He explained that the machine will also clean the room of viral particles and only supply purified air to the patient. The patient can self-care, releasing specialist nurses for other duties. Murray reported that robots that can help fight coronavirus have now been developed. Production has been accelerated, and it now takes less than a day to make one robot at their Odense facility in Denmark's third largest city and home to a growing robotics hub. Glowing like light sabers, eight bulbs emit concentrated UV-C ultraviolet light which destroys bacteria, viruses, and other harmful microbes by damaging their DNA and RNA, so they cannot multiply, and it is also hazardous to humans. However, there has been no specific testing to prove the robot's effectiveness against coronavirus, but the researchers are confident it will work.[45]

---

[44] "Coronavirus: The New Invention Inspired by A Pandemic," BBC News, 2020, Accessed April 28, 2020, https://www.bbc.com/news/uk-wales-52008745.

[45] Adrienne Murray, "Coronavirus: Robots Use Light Beams to Zap Hospital Viruses," *Technology of Business*, 2020, Accessed April 28, 2020, https://www.bbc.com/news/business-51914722.

Africa's Fight against COVID-19

With regard to COVID-19 that continues to rampage all the continent of the world, Colin Dwyer observed that countries on the African continent have largely managed to dodge its brunt, even as the global pandemic has besieged medical centers in the US and Western Europe; however, the global health authorities fear this will not continue forever. Dwyer cited the United Nations Economic Commission for Africa who claimed that anywhere between 300,000 and 3.3 million African people could lose their lives as a direct result of COVID-19, depending on the intervention measures taken to stop the spread.

According to the UN agency, the problem rests partly with the layout and infrastructure of some of the biggest cities on the continent where the majority of the urban population lives in over-crowded neighborhoods without reliable access to handwashing facilities. Couple that with relatively low supplies of hospital beds and the fact that 71 percent of the continent's workforce is "informally employed," according to the UNECA, without alternatives to work from home in the case of an outbreak, it becomes clear that "the continent is vulnerable."

Furthermore, the commission calculated the impact of the virus in Africa through a computer model collected by researchers at Imperial College London—whose grim outlooks on the possible effects in other parts of the world have already proven widely influential and in a worst-case scenario in which governments do not intervene with preventative measures such as large-scale social distancing—Africa may see more than 22 million people require hospitalization and some 3.3 million die of COVID-19.[46]

Additionally, Vera Songwe indicated that $100 billion is needed to "urgently and immediately provide fiscal space to all countries to

---

[46] Colin Dwyer, "U.N. Agency Fears 'Vulnerable' Africa May Suffer at Least 300,000 COVID-19 Deaths," NPR, 2020, Accessed April 25, 2020, https://www.npr.org/sections/coronavirus-live-updates/2020/04/17/836896562/u-n-agency-fears-vulnerable-africa-may-suffer-at-least-300-000-covid-19-deaths.

help address the immediate safety net needs of the populations." Already, Songwe had implied that countries in Africa have been suffering under the virus's fiscal effects, even if the physical ones had not yet made their full impact felt.[47]

With regard to the surpassing thousands of deaths that the Western nations have witnessed during COVID-19 pandemic despite their state-of-the-art technology and renowned public health system in comparison to Africa where the challenge is so demanding with no capacity and resources to flatten the curve, many have wondered how Africa will survive the pandemic. It might be true that Africa does not have the capacity to survive COVID-19 because of the lack of "state-of-the-art" technology and upgraded public health system that could meet the world's standard. Still, some African nations are more resilient in curtailing the surge in COVID-19 cases and death in comparison to the Western nations.

Africa has always shocked and surprised the world, even during the last Ebola pandemic. This can only be attributed to the depth of Africa's incomparable faith in God. African Christians know how to activate and deploy divine weapons of mass destruction through effective and fervent prayers of the righteous man (Jesus Christ) coupled with fasting and praise. The Almighty God knows Africa does not have the capacity to deal with COVID-19 pandemic, but they have a strong faith in God to do the best they can and repose their trust in God to grant them great deliverance from COVID-19 pandemic.

Timothy Tennent advocated that for those of us steeped in the Western traditions, it is not enough to simply celebrate the emergence of African indigenous theologizing, but we must come to realize how much we need to learn from their theological reflections, and that does not mean African Christians would not continue to benefit from Western, Asian, and Latin American reflections. He buttressed

---

47 Vera Songwe, "Without adequate protection, estimates show that over 300,000 Africans could lose their lives due to COVID-19—ECA Report," UNECA, 2020, Accessed April 25, 2020 https://www.uneca.org/stories/without-adequate-protection-estimates-show-over-300000-africans-could-lose-their-lives-due.

that this celebration of particularity should not be allowed to disintegrate into theological fragmentation. He noted that the Gospel has flourished the most in Africa when God was presented not as an imported deity from Europe but as the God who was already there, although known and worshipped only dimly and needing the full revelation of the person and work of Christ as revealed in Scripture.

Tennent confirmed that the church of Jesus Christ is growing in unprecedented ways in parts of the world once only regarded as the mission field and where 43,000 people were leaving the church every day in Europe and North America, 16,500 are coming to faith each day in Africa, and those from the older northern churches of Christendom must listen attentively to these new southern Christians as the Western nations are no longer the only central players on the field. He added that the West was not accustomed to living in a world where the heartlands of Christianity are located in Africa, Latin America, and Asia, twenty-first-century Christianity will largely be determined by the faithfulness of those outside the primary sphere of influence because the theology that matters the most is wherever the most Christians are located.

Tennent maintained that we must rejoice that in God's sovereignty, He has given us the opportunity to serve in new and exciting ways alongside our brothers and sisters from around the world, and as global Christians, we have "been to the mountaintop" and have captured a glimpse of some of the great things God is doing around the world today. But together, with all Christians in all times and places, we must surely recognize that the best theological enquiry anywhere in the world or during any time in history always serves to pull the entire church forward into that great eschatological fact of Jesus Christ.[48]

Kiera Butler reported that the task of preparing an entire African continent for a global pandemic is daunting. Kierra further reported that many of the aid groups secret weapon in the neediest communities was a lesson from the laid groundwork from the Ebola

---

[48] Timothy C. Tennent, *Theology in the Context of World Christianity, How the Global Church Is Influencing the Way We Think About and Discuss Theology* (Grand Rapids: Zondervan, 2007), 264–272.

outbreak of 2014–2016, which resulted in 28,600 cases and 11,325 deaths worldwide.

Butler cited Linda Venczel who recognized that there had been missteps from past outbreaks which serve as important lessons during the coronavirus outbreak. She recognized that during Ebola, some health centers sent test results to the government but never let local health officials know who had tested positive. Venczel added that her team worked hard to make sure that the system for the coronavirus will close that loop so that health care workers can easily and quickly get in touch with those who test positive, and their families and could advise them to quarantine.

However, she noticed that sustaining the public health infrastructure of communities once the crisis has passed has been a potential problem because between outbreaks, funding for infectious disease control in the developing world tends to dry up, and the developing world will turn their backs. Venczel warned that this outbreak will not be the last because of increased world travel and climate change and that infectious disease will be a recurring problem over the decades to come. She explicated that a one-off for an emergency is helpful, but what is really needed is sustained funding.[49]

The historical suppression of Africa through slavery led to Africa's underdeveloped systems, Robinson Milwood explained that it was part and parcel of Britain's strategy and engagement with their brutal methodology of decivilization, dehumanization, deculturalization, inferiorization, and animalization of Africans compounded with avariciousness has produced the Christianization of Africans with semantic cultural Christianity overlaid with the blatant absence of morality and social equality of Africans.

Milwood explained that it was Britain's intention through the merchants, planters, slave masters, traders, and slavers, who were indeed the ministers of religion and priests of Western European and

---

[49] Kiera Butler, "Using Lessons Learned from Ebola, Experts Are Preparing for a Coronavirus Outbreak in Africa," Mother Jones, 2020, Accessed May 9, 2020, https://www.motherjones.com/politics/2020/03/using-lessons-learned-from-ebola-experts-are-preparing-for-a-coronavirus-outbreak-in-africa/.

British cultural Christianity, to plan a plot that would keep African slaves in perpetual ignorance and uncivilized. Milwood quoted Henry Berry as saying, "We have as far as possible, closed every avenue by which light may enter the slaves' mind. If we could extinguish the capacity to see the light, our work would be complete; they would then be on a level with the beast of the field and we should be safe."

Milwood indicated that this thesis was on the exposure of Western European and British barbarity, savagery, brutality, racism, and sadism toward Africans, which has become a perpetual intellectual suppression of African history and intellectual powers. He highlighted that African slaves were oppressed and exploited by the actions and deeds of forced deracination and enslavement to the intent that the "unsafeness" will continue for everyone attempting to extinguish the African and African descendants' capacity to see the light that had been hidden from the black race for so many centuries and that there will never be a peroration until Africa has political unification, economic liberation from Europe, the West, and Britain and reparation from these countries and all the churches.[50]

Presently, the continent of Africa is still upholding certain levels of spiritual, social, and moral tenets to a greater degree that God honors which always attracts the mercy and goodness of God to Africa. With regard to the Judeo-Christian heritage of the Bible, Abraham, the father of faith, was enriched in Egypt that was in the continent of Africa (Gen. 12:16). Isaac was richly blessed when he visited Africa (Gen. 26:1–3). Jacob was greatly enriched while he was in Africa during a global famine (Gen. 46:1–8). It was in Africa that Joseph became the prime minister (Gen. 41:41–46), and it was in Africa that the twelve sons of Jacob were spared and also multiplied greatly during the famine that struck the whole earth.

We must remember that Moses, the savior of the Old Testament church, was born in Africa (Ex. 2:1–10) and became great in the

---

[50] Robinson Milwood, *Western European and British Barbarity, Savagery and Brutality in the Transatlantic Chattel Slave Trade: Homologated by the Churches and Intellectuals in the Seventeenth–Nineteenth Century, A Critical Study* (USA: Xlibris Corporation, 2013), 199.

continent before God used him to liberate the nation of Israel (Ex. 12:51). It was in Africa that Israel obtained wealth in silver and gold that was later used to build the tabernacle of God (Ex. 12:36). Africa became a place of refuge for our precious Lord, Jesus Christ, when Herod hunted for his dear life (Matt. 2:13).

There are so many biblical treasures and blessings of God on the continent of Africa. The continent of Africa is on God's agenda for His next move during this end-time harvest of souls into the kingdom of God. Historically, there has been so much pain, rejection, sufferings, slavery, and backwardness of Africa, just like it was for the Jews of God. This has made Africa to be stronger and better prepared for what God is about to do.

Hagar, the Egyptian concubine of Abraham, received a revelation of the name of God (Gen. 16:13). She had an encounter with God in the form of an angel and was given a promise that her progeny shall become a great nation (Gen. 21:18). Keturah, the wife of Abraham, was from Africa (Gen. 25:1, 4; 1 Chron 1:32–33); Jethro, Moses' father in-law who gave a plausible advice to Moses, was from Africa (Ex. 3:1, 4:18, 18). Moses' Cushite African wife aroused the bitter jealousy of his sister, Miriam (Num. 12:11–16). Initially, she and her family had received the exiled Moses for forty years who served her father as a shepherd in Sinai.

Zipporah had a better understanding of the importance of circumcision and performed the ritual on her sons (Ex. 4:25). When the Israelites settled in the land of Canaan, there were Africans among them (Ex. 12:38; Neh. 13:3). The bride in the Song of Solomon is "black and beautiful" (Song of Sol. 1:5), and as earlier mentioned, a Cushite who possessed tact, discretion, and a high position in the royal court appeared as a trusted courtier and was sent to tell David about news of Absalom's death (2 Sam. 18:19–32).

Solomon married an Egyptian princess (1 Kings 9:16, 24; 2 Chron. 8:11) and received the Queen of Sheba from Africa (1 Kings 10:1–13; 2 Chron. 9:1–2), an influential queen who ruled the dark-skinned people on both sides of the Red Sea. She had tested Solomon with hard questions while she poured unto Solomon all that was in her heart. Tirhakah, king of Ethiopia in Africa, came to the aid of Hezekiah when Jerusalem was besieged (2 Kings 19:9; Isa. 37:9). Ebedmelech, a confidential adviser of the king, identified as a Cushite (Jer. 38:7, 10, 12, 39:16) believed the words of Jeremiah from the Lord to Judah and risked his life to rescue the prophet from the dungeon. Jeremiah commends Ebedmelech's faith (Jer. 39:15–18) and decrees God's special covenant of protection to him. The prophet Zephaniah, a descendant of Hezekiah, the son of Cushi, prophesied about Cush (Zeph. 1:1). Zephaniah 3:10 declares, "From beyond the rivers of Ethiopia my suppliants, even the daughter of my dispersed shall bring mine offering."

Jehudi, the courtier sent to bear Jeremiah's message from Baruch to King Zedekiah, appears to have had a Cushite ancestor (Jer. 36:14). Simon of Cyrene was moved to carry the cross of Jesus when he came as a devout Jew for the feast of Passover in Jerusalem. He bore Jesus's cross on his way to Golgotha (Mark 15:21). Simon touched the cross of Jesus Christ and thus significantly and prophetically united Africans to the Christ achievements of carrying the cross where the penalty for man's sins was duly meted out. Simon must have been a believer, and his sons known to the Christian community (Mark 15:21; Rom. 16:13). Certain prophets and teachers at the church in Antioch gathered to minister to the Lord, and among them were two Africans, Lucius of Cyrene and Simon called Niger (Acts 13:1–2). "Niger" is a Latin word for "black," and the Simon here could have been this same Simon of Cyrene.

The kingdom of Cush continues to play a major role in the New Testament where we read of the conversion of Candace's Ethiopian treasurer (Acts 8:26–39). Candace was the royal title of the Queen Mother of Nubia, a powerful African nation located principally in what is now known as Sudan. God has started to use Africa as a source of blessing to the whole world. Africa is steadily rising up to take her place in God's ultimate end-time agenda, and thus, Africa rejects becoming the COVID-19 epicenter.

Africa is like the Cushite who began the race of bearing good news to David the king, and while he started running, he was overtaken by Ahimaaz (2 Sam. 18:19–32). But Ahimaaz had to step aside for Cushi because he has not seen the end of the battle and thus has no real message for the King of kings and Lord of lords. He is only running zealously without the solution. His response, according to 2 Samuel 18:29–33, was, "[I] saw a great tumult, but I knew not what it was. And the king said unto him, turn aside, and stand here. And he turned aside and stood still."

The "Ahimaaz" of this world have had their own day of out-running Cushi in the race of life. But the watchmen upon the walls (intercessors) are seeing another man running in the person of Cushi (Africa). They are the one that have the "now" and the "real" message for the King of kings and Lord of lords. Cushi's message was defi-nite, impactful, conclusive, and clear. The message was that all the enemies of the King have been placed under His feet, including the last enemy which is death. Second Samuel 18:32 declares, "And the king said unto Cushi, is the young man Absalom safe? And Cushi answered, the enemies of my lord the king, and all that rise against thee to do thee hurt, be as that young man is."

Christians' Post-COVID-19 Fight

God's eternal life plan is fabulous. It is free because Jesus had already paid for it. All it costs is our faith in God's Word to live and not die and to declare the glory of God in the land of the living (Ps. 118:17, 25). If we want to stay well, our faith in God's Word must be strong because Satan will try to challenge us. That is why Christians must adopt the following spiritual lockdown rules which should continue to be practiced, even though the coronavirus physi-cal lockdown is over. These include:

Constantly wash our hearts with the blood of Jesus Christ (Ps. 66:18, 73:1; Heb. 9:13–14):

> If I regard iniquity in my heart, the Lord will not hear me.
>
> Truly God is good to Israel, even to such as are of a clean heart.
>
> For if the blood of bulls and of goats, and the ashes of an heifer sprinkling the unclean, sanctifi-

eth to the purifying of the flesh. How much more shall the blood of Christ, who through the eternal Spirit offered himself without spot to God, purge your conscience from dead works to serve the living God?.

Constantly keep social distance from evil (Job 28:29; Ps. 34:14, 37:27; Prov. 16:6):

And unto man he said, Behold, the fear of the Lord, that is wisdom; and to depart from evil is understanding.

Depart from evil, and do good; seek peace, and pursue it.

Depart from evil, and do good; and dwell for evermore.

By mercy and truth iniquity is purged: and by the fear of the Lord men depart from evil.

Constantly avoid the crowd of wickedness and wicked people (Ps. 1:1, 101:4):

Blessed is the man that walketh not in the counsel of the ungodly, nor standeth in the way of sinners, nor sitteth in the seat of the scornful.

A froward heart shall depart from me: I will not know a wicked person.

Constantly cover your mind with the shield of the cross of Jesus so as not be infected from those who sneeze out sin and hatred (Lev. 19:17; Gal. 6:14; 1 John 2:9, 2:11, 3:15, 4:20):

Thou shalt not hate thy brother in thine heart: thou shalt in any wise rebuke thy neighbour, and not suffer sin upon him.

But God forbid that I should glory, save in the cross of our Lord Jesus Christ, by whom the world is crucified unto me, and I unto the world.

He that saith he is in the light, and hateth his brother, is in darkness even until now.

But he that hateth his brother is in darkness, and walketh in darkness, and knoweth not whither he goeth, because that darkness hath blinded his eyes.

Whosoever hateth his brother is a murderer: and ye know that no murderer hath eternal life abiding in him.

If a man say, I love God, and hateth his brother, he is a liar: for he that loveth not his brother whom he hath seen, how can he love God whom he hath not seen?

Constantly avoid shaking hands with abomination (Deut. 25:16; Prov. 11:1, 15:8, 26, 16:5, 17:15):

For all that do such things, and all that do unrighteously, are an abomination unto the Lord thy God.

For the froward is abomination to the Lord: but his secret is with the righteous.

A false balance is abomination to the Lord: but a just weight is his delight.

The sacrifice of the wicked is an abomination to the Lord: but the prayer of the upright is his delight.

The thoughts of the wicked are an abomination to the Lord: but the words of the pure are pleasant words

> Every one that is proud in heart is an abomination to the Lord: though hand join in hand, he shall not be unpunished.
>
> He that justifieth the wicked, and he that condemneth the just, even they both are abomination to the Lord
>
> Divers weights, and divers' measures, both of them are alike abomination to the Lord.

Constantly avoid hugging heresies and false teachings (2 Pet. 2:1; Titus 3:10; 2 John 10–11):

> But there were false prophets also among the people, even as there shall be false teachers among you, who privily shall bring in damnable heresies, even denying the Lord that bought them, and bring upon themselves swift destruction.
>
> A man that is an heretick after the first and second admonition reject.
>
> If there come any unto you, and bring not this doctrine, receive him not into your house, neither bid him God speed. For he that biddeth him God speed is partaker of his evil deeds.

Constantly maintain staying safe and being saved (Jer. 17:14; 2 Cor. 13:5):

> Heal me, O Lord, and I shall be healed; save me, and I shall be saved: for thou art my praise.
>
> Examine yourselves, whether ye be in the faith; prove your own selves. Know ye not your own selves, how that Jesus Christ is in you, except ye be reprobates?

Constantly sanitize your hands with God's Word (Lev. 8:10; John 17:17; 1 Thess. 4:3; James 4:8):

> And Moses took the anointing oil, and anointed the tabernacle and all that was therein, and sanctified them.
>
> Sanctify them through thy truth: thy word is truth.
>
> For this is the will of God, even your sanctification, that ye should abstain from fornication.
>
> Draw nigh to God, and he will draw nigh to you. Cleanse your hands, ye sinners; and purify your hearts, ye double minded.

Constantly seek immediate restoration whenever you observe any symptoms of sin or you are overtaken in a fault (Gal. 6:1; James 5:15, 20; 1 John 5:16; Jude 1:23):

> Brethren, if a man be overtaken in a fault, ye which are spiritual, restore such an one in the spirit of meekness; considering thyself, lest thou also be tempted.
>
> And the prayer of faith shall save the sick, and the Lord shall raise him up; and if he have committed sins, they shall be forgiven him.
>
> Let him know, that he which converteth the sinner from the error of his way shall save a soul from death, and shall hide a multitude of sins.
>
> If any man see his brother sin a sin which is not unto death, he shall ask, and he shall give him life for them that sin not unto death. There is a sin unto death: I do not say that he shall pray for it.
>
> And others save with fear, pulling them out of the fire; hating even the garment spotted by the flesh.

Constantly boost your immunity with God's Word, fasting and prayer, and the power of the Holy Spirit (Job 23:12; Jer. 15:16; Zech. 4:6; Mark 9:29; Luke 4:4; Rom. 8:26):

> Neither have I gone back from the commandment of his lips; I have esteemed the words of his mouth more than my necessary food.
>
> Thy words were found, and I did eat them; and thy word was unto me the joy and rejoicing of mine heart: for I am called by thy name, O Lord God of hosts.
>
> Then he answered and spake unto me, saying, This is the word of the Lord unto Zerubbabel, saying, Not by might, nor by power, but by my spirit, saith the Lord of hosts.
>
> And he said unto them, This kind can come forth by nothing, but by prayer and fasting.
>
> And Jesus answered him, saying, It is written, That man shall not live by bread alone, but by every word of God.
>
> Likewise the Spirit also helpeth our infirmities: for we know not what we should pray for as we ought: but the Spirit itself maketh intercession for us with groanings which cannot be uttered.

Superimposing Secular Education with Spiritual Education

Hidden in 2 Peter 3:8 is the scientific fact of Einstein's theory of relativity that time dilates or gets slower as speeds approach the speed of light. It reads, "But, beloved, be not ignorant of this one thing, that one day is with the Lord as a thousand years, and a thousand years as one day."

That the earth is round is revealed clearly in Isaiah 40:22, "It is he that sitteth upon the circle of the earth, and the inhabitants thereof are as grasshoppers; that stretcheth out the heavens as a curtain, and spreadeth them out as a tent to dwell in."

Thomas Strouse deduced that Albert Einstein had rejected the biblical truth that the earth is at rest (and therefore that the Scriptures and their Author are not absolute), and he rejected the Copernican Principle that the ether is at rest (with the earth supposedly translating through the absolute ether). Strouse emphasized that he actually denied that there was any ether since the earth could not be detected as having moved through it, and he cleverly shifted the frame of reference from the earth to the "observer" and the "absolute" from the motionless ether to the speed of light.

Strouse highlighted that Einstein actually recognized that if light is the only absolute and its speed is finite (186,000 miles per second), the observer must be the frame of reference, which then allows for multiple frames of reference at any time. He footnoted that this humanistic subjectivism is the basis for the ultimate solipsism which states "I only exist." Therefore, the outworking of Einsteinian physics is that everything is relative to me as the creator of my own universe. He warned that it is a non sequitur that the unredeemed world of physicists would discern the lie of the pseudoscience about which Paul warned Timothy in 1 Timothy 6:20, "O Timothy, keep that which is committed to thy trust, avoiding profane and vain babblings, and oppositions of science falsely so called."

However, it is a spiritual tragedy that Christian creationists are willing to countenance part of the lie and denounce the rest of it. He also cited Karen Wright who inferred that Einstein got it wrong not once, not twice, but countless times and that he made subtle blunders, he made outright goofs, his oversights were glaring, and that error infiltrated every aspect of his thinking. He was wrong about the universe, wrong about its contents, wrong about the inner workings of atoms. Furthermore, in 1911, Einstein predicted (by relativity) how much the sun's gravity would deflect nearby starlight and got it wrong by half. It was also stated that he rigged the equations of general relativity to explain why the cosmos was standing still when it wasn't, and beginning in the mid-1920s, he churned out faulty unified field theories at a prodigious rate.[51]

Second Timothy 2:15 indicates, "Study to shew thyself approved unto God, a workman that needeth not to be ashamed, rightly dividing the word of truth." It is obvious that Christians pay more attention to secular education at the expense of the light of God's Word by the Holy Spirit. Word-based education or spiritual education can only be acquired by being born again, studying the Word of God, and living by faith. We will experience a balanced learning if we superimpose secular education with the unparalleled spiritual education.

While secular education is extremely very important, it must submit to Christ-centered theological education. Paul states in 1 Corinthian 15:46, "Howbeit that was not first which is spiritual, but that which is natural; and afterward that which is spiritual."

Secular education will enable the Christian to be able to read and understand the Bible from which we get our spiritual education. Furthermore, secular education gives us an understanding of the physical visible creation, which God uses as an analogy to teach us about invisible spiritual realities. Paul explained in Romans 1:20, "For the invisible things of him from the creation of the world are clearly seen, being understood by the things that are made, even his eternal power and Godhead; so that they are without excuse."

Jennifer Shepard Payne in the *Journal of Religion and Health* from the US National Library of Medicine, National Institutes of Health (NIH), asked whether a pastor will refer to a mental health center; however, if they feel qualified to intervene themselves, they may not. This is because pastors are known to always provide grief counseling, and it is important to understand the decisions they make when intervening with depressed individuals.

According to Shepard Payne in a random sample of 204, Protestant pastors completed surveys about their treatment practices

---

[51] Thomas M. Strouse, "Einstein Versus the Bible," Bible Baptist Theological Seminary 3:11, 2011, Accessed May 7, 2020, http://www.bbc-cromwell.org/Seminary_Articles/Einstein%20Versus%20the%20Bible.pdf.

for depression. Fisher's exact analyses revealed that more pastors with some secular education yet no educational degree felt that they were the best person to treat depression than pastors who had no secular education or pastors who had at least a secular bachelor's degree. However, the level of theological education did not influence beliefs about the pastor being the best person to treat depression. In addition, neither secular nor theological education level influenced the pastors' views on referring people to mental health centers for depression treatment.

Shepard Payne cited some of the published empirical literature that discusses clergy involvement in mental health which alludes to certain untested assumptions, and some of the assumptions were that most pastors are uneducated (or, at the very least, antiquated in their thinking). Pastors with education primarily have theological educational backgrounds only. Clergy with a theological education (even with a graduate school education) are not equipped to make decisions about mental health in general and depression specifically and so do not understand when to refer someone out to a mental health center or a professional. They do not realize that they should not be handling depressed cases and that they are more likely to be against a medical model of treatment than for it while pastors with secular education degrees are more likely to make referrals to mental health centers than those without secular degrees (especially if their secular degrees were in a health or counseling-related field).

She suggested that researchers need to complete additional empirical studies in order to confirm or refute these assumptions, and based on the assumptions, it would be logical that the higher the level of secular education, the more likely the pastors will be open to referring to mental health centers. Additionally, a logical deduction based on assumptions would be that more counseling-related training would cause pastors to agree with mental health referral more readily. However, if no significant differences exist or if other factors besides secular education influence differences, then there is a need for these untested assumptions to be reexamined. She highlighted that results from this study may inform best practices in training pastors on mental health topics such as depression.[52]

God's Word is Jesus Christ personified, for the Word was made flesh and dwells among us (John 1:14). It is the source out of which all truth evolved—whether spiritual, scientific, historical, organizational, political, cultural, moral, sociological, economic, psychological, educational, natural, or legal—originates. All things, visible and invisible, were created were created and upheld by God's Word (Heb. 1:3, 11:3). John states in John 17:17, "Sanctify them through thy truth: thy word is truth." Most men are only accustomed to the physical but are not aware of the spiritual realm that encompasses the subconscious and the psychological realms.

Spiritual things are concealed or imperceptible to the physical senses or equipment but are tangible as they have a material effect on physical things: for instance, psychological (spiritual) forces that cannot be seen, perceived by the eyes or physical senses, or measured physically like fear—COVID-19 and other viruses, bacteria, anxiety, joy, peace—have a physical effect on your heart, blood pressure, and general health and can be measured physically.

On the other hand, science is the cerebral and sensible activity embracing the methodical study of the structure and behavior of the physical and natural world through observation and experiment research. According to NASA Science, Space Exploration, "Science consists of observing the world by watching, listening, observing, and recording. Science is curiosity in thoughtful action about the world and how it behaves."[53]

Using the Bible as the final and "only" authority, we can study the character and power of God through revelation of the reality of spiritual things; therefore, science is limited to physical truth, but God's Word divulges both physical and spiritual truth to us. No true

---

[52] Jennifer Shepard Payne, "The Influence of Secular and Theological Education on Pastors' Depression Intervention Decisions," *Springer Journal of Religion and Health*, 53(5?):1398–1413, 2014, Accessed July 13, 2020, https://www.ncbi.nlm.nih.gov/pmc/articles/PMC4138430/.

[53] "What Is Science?" NASA Science, Space Place, Accessed May 7, 2020, https://spaceplace.nasa.gov/science/en/.

scientific truth must cross the boundary of opposing God's Word, but rather it, should enhance it.

Craig Rusbult stated that scientism begins with a good idea that, when exaggerated, becomes a bad idea and that science has earned our trust because it has been useful for understanding many aspects of physical reality and for developing technology. He explained that this trust should not be extended into areas where it is not justified and where science is not useful. We can trust science for some things and not others. He added that when confidence in science is misplaced and becomes scientism, it can lead us to wrong conclusions.[54]

Johannes Kepler—the German mathematician and astronomer who discovered the laws of planetary motion which later served as one of the foundations for Isaac Newton's theory of universal gravitation—is considered to be one of the founders of the field of astronomy, and as of the late sixteenth century, there was no scientific community schooling in Germany or elsewhere. It was under the control of church institutions, whether Roman Catholic or Protestant, and local rulers who used the churches and the educational systems as a means to consolidate the loyalty of their populations.[55] God's Word, the Bible, states that the heavens are being "stretched." NASA, in modern astronomy, had observed in the 1990s the expansion of the universe. It might have enough energy density to stop its expansion and re-collapse; it might have so little energy density that it would never stop expanding, but gravity was certain to slow the expansion as time went on. NASA Universe stated that supposedly, the slowing had not been observed, but theoretically, the universe had to slow whereas the universe is full of matter and the attractive force of gravity pulls all matter together. Then came 1998 and the Hubble Space Telescope (HST) observations of very distant supernovae that

[54] Craig Rusbult, "How Should We Interpret the Two Books of God in Scripture & Nature," 2004, Accessed May 7, 2020, https://www.asa3.org/ASA/education/origins/two-books.htm.

[55] Robert S. Westman, "Johannes Kepler, German Astronomer," *Encyclopedia Britannica*, Accessed May 7, 2020, https://www.britannica.com/biography/Johannes-Kepler.

showed that a long time ago, the universe was actually expanding more slowly than it is today.

NASA explained that the expansion of the universe has not been slowing due to gravity as everyone thought, but it has been accelerating although no one expected this, and no one knew how to explain it. But something was causing it. NASA clarifies that eventually, theorists came up with three sorts of explanations what this might be because it was a result of a long-discarded version of Einstein's theory of gravity, one that contained what was called a "cosmological constant," or there was some strange kind of energy-fluid that filled space. And if that was not the case, it might be because there was something wrong with Einstein's theory of gravity and a new theory could include some kind of field that created this cosmic acceleration. NASA stressed that theorists still do not know what the correct explanation is, but they have given the solution a name: dark energy.

Their explanation is that more is unknown than is known and that the amount of dark energy there is known because how it affects the universe's expansion is known; and other than that, it is a complete mystery.[56] Psalms 104:2 states, "Who coverest thyself with light as with a garment, who stretchest out the heavens like a curtain." Likewise, Job 9:8 corroborates, "Which alone spreadeth out the heavens, and treadeth upon the waves of the sea."

Recently, Max Planck Society documented that the star Kepler-160 and its companion, KOI-456.04, are more reminiscent of the Sun-Earth system than any previously known exoplanet-star pair, and among the more than four thousand known exoplanets, KOI-456.04 is something special, which is less than twice the size of Earth and orbits a sun-like star. It does so with a star-planet distance that could permit planetary surface temperatures conducive to life. The object was discovered by a team led by the Max Planck Institute for Solar System Research in Göttingen. Its host star, called Kepler-160, actually emits visible light. The central stars of almost

---

[56] "Dark Energy, Dark Matter," NASA Science, Share the Science, Accessed May 7, 2020, https://science.nasa.gov/astrophysics/focus-areas/what-is-dark-energy/.

all other exoplanets, on the other hand, emit infrared radiation and are smaller and fainter than the sun and therefore belong to a class of red dwarf stars.

Planck Society indicated that the red dwarf stars are known for their extremely long lifetimes, and life on an exoplanet in orbit around an old red dwarf star could potentially have had twice as much time than life on Earth to form and evolve.[57]

Isaiah 42:5 indicates, "Thus saith God the Lord, he that created the heavens, and stretched them out; he that spread forth the earth, and that which cometh out of it; he that giveth breath unto the people upon it, and spirit to them that walk therein."

Jeremiah 10:12 infers, "He hath made the earth by his power, he hath established the world by his wisdom, and hath stretched out the heavens by his discretion."

There is no way we can deny God's Word as the final and "only" authority over the physical and spiritual world. There is overwhelming evidence of an intelligent and powerful Creator in the physical as seen both in the heavens and in the physical body. Psalms 19:1–4 declares:

> The heavens declare the glory of God; and the firmament sheweth his handywork. Day unto day uttereth speech, and night unto night sheweth knowledge. There is no speech nor language, where their voice is not heard. Their line is gone out through all the earth, and their words to the end of the world. In them hath he set a tabernacle for the sun.

That is why we must all praise God for our being fearfully and wonderfully made because through the visible creation, God has

---

[57] Max Planck Society, "'Mirror Image' of the Earth and Sun Discovered 3,000 Light-Years Away," *SciTechDaily*, 2020, Accessed June 9, 2020, https://scitech-daily.com/mirror-image-of-the-earth-and-sun-discovered-3000-light-years-away/.

shown us the invisible existence of His power. Psalm 139:14 states, "I will praise thee; for I am fearfully and wonderfully made: marvelous are thy works; and that my soul knoweth right well."

Paul stated in Romans 1:19–20:

> Because that which may be known of God is manifest in them; for God hath shewed it unto them. For the invisible things of him from the creation of the world are clearly seen, being understood by the things that are made, even his eternal power and Godhead; so that they are without excuse.

Scientists had come up with genetic keys while nutritionists proclaimed that some certain foods guarantee long healthy lives to those who eat them. Fitness experts had also invented exercise plans that promise to keep us young, slim, and agile at any age. Although good nutrition and exercise really do help, most people are yet to come up with a guaranteed life youth-renewing plan that provides people in their eighties, nineties, hundreds, and beyond the strength and the vitality of people half their age, except Moses.

Peter D'Adamo specified that evolution is very subtle, and human being genetic makeups and that of their progeny continue to alter infinitesimal and in unknown ways of which humans are completely unaware of. He observed that there have been recent outbreaks of rare viruses and infectious diseases as we press into the remaining untouched jungles of this planet. He stresses that these diseases defy medical intervention and wonders whether the human body will ever produce answers to the challenges posed by the unknown, and these challenges include increasing ultraviolet radiation caused by the depletion of the ozone layer, increased pollution of air and water, increased food contamination, overpopulation and famine, infectious diseases beyond our power to control, and unknown plagues emerging from all of the above.

D'Adamo remarked that the human race will survive all of these, although we might now not know how to survive. He suggested that a new blood type will emerge that is called Type C, which will be able to create antibodies to fend off every antigen that exists today and any future permutation of antigens that develops. He advocated that in an overcrowded and polluted world with few natural recourses left, the new Type Cs will come to dominate their societies, and the antiquated blood types will begin to die off in an increasingly hostile environment for which they are no longer suited, and the Type C blood type will finally rule.[58]

Some had claimed that sudden and untimely death is natural, and they believe it is part of God's plan and that we should embrace it. But the Bible presents a different picture. It tells us that death was not a part of God's original design. It was not included in His perfect will. In fact, He specifically commanded Adam and Eve not to open the door to it. But Adam and Eve disobeyed. They bowed the knee to Satan by succumbing to his temptation. Through their sin, they introduced death into God's beautiful world.

---

[58] Peter D'Adamo, *4 Blood Types, 4 Diets, Eat Right for Your Type. The Individualized Diet Solution to Staying Health, Living Longer & Achieving Your Ideal Weight* (Canada: G. P. Putnam's Sons, 1996), 324–326.

CHAPTER 4

Globalization: COVID-19 Global Advantages and Catastrophes

COVID-19 had drastically changed our understanding of the world around us. It has confronted our previous ideologies ranging from capitalism to neo-liberalism, from the over-significance of work to realizing work-life balance and spending time with immediate family, and from globalization to nationalization. The world we live in is progressively interconnected and, subsequently, interdependent. Our initial understanding was that a categorized but interconnected world was the best system for launching every advancement.

But this, our strength, can also be a source of our weakness. Our interconnectedness has made us more vulnerable as the very potency that makes us proud to be members of a global village has occasioned the spread of coronavirus through cross-border infection. Our interdependence now predisposes us to a greater risk. The closure of borders of several countries as coronavirus pandemic spreads like wildfire globally has impacted the flow of people and goods across the borders and has left many thinking about the negative impact of COVID-19 on the international system of trade and travel.

However, COVID-19 has not come to degenerate or annihilate globalization but has only changed and enhanced its mechanisms. While globalization had survived the 1918 Spanish flu, SARS in 2003, H1N1 in 2009, the two world wars and war on terrorism, it will also survive COVID-19 and come out strong with a brand-new configuration.

Thomas Friedman, on differentiation of globalization, explains that globalization has gone into a whole new level as he identified that there have been three great eras of globalization. He classified the first that lasted from 1492 to 1800 when Columbus set sail, opening trade between the Old World and the New World, which he called Globalization 1.0 that literarily shrank the world from a size medium.[59] Accordingly, Globalization 1.0 was about countries and muscles that embrace the key agent of change, the dynamic force driving the process of global integration with how much brawn, muscle horsepower, wind power, or later steam power that particular country had or how creative one could deploy it. He stated that the focus in Globalization 1.0 was, "Where does my country fit into global competition and opportunities? And how can one go global and collaborate with others through my country?"[60]

Nevertheless, Friedman explained that in the second great era, Globalization 2.0, which lasted from 1800 to 2000, interrupted by the great depression and World Wars I and II, was an era that shrank the world from a size medium to a size small. The key agent of change during this era and the dynamic force driving global integration was multinational companies. He noted that these multinationals went global for markets and labor, spearheaded first by the expansion of the Dutch and English joint-stock companies and the Industrial Revolution. Friedman narrated that in the first half of this era, global integration was powered by falling transportation cost, the steam engine and railroad, while the second half was characterized by falling telecommunication costs, telephones, the PC, satellites, fiber-optic cable, and the early version of the World Wide Web.[61]

Friedman explained that this era witnessed the birth and the maturation of a global economy that fosters enough movement of goods and information from continent to continent for there to be a global market with global arbitrage in products and labor. He

---

[59] Thomas L. Friedman, *The World Is Flatt. A Brief History of the Twenty-first Century* (New York: Farrar, Straus and Giroux, 2006), 8–11

[60] Ibid., 9.

[61] Ibid., 9.

postulated that the dynamic forces behind this era of globalization were breakthroughs in hardware from steamships and railroads in the beginning to telephones and mainframe computers toward the end. He argued that around the year 2000, we entered a whole new era which is called Globalization 3.0, and Globalization 3.0 is shrinking the world from a size small to a size tiny and flattening the playing field at the same time.[62]

Additionally, he postulated that Globalization 3.0 differs from the previous eras not only in how it is shrinking and flattening the world and in how it is empowering individuals but the fact that Globalization 1.0 and 2.0 were driven primarily by European and American individuals and businesses, although actually having the biggest economies in the world in the eighteenth century where in the Western countries, companies, and explorers were the ones doing most of the globalizing and shaping the system. But going forward, this will be less and less true, and they will no longer be the major actors because of the flattening and shrinking of the world and as Globalization 3.0 is going to be more and more driven not only by individuals but also by a much more diverse non-Western and non-white group of individuals, individuals from every corner of the flat world that are being empowered. Globalization 3.0 has therefore made it possible for so many people to plug in and play.[63]

In a way, many have placed much denunciation on globalization as a fuel that added fire to the COVID-19 pandemic, having ignored the fact that viruses have been a part of the world since the fall of Adam in the Garden of Eden. Many have been sidetracked to think because the virus began from China, which then spread like fire across the world, it was due to globalization and thus imposing disconnection to international travels to curb the pandemic. While this could be detrimental, the COVID-19 pandemic has provided several layers of innovations. As a result of COVID-19, there has been increased teleworking and refurbishment of the world health care systems. Just as the 9/11 terrorist attacks launched the United

---

[62] Ibid., 10.
[63] Ibid. 11.

States and the Western world into "war or terror" and mandated an overhaul of airport security, COVID-19 will gradually introduce health screenings at every port of entry in all nations of the world.

What happens when the world is not moving anywhere at the same time? Some geologists have observed that the slowdown in human activity is literally stabilizing the earth's crust, causing the world to have less geological shaking known as ambient seismic noise, such as the vibrations generated by cars, trains, buses, planes, and people tramping on the earth, and in this moment of quietness, it is helping geologists to detect earth's smaller quakes. Less traffic during the lockdown has led to less atmospheric pollution. Insurance premiums have gone down while road accidents have drastically reduced since many people now work from home.

Victor Tangermann cited Thomas Lecocq, a geologist and seismologist at the Royal Observatory in Belgium. He acknowledged that once-crowded city streets were now empty, and the unlikely beneficiary of the coronavirus lockdown has made the planet highway traffic to slow down to a minimum. Also, fewer and fewer people can be found milling about outside. Lecocq observed that the global containment measures to combat the spread of coronavirus have seemingly made the world much quieter. And in the absence of the noise, the earth's upper crust is moving just a little less.[64]

Tangermann adds, "Regardless, a significant drop in seismic noise also shows that we are at least doing one thing right during the current pandemic, staying in the safety of our own homes as we wait for the virus to run its course."[65] And since COVID-19 has no respect for border, it must not be a tool to annex and suffocate globalization but must be a tool that must be used to enhance international cooperation; otherwise, the virus might be defeated in one location while it resurfaces at another, thereby ruining whatever accomplishment a country might have previously achieved.

---

[64] Victor Tangermann, "Earth Is Vibrating Substantially Less Because There's So Little Activity Right Now," Science Alert, 2020, Accessed April 20, 2020, https://www.sciencealert.com/the-earth-is-moving-substantially-less-because-of-the-global-pandemic.

[65] Ibid.

James Le Duc and Neal Nathanson states, "The human population is growing inexorably, and is becoming urbanized even faster. As a result, there are an increasing number of large-crowded cities, which provide an optimal setting for the rapid spread of any newly emergent infectious agent."[66] They studied the "emergence" of a viral disease represents the first identification of the cause of a well-recognized disease. They cited La Crosse virus, a mosquito-transmitted bunya virus that was first isolated from a fatal case of encephalitis in 1964. Furthermore, they mentioned Hantavirus pulmonary syndrome which is another example of the "emergence" of an existing but previously unrecognized disease.[67]

They substantiated that in 1993, in the four corners area of the southwestern United States, there occurred a small outbreak of cases of acute pulmonary illness with a high mortality. Epidemiologic and laboratory investigation rapidly identified the causal agent, a previously unknown hantavirus now named Sin Nombre virus (SNV) which is an indigenous virus of deer mice (*Peromyscus maniculatus*) that are persistently infected and excrete the virus. Apparently, deer mice produce virus-infected excreta, and when they infest human dwellings, aerosolized fomites can result in occasional human infections. They concluded that the 1993 outbreak is thought to reflect a transient rise in deer mouse populations associated with an unusual crop of pine nuts, a major food source for these rodents. This recognition of SNV soon led to the discovery of other unrecognized hantaviruses in North, Central, and South America, many of which also cause serious human disease.[68]

They further specified that a virus that is already widespread in a population can emerge as a cause of epidemic or endemic disease due to an increase in the ratio of cases to infections. Such an increase can be caused by either an increase in host susceptibility or enhance-

---

[66] James W. Le Duc and Neal Nathanson, "Viral Pathogenesis. Emerging Viral Diseases: While We Need to Worry about Bats, Camels, and Airplanes," *Elsevier Public Health Emergency Collection*, 215–231, 2016, Accessed April 30, 2020, https://www.ncbi.nlm.nih.gov/pmc/articles/PMC7170184/.

[67] Ibid.

[68] Ibid.

ment of the virulence of the virus. Although counterintuitive, there are some dramatic instances of such phenomena.[69]

They also explained that a virus that is endemic in a population may "fade out" and disappear because the number of susceptible has fallen below the critical level required for perpetuation in that population, and if the population is somewhat isolated, the virus may remain absent for many years. They clarified that a virus can enter and spread in a region where it had never previously circulated, leading to the emergence of a disease new to that locale such as the emergence of West Nile virus (WNV) in the United States, beginning in 1999, that was confined to a finite geographic area based on the range of its vertebrate reservoir hosts and permissive vectors.[70]

Le Duc and Nathanson, who also studied the zoonotic infections of animals that can be transmitted to humans and are a major cause of emerging virus diseases of humans, elucidated that these viruses are transmitted by direct contact by virus-laden droplets or aerosols or by insect vectors and that all zoonotic viruses have one or more animal reservoir hosts which play an important role in the epidemiological dynamics of human infections.[71]

They specified that though many zoonotic viruses can be transmitted to humans on occasion, their relative ability to spread from human to human determines whether or not they emerge as significant new virus diseases of mankind, and because most zoonotic viruses that are transmitted to humans cannot be spread directly from person to person, humans are considered to be "dead-end hosts."[72] They indicated that there are more than 500 viruses belonging to several virus families that are also classified as arboviruses (arthropod-borne viruses) based on a vertebrate-arthropod maintenance cycle in nature. Arboviruses replicate in both the vertebrate host and the arthropod vector (mosquitoes, ticks, sandflies, and others), and transmission occurs when the vector takes a blood meal.[73]

---

[69] Ibid.
[70] Ibid.
[71] Ibid.
[72] Ibid.
[73] Ibid.

Le Duc and Nathanson reviewed the 2002 outbreak of severe acute respiratory disease (SARS) which began in Guangdong Province in southeast China near the Hong Kong border and identified the first cases that were concentrated in food handlers who then spread the virus to the general population in that region. Moreover, the Middle Eastern Respiratory Syndrome (MERS) was also an acute respiratory disease of humans first recognized in 2012 when a novel coronavirus (MERS-CoV) was isolated from two fatal human cases in Saudi Arabia and Qatar.[74]

They appraised the 2014/15 Ebola hemorrhagic fever which riveted the world's attention that the international health community failed to control and evaluated that the Ebola was a filovirus indigenous to Africa maintained in one or more reservoir species of wild animals among which bats are a likely host. They inferred that although the transmission cycle is not well-documented, still it is thought that humans get infected either by direct contact with bats or while slaughtering infected wild animals who may have acted as intermediate hosts. They noted that Ebola virus was first isolated in 1976 in an outbreak near the Ebola River in the Democratic Republic of the Congo (then called Zaire), and almost concurrently, the second outbreak occurred in southern Sudan.[75]

It must be clear that when humanity provokes God, no nation on earth can defend them from the consequences. COVID-19 has been designed not to cripple globalization but to enable the world to turn to God who alone is our defense and protection from the present and future pandemics. The only superpower that be is God Almighty. Coronavirus, as it were, does not discriminate based on political views or on intellectualism. It has sets in an unprecedented time that will be remembered for decades where grocery stores were emptied, the market sank, and everyone was stuck in their homes.

---

[74] Ibid.
[75] Ibid.

Global Awakening

As the coronavirus (COVID-19) sweeps across many countries of the world, some have concluded that we are on the verge of a spiritual awakening and revival. The pandemic has enabled many to start to spend time with families, share meals, communicate to neighbors, help one another, and take long walks outside while at the same time maintain social distancing.

Just like it was difficult to purchase Bibles at the Dollar Store in most US cities during the 9/11 terrorist attack, so also it is becoming difficult to find basic cleaning supplies like Lysol and Clorox. Many people are focusing on being clean on the outside, and that is very commendable, but we must remember that God looks on the inside deeper, and so we must commit ourselves to being clean on the inside. We must be holy as our God is holy (1 Pet. 1:15–16). Outward cleanliness might be good, but inward cleanliness is much more important (Matt. 23:25, Luke 11:39). God is using the COVID-19 pandemic to call us to examine ourselves and repent so He can reveal where we need that inner cleansing. This is not about condemning anyone but making a 180-degree turn from sin and iniquity. We have to use this time to prepare for the expected revival and reawakening. This cannot be a wasted time but a time to clean up and redeem the time so as to be a beneficiary of the blessings that are ahead.

Thomas G. Long observes, "The inability to make some kind of sense of the actions and will of God in a world of suffering and evil puts pressure on people of faith…to abandon the biblical claim that God is a God of history, of time, of material embodiment and actual circumstances, in favor of a mystical God of nature and spirituality."[76]

The COVID-19 pandemic led to the shutdown of some distilleries stepping in and producing hand sanitizer instead of booze just as the Scriptures confirm, "They will beat their swords into plowshares" (Isaiah 2:4). Although there has been an unthinkable tragedy of people dying every day from COVID-19, it is this very thing, the

---

[76] Thomas G. Long, *What Shall We Say? Evil, Suffering, and the Crisis of Faith* (Grand Rapids, MI: Eerdmans, 2011), 34.

fear of death, the acknowledgement of the fragility of life that has been a wakeup call for many. Indeed, the COVID-19 pandemic has created an awakening.

COVID-19 is a demonic bondage already defeated by Jesus Christ. Neil Anderson analyzed common misconceptions about bondage to be demons that were active when Christ was on the earth, but their activity has subsided. What the early church called demonic activity we now understand to be mental illness, which statements underline the credibility of Scripture that some problems are psychological, and some are spiritual. Even though Christians cannot be affected by demons, demonic influence can be evident in extreme or violent behavior and gross sin. Thus, freedom from spiritual bondage is the result of a power encounter with demonic forces.

Anderson explained that the Western world is experiencing a massive paradigm shift in its worldview best seen in the rise of the New Age movement—the acceptance of parapsychology as a science, the growing popularity of the supernatural, and the increasing visibility of satanism in our culture. He added that New Age mysticism, which gathered its greatest strength with the influx of Eastern religions in the 1960s, has been popularized by a host of celebrities, businesses, education, and even in religion across the nation.[77]

But with the advent of this already defeated demonic bondage called COVID-19, several politicians now think of their constituents while some countries now realize the importance of God. With the entrance of coronavirus, many people are learning how to work on their mannerisms. It has taught humans the importance of proper hygiene and safety precautions, such as how to sneeze, yawn, and cough publicly. Many are realizing that all humans are equal and that there is no country that is superior. There are many people from the West who now desire to make Africa their home. Due to COVID-19, many have been brought back to their Creator because humanity and morals have failed. Now we realize that God is our only healer and physicians working in and through the medical doctors.

---

[77] Neil Anderson, *The Bondage Breaker* (Eugene OR: Harvest House Publishers, 2000), 19–28.

The bars, nightclubs, brothels, and casinos have been forced to close down. Coronavirus has brought interest rates down and brought families together like never before. Many people have stopped eating dead and forbidden animals. There have been great advances in telecommunication, even at a faster rate, and the world is more networked than ever through teleworking.

Students in different parts of the world are now engaged in virtual learning experiences as COVID-19 has brought real changes to their learning world. Educational tech and digital transformations have connected more people in their homes although it also revealed inequalities with regard to who has devices and bandwidth, who has the skills to self-direct their learning, and how much time parents have to navigate their children in their learning process. Students can now take ownership over their learning, they can personalize their learning, understand more about how they learn, and what support they need. The COVID-19 pandemic has become a tool that revolutionizes the world's educational and economic systems in terms of rising unemployment and recession.

Rana Chakrabarti explained that the lockdown following the COVID-19 pandemic created an overnight change from learning in the physical to digital world. Even though a sense of place is important to learning, the social experience is priceless. She observed that while listening happens in class, real learning happens outside when we process the learning experience with our mates in cafes or on walking routes. Furthermore, the heart of all learning is the process of learn-do-reflect, labs, and projects which fulfills the hands-on portion. Also, reflection happens when the educator gives feedback, which virtual has dismantled the entire mechanism.

This is why in a post-COVID world, there is an even bigger change at hand with the big flip being the reversal of power from the educator to the learner. Additionally, she explained that in a post-COVID world, with mostly prerecorded and few live sessions, an educator will no longer strictly control the sequence of learning because the learners will start where it interests them, learn at the pace, and for the duration, they can and do it out of sight of the educator. Therefore, they will have to craft attention rather than curriculum.

Chakrabarti noted that the best teaching experience will be a production that will be delivered as a performance, and since the medium is a screen, educators will learn from television shows and scriptwriters on how to produce episodic learning experiences. She stated that there will be a break away from the tyranny of the flat screen and that our ability to create virtual worlds will transform both learning and teaching in a post-COVID world. The now-affordable headsets for virtual, augmented, and mixed reality (together called XR or extended reality) will make it possible for us to experience instead of just listen to a lesson.

Furthermore, she clarified that storytelling and simulation in the form of scenes and situations that propel learners' curiosities will become the central device to facilitate learning and learning in a post-pandemic world will be about mastering by doing rather than mastering by knowing.

She elucidated that automation and artificial intelligence will eliminate most repetitive jobs that can be precisely specified, and companies will increasingly present applicants with real-life challenges and gauge how they respond. She concluded that learners who focus on mastery and deliberate practice, applying what they have learn to changing contexts, will be set apart while educators and learners alike are bound to struggle with the transition, which needs to happen slowly with plenty of handholding for both. Chakrabarti explains, "Educators who really want to empower their students will be the first ones to try this out."[78]

Christine Romans explored the depression that was labelled as a bad recession. She cited Kevin Hassett who compared the coronavirus collapse in the US economy to the Great Depression. Hassett states, "This is the biggest negative shock that our economy, I think,

---

[78] Rana Chakrabarti, "What Will Learning Look Like in a Post Pandemic World?" Forbes: SAP BrandVoice Innovation, 2020, Accessed June 15, 2020, https://www.forbes.com/sites/sap/2020/06/11/how-covid-19-changes-gen-z-approach-to-the-workplace/#4c66966742ea.

has ever seen. We're going to be looking at an unemployment rate that approaches rates that we saw during the Great Depression." Hassett noted that during the Great Recession, America lost 8.7 million jobs, but during COVID-19, the nation is losing many jobs about every ten days, and he decries that a depression is essentially a really bad recession and that this one is just what it is.

Romans analyzed from a bit of the Great Depression history that it encompasses two downturns, and from the National Bureau of Economic Research, the official bookkeeper of booms and busts in the economy, a sharp downturn from 1929 to 1933 was discovered when GDP fell 27 percent and again from 1937 to 1938, but most economists did not believe that the economy returned to something considered "normal" until 1940 or 1941. However, there is an important difference today, and that is America has a safety net this time, and how well it works will decide if this is a depression in name only, given Congress had spent trillions of dollars in rescue and bailout funds.[79]

Zachary Mack acknowledges the clearer studies and research evolving from doctors' understanding of how to treat severe cases of incoming coronavirus patients; however, it is being discovered that the disease is taking a greater toll on the body than originally envisaged because of the horrific side effects and complications. He elucidated that medical experts have started raising concern over COVID-19 survivors developing post-traumatic stress disorder (PSTD) that could affect them for years to come. Mack cited BBC, who commented on administrators from Britain's National Health Service initiating calls for all physicians to automatically screen COVID-19 patients for PSTD before discharging them from the hospital. This is because the effects of the disease, which can include intense nightmares and vivid flashbacks, can potentially last for life if they are not properly addressed and treated.

---

[79] Christine Romans, "Great Depression Comparisons Are Depressing, but this Time Is Different," HBJ Hartford Business, 2020, Accessed May 2, 2020, https://www.hartfordbusiness.com/article/great-depression-comparisons-are-depressing-but-this-time-is-different.

Mack cited the report published in the medical journal, *Global Health Research and Policy*, in relation to treatment of PTSD in coronavirus survivors. There, researchers observed the case rates of PTSD in survivors of previous disease outbreaks, including the 2003 SARS outbreak, H1N1 flu epidemic of 2009, and the Ebola outbreak of 2015. They found "a rather high prevalence of mental health problems among survivors, victim families, medical professionals, and the general public after an epidemic of infectious disease," and the authors conclude that it's "urgent to provide mental health service targeted at prevention of PTSD to survivors and other people exposed to COVID-19."

Moreover, experts are continuing to look ahead and raise awareness about the mental health implications of the pandemic because failure to do so could have long-term consequences.[80] Additionally, one third of military and government expenditure have been diverted to health care. Many Arab countries have banned "shisha," which according to Rolando Fuertes Jr. is an exotic water pipe also known as "hookah" to smoke fruit-flavored tobacco, talk, and watch the world pass, which has become an almost integral part of the Arabs' social lives and their culture, and it is rapidly gaining popularity all over the world.[81]

In another instance, more people are learning to pray due to coronavirus, and virtual church attendance has increased. Coronavirus undermines dictators and their powers, and many are elevating God rather than personal ambition, progress, and technology. Coronavirus has set many prisoners free and has forced authorities to look at its prisons and prisoners. Coronavirus is now making us stay at home, living simple lives, and get the much-needed rest that is needed. Many are spending less while the governments are

---

[80] Zachary Mack, "One Horrifying Way COVID-19 Could Affect You for Years, Warn Doctors. Doctors Are Raising the Alarm on this Potential Side Effect that Can Affect Survivors for Life." BESTLIFE Health, 2020, Accessed July 2, 2020, https://bestlifeonline.com/covid-19-affect-for-years/.

[81] Rolando M. Fuertes Jr., "Middle East and Africa, Shisha: An Arab Delight, a Taste of Home," *The Seoul Times*, 2020, Accessed April 29, 2020, https://theseoultimes.com/ST/?url=/ST/db/read.php%3Fidx=900.

giving out stimulus checks. No more sport betting since all sporting activities have been postponed till further notice. There is no excuse for husbands not to stay at home again and using the job as an excuse.

Most importantly, it has paved the way for children of God to draft in many unbelievers into the fold and for us to reflect and thank God for waking us up to this new reality of social distancing and not social isolation from the Lord and from one another.

Barroso and Kochhar stated that COVID-19 is proving to be not only a public health crisis but also an economic crisis because the call for social distancing has negatively impacted service sector jobs that depend on customer-provider interactions or involve the congregation of large numbers of people. Barroso and Kochhar buttressed that workers in industries, such as restaurants, hotels, childcare services, retail trade, and transportation services are at a higher risk of losing their jobs.

They detailed from a Pew Research Center of government data that nearly one in four US workers, which is about 38.1 million out of 157.5 million, are employed in the industries most likely to feel an immediate impact from the COVID-19 outbreak, and among the most vulnerable of this are workers in retail trade (10 percent of all workers) and food services and drinking places (6 percent) with these two industries employing nearly twenty-six million Americans in total. And based on the demographics of workers in higher-risk industries, young people in particular are set to be disproportionately affected by virus-related layoffs. Among the 19.3 million workers aged sixteen to twenty-four in the economy overall, 9.2 million or nearly half are employed in service sector establishments. Younger workers make up 24 percent of employment in higher-risk industries overall, and many establishments in these industries are facing a high likelihood of closure in areas with more severe COVID-19 outbreaks.

Barroso and Kochhar added that employment outcomes in retail trade, which employs 16.2 million workers, are more uncertain. While brick-and-mortar operations are at higher risk because some are closed by government mandate, and shoppers are otherwise encouraged to stay home, this has greatly enabled electronic shopping providers to benefit.[82]

Adam Kuczynski and Jonathan Kanter explained that staying away from each other to fight the spread of coronavirus is a hard pill. But this hard pill comes with a side effect. However, the side effect cannot be compared with the benefit that comes with this practice. Realistically, in times of stress and illness, being deprived of social connection can create more stress and illness.

Among many things we can do to mitigate the downside of social distancing and isolation that are in effect is to let people know how much you care about them through a phone call with a real voice, which is better than text. Kanter and Kuczynski stated that what you say when connecting also matters. Your task might be to just listen and convey that you understand their feelings and really accept them. Additionally, they stated that we should be able to embrace others by expanding how we feel we define our group identities. They advised that we must be generous and realize that maintaining social distance does not hinder building a foundation of healthy coping, maintaining awareness of the side effects of our necessary societal changes, and staying connected to our values and to each other. This is because human beings have great capacity for empathy and caring in times of suffering.[83]

According to Charles Goldman and Rita Karam, the college experience in America might never look the same as COVID-19 is threatening to upend the models that both public and private higher education depend on in the United States. Previously, colleges and universities have been increasing their use of online learning for years, but COVID-19 has accelerated that change, forcing students and faculty across the country to adapt to online methods.

---

[82] Ibid.

[83] Adam Kuczynski and Jonathan Kanter, "Social Distancing Comes with Social Side Effects—Here's How to Stay Connected," The Conversation, Academic Rigor, Journalistic Flair, 2020, Accessed May 17, 2020, https://theconversation.com/social-distancing-comes-with-social-side-effects-heres-how-to-stay-connected-133677.

Some colleges have thus replaced all in-person instruction, labs, and exams with online delivery. They continued that many private (and some public) universities attract significant numbers of foreign students who pay full tuition, but many of those students may not be able to come to the United States for now or may choose to stay home or go to countries with fewer COVID-19 cases. This will result into additional serious financial blow to some colleges and universities, especially private ones. But if the effect is only a year or so, colleges can probably navigate it with some significant short-term pain. However, if the effect lasts longer, it could push some private colleges into insolvency.

Goldman and Karam stated that low-income students might seek to defer their admission or drop out to take a job to support their families due to the financial pressures caused by the COVID-19 shutdowns. The advantage of face-to-face learning and residential education is in providing a rich experience that helps students and faculty form supportive networks and learn valuable social and behavioral skills while online delivery provides valuable access to higher education if it is delivered well. But much depends on whether each college designs and implements high-quality online courses.

The long-term shifts sparked by COVID-19 have threatened the traditional business models of public and private colleges and universities, and as a result, the remaining institutions capable of face-to-face education and a true campus living experience will become the province of students with high family incomes or outstanding academic ability.[84]

Alternatively, coronavirus pandemic has created opportunities for individuals, married couples, and families to quarantine with the Lord Jesus and to ask for His mercy and help for now and the future.

---

[84] Charles Goldman and Rita Karam, "College in America Could Be Changed Forever," CNN Business Perspectives, 2020, Accessed July 9, 2020, https://us.cnn.com/2020/07/07/perspectives/higher-education-pandemic/index.html?utm_source=WhatCountsEmail&utm_medium=RAND%20Policy%20Currents+AEM:%20%20Email%20Address%20NOT%20LIKE%20DOT-MIL&utm_campaign=AEM:631600804.

According to 1 Kings 19:9, 13, it has brought us to a cave where we can quarantine with God and commune with Him like never before:

> And he came thither unto a cave, and lodged there; and, behold, the word of the Lord came to him, and he said unto him, What doest thou here, Elijah?
>
> And it was so, when Elijah heard it, that he wrapped his face in his mantle, and went out, and stood in the entering in of the cave. And, behold, there came a voice unto him, and said, What doest thou here, Elijah?

The lockdown in several nations has enabled families to pray and seek God's face for themselves and the world. We are seeing more families praying prayer of agreement. Jesus proclaimed in Matthew 18:19–20:

> Again I say unto you that if two of you shall agree on earth as touching anything that they shall ask, it shall be done for them of my Father which is in heaven. For where two or three are gathered together in my name, there am I in the midst of them.

Many have testified how praying together during COVID-19 lockdown has saved their marriage and family. Prayer is known to solve any problem, and it can bring down any mountain in marriage and in the family. Brother James declares in James 5:13, "Is any among you afflicted? let him pray. Is any merry? let him sing psalms."

We know that couples that stay connected in prayers live happier and healthier, including their children. Families that are not used to praying in their home are now praying and having church in their homes, thereby overcoming the challenges of quarrelling, nagging, unnecessary arguments, hatred, lack of respect, selfishness, and insensitivity. Love and respect for each other is becoming the product of family altars. Most couples and their respective families now have emotional security and confidence in each other. Through family prayers, impossible situations and difficult issues of life are being solved. Many couples have used the lockdown and restrictions as a platform to strengthen their relationships and thus emerging as better couples.

CHAPTER 5

Gleanings from COVID-19 and True-Life Chronicles

Our perception of being independent has been endangered by COVID-19 global pandemic. It has derided the medical, technological, military, and nearly every other sophisticated system the world has created for protection. COVID-19 has grown and mutated into an economic and social crisis at an unprecedented rate in several parts of the world among the rich and poor, the powerful, and the marginalized, including the disenfranchised—all are very apprehensive as they face the reality of the unknown.

The post-COVID-19 world will be battling with uncertainty of human existence and vulnerability of human life. It has emphasized the danger of snubbing our interdependence and the importance of global cooperation. We have learned the foolishness of pretending that we can achieve security in isolation within the borders of our nation, culture, class, or religion. The COVID-19 pandemic has revealed to us that we might not be able to return to "business as usual." The world has learned that we need early warning systems for future crises. COVID-19 highlights the need for vigilance, for new narratives, and reformed governance institutions. We must dramatically reorganize our set of priorities and engagements. Digital access must now be seen as a utility, such as electricity, water, and gas.

COVID-19 placed billions of people in lockdown and has made every act of physical contact and every expression of physical loving-kindness and compassion susceptible to illness and death.

Now we have learned that we can no longer ignore our vulnerability by pretending that we are in control of our destinies. The COVID-19 pandemic has demonstrated to us how we ought to appreciate the sacredness of life and the value of freedom. We cannot continue to take for granted the freedom to move and of being around our loved ones.

The COVID-19 pandemic has revealed to us the importance of recognizing the true purpose of all our businesses, economies, political leaders, and governments, which is primarily to serve human needs and purposes. The COVID-19 pandemic demonstrates to us that our economic, political, and social systems can serve our needs and purposes only when they stimulate us to cooperate at the appropriate scale.

Rakesh Kochhar indicated that the economic fallout from COVID-19 has not only taken jobs away from many American workers but has also put in doubt the economic fortunes of many business owners who employ them. He described the economic risk to business owners as one that varies by the demographic groups to which they belong. He also indicated that men, white or Asian entrepreneurs, people aged fifty-five and older, and college graduates are more likely to be business owners compared with their shares in the workforce overall according to a Pew Research Center analysis of federal government data.

At the same time, women, Asians, and foreign-born entrepreneurs have a greater presence in higher-risk industries than in the economy overall. Kochhar explained that business owners are both older and more educated than the US workforce, whether across all industries or in higher-risk industries. About half of business owners are either fifty-five or older or have graduated from college. By comparison, only 23 percent of employed workers overall are fifty-five or older, and 40 percent are college graduates. He elucidated that it is yet unknown, which businesses will survive the economic fallout from the COVID-19 outbreak or the extent to which government-lending programs will keep them afloat. What matters most is the duration of the economic slide and whether it resembles the aftershock of a natural disaster or a deep cyclical downturn.[85]

Beachum, et al., stipulated that as Americans show more signs of quarantine fatigue and many face pressures to ease coronavirus restrictions, Anthony Fauci had cautioned that a second wave of infections is inevitable in the United States. They specified that Fauci had proposed that the US might be in for a bad fall in the year 2020 and even a bad winter if the right countermeasures are not put in place. They acknowledged Fauci's anticipation about COVID-19 that it will not necessarily go away due to how contagious it is and its reach around the world.[86]

This is why we have to understand that no human being can be indomitable nor infallible without the absolute control of Jesus Christ over that life. Without Jesus Christ, we are most vulnerable to all the wiles and attacks of the devil, but if God be for us, who can be against us (Rom. 8:31). The answer to this question can clearly be seen in Psalms 56:9, "When I cry unto thee, then shall mine enemies turn back: this I know; for God is for me." Our enemies must turn back when we cry to God for mercy in genuine repentance and humility.

COVID-19 did not exempt anyone and has become a teachable encounter that must never be wasted. Many did volunteer to pack food and other needed items for those who desperately needed it. Several youths in different nations stepped out by dispensing groceries for those who needed assistance, and some created public service announcements to help inform others about its dangers. COVID-19 made us to appreciate the true value of many people whose roles in society tended to be undervalued from the nurses to the emergency

---

[85] Rakesh Kochhar, "The Financial Risk to US Business Owners Posed by COVID-19 Outbreak Varies by Demographic Group," Pew Research Center, *Fact Tank News in the Numbers,* 2020, Accessed May 18, 2020, https://www.pewresearch.org/fact-tank/2020/04/23/the-financial-risk-to-u-s-business-owners-posed-by-covid-19-outbreak-varies-by-demographic-group/.

[86] Beachum, et al..., "The Second Wave of Coronavirus Is Inevitable," *The Washington Post,* 2020, Accessed April 29, 2020, https://thehill.com/changing-america/resilience/natural-disasters/495211-fauci-says-second-wave-of-coronavirus-is.

responders to the people sitting at the checkout counters in super-markets, the delivery personnel, and the many nameless strangers who suddenly offered help to the old and vulnerable. The pandemic has revealed a vast sea of kindness and benevolence in our communities around the world. It has led to countless acts of selfless heroism in hospitals and care homes. It has impelled many of us to use our greatest strengths to serve our greatest purposes, suddenly giving our lives new inspiring meaning.

COVID-19 had become the instrument that the Lord used for human beings to begin to give, help, donate, and serve like never before in history. This servant-leadership sacrifice will definitely metamorphosize and modify the way people—especially young people—view leadership. The liberal and beautiful nature of humanity that emerged during the COVID-19 pandemic will continue to exemplify the courageous and selfless leadership we need during any other foggy season in decades to come.

Transitioning from "Self" to "Us" Mentality

COVID-19 taught us how to transition from focusing on "self-mentality" to focusing on "us ideological approach." We have must realize that all people were created in the image of God, and everyone on earth is worthy of respect and care. We must shift from "self-nationalism" to a globally effective response to the COVID-19 pandemic because we are social creatures, suited primarily for cooperation in social groups of limited size. Our national affiliations must now be augmented to a global affiliation to our common humanity that must overcome this pandemic together. Political governments around the world must now rally around our institutions of multilateral cooperation and ensure that national and multilateral goals complement one another as we live in the post-COVID-19 world era. The pandemic has shown us that we must begin to deal with challenges from the ground up.

Our objectives are to contribute to the fulfillment of human needs and purposes which will enable us to deal with local challenges locally, community challenges at a community level, state challenges at a state-wide level, national challenges nationally, and now global challenges globally.

COVID-19 might be a novel challenge, but it is never the first large-scale health crisis to show us why we need to make this world a better place to live and experience righteousness, joy, and peace of God in the Holy Ghost (Rom. 14:17). The pandemic has revealed humanity's weaknesses in how we think about God and His Word. It has shown us about the importance of global health and how we prepare for disease through obedience to God's Word (Exo. 23:25–27). Many questions about COVID-19 still remain, such as, how could we have avoided such a global pandemic in this age? And are there any safe places to hide? It is only by answering these questions and by learning the lessons of challenges of COVID-19 that we can build a world that is less vulnerable to global health crises like what we now face.

Aaron Gulley examined that New Zealand, the island nation, chose strict lockdowns and austerity because of COVID-19 which forced the country to close her landscapes as well as its borders. The country began mandatory quarantine for all visitors, one of the strictest policies in the world at the time, even though there were just six cases nationwide, and just ten days later, it instituted a complete countrywide lockdown, including a moratorium on domestic travel. The Level 4 restrictions meant grocery stores, pharmacies, hospitals, and petrol stations were the only commerce allowed while vehicle travel was restricted and social interaction was limited to within households.

Gulley cited Prime Minister Jacinda Ardern, "We must fight by going hard and going early… We have the opportunity to do something no other country has achieved, elimination of the virus." Ardern mentioned a few days after the lockdown that instead of just slowing the transmission of the virus, New Zealand had set a course of eradicating COVID-19 from its shores by cutting off the arrival of new cases and choking out existing ones with the restrictions. The plan seems to have worked as the daily infection rate in the island nation of 4.9 million people steadily dropped from a maximum of

146 in late March 2020 to just a few cases a day by mid-April 2020. This low number of new cases gave the government the confidence to ease its social distancing restrictions to Level 3. On April 28, 2020, Ardern pronounced COVID-19 eliminated and clarified that elimination does not necessarily mean zero cases.

Gulley clarified that New Zealand might be sounding confident about ridding itself of COVID-19. Success might not yet be guaranteed as countries like Singapore that seem to have the virus under control and have since struggled with a second wave of infections, including China which appeared to have stopped the spread completely, but afterward contended with flare-ups. However, even if New Zealand manages to snuff out COVID-19, the road ahead will be rough because once the country is virus-free, it will need to maintain the total halt on arrivals until a vaccine is developed and widely disseminated or risk the threat of reinfection. This will then be a tough prospect for a country like New Zealand where tourism is the largest export industry in terms of foreign exchange earnings that accounts for 10 percent of GDP and nearly 15 percent of the workforce. Hundreds of thousands of jobs will be endangered, and the forecasts already suggest the Kiwi economy will not recover until at least 2024.[87]

Sophie Cousins documented on May 9, 2020, that an aggressive approach has enabled New Zealand to end community transmission of SARS-CoV-2. Cousins reported that New Zealand recorded its first day of no new cases of coronavirus disease more than a month after its strict lockdown began. On March 23, a month after the country had recorded its first case, New Zealand committed to an elimination strategy. A few days later, Prime Minister Jacinda Ardern announced a strict national lockdown when it only had 102 cases and zero deaths. Her swift decision had made her to win international praise, including from the World Health Organization.

---

[87] Aaron Gulley, "New Zealand Has 'Effectively Eliminated' Coronavirus. Here's What They Did Right." *National Geographic* Coronavirus Coverage, 2020, Accessed May 9, 2020, https://www.nationalgeographic.com/travel/2020/04/what-new-zealand-did-right-in-battling-coronavirus/.

Cousins explained that New Zealand's decision to pursue an elimination approach was a vastly different approach to usual pandemic planning, which has historically been based on a mitigation model that focuses on delaying the arrival of a virus followed by a range of measures to flatten the curve of cases and deaths.

Cousins cited Michael Baker, who has been advising the New Zealand Government on its response and who projected implementing a full lockdown involving the closure of schools and nonessential workplaces, a ban on social gatherings, and severe travel restrictions that enabled the country to consider elimination, and while the strategy has had its critics, the evidence was overwhelming that elimination could be achieved. Baker indicted that full lockdown did allow the country to get key systems up and running to effectively manage borders and do contact tracing, testing, and surveillance.

Cousins inferred that as New Zealand now eases its restrictions and its economy slowly reopens, there are discussions about how it can open up its borders while ensuring that everyone is protected, particularly susceptible populations. Officials have pleaded for vigilance as breaches of the shutdown rules continue to rise.[88]

DW.com reported that New Zealand will lift restrictions now that the last-known COVID-19 patient has recovered. Prime Minister Ardern said although transmission of the virus has been "eliminated," it will take work to keep it that way. DW.com cited the country's director-general of health, Ashley Bloomfield—who proclaimed that the last remaining patient from Auckland had been symptom-free for forty-eight hours and is regarded as recovered and was now able to leave isolation—said that having no active cases for the first time since February was "a significant mark in our journey."

Social distancing measures have been dropped due to the fact that New Zealand's last known COVID-19 patients has recovered. However, the country's strict border restrictions will remain in place, including managed isolation and quarantine for travelers. But the

---

88 Sophie Cousins, "New Zealand Eliminates COVID-19," *The Lancet*, 395:10235, P1474, 2020, Accessed June 8, 2020, https://doi.org/10.1016/S0140-6736(20)31097-7.

rest of the country's coronavirus measures will be lifted by midnight on Monday, June 8, 2020 (12:00 UTC), meaning that public and private events can resume without curbs while the retail and hospitality industries can operate without social distancing measures.[89]

God has empowered His children by His Holy Spirit to overcome this virus and any other future pandemic through His wisdom revealed by His Word (Luke 10:19). We are the salt and the light of the world (Matt. 5:13–14). However, we are living in a world that lies in wickedness. Apostle John declares in 1 John 5:19, "And we know that we are of God, and the whole world lieth in wickedness." This is the reason why we cannot afford to lose the sweetness of our salt or let our light be hidden under the bushel. You can know how the world tastes by checking the salt content. You can see clearly when the light of the world begins to shine in gross darkness (Isa. 60:1–2).

We must tenaciously turn to the Lord who mercifully protected the Israelites from the plagues in Egypt and who also heard King David's prayer for mercy when pestilence was attacking Israel and Judah (2 Sam. 24:10–25). God wants us to turn to him in mercy, grace, and love. Those afflicted with COVID-19 are not more sinful than the rest of humanity. The Word of God specified in the Gospel of Luke 13:1–3:

> There were present at that season some that told him of the Galilaeans, whose blood Pilate had mingled with their sacrifices. And Jesus answering said unto them, suppose ye that these Galilaeans were sinners above all the Galilaeans, because they suffered such things? I tell you, Nay: but, except ye repent, ye shall all likewise perish.

Did the Lord allow the devil to send just one virus out of zillions of viruses in his possession to discombobulate the earth? Why

---

[89] Made for Minds, "New Zealand Declares Itself Coronavirus-Free After Last Case," DW.com, 2020, Accessed June 8, 2020, https://www.dw.com/en/new-zealand-declares-itself-coronavirus-free-after-last-case/a-53723603.

is it that the world superpowers who have stockpiled countless thermonuclear weapons cannot deal with this coronavirus? COVID-19 has revealed to us the need for the merging of both left-wing ideologies that encompasses protecting the poor and disadvantaged from exploitation and right-wing ideologies that focus on the importance of freedom. This will help businesses, corporations, and governmental agencies to manage risk in order to serve the public interest.

Scientists have informed us that coronavirus could not be synthesized or created from the lab, and not only that, it is virtually impossible. Mary Beusekom stated that the virus does originate from nature, and there is no evidence or data that connects this to a lab. She cited Kristian Andersen who clarified that the virus's receptor binding domain, which makes it an efficient human pathogen, is also found in coronaviruses in pangolins, scaly anteaters proposed as an intermediary host between bats and humans. Andersen indicated that it is something that is completely natural and not something that happens in tissue culture.[90] But while this virus does not originate from God, God knew about it, and at the end of it all, He will make it to work together for the common good of all those who love God and those who are the called according to His purpose (Rom. 8:28).

Although the virus started from China, we have to understand that God also loves the Chinese people just as He loves the Italians, Koreans, Africans, and Americans. He loves the elderly and those with preexisting conditions just as He loves the young and the healthy. God has never left us alone to face this crisis by ourselves. He is with health care workers as they risk their lives to care for patients. He is with grocery workers and delivery drivers as they serve those who can stay safely at home because of their sacrifice. He is with those who are unemployed because of the COVID-19 pandemic and those who would shelter at home if they had one. He is with patients

[90] Mary Van Beusekom, "Scientists: 'Exactly Zero' Evidence COVID-19 Came from Lab," Center for Infectious Disease Research and Policy (CIDRAP), 2020, Accessed May 14, 2020, https://www.cidrap.umn.edu/news-perspective/2020/05/scientists-exactly-zero-evidence-covid-19-came-lab.

who suffer and families who have lost their loved ones. There has been an outpouring of financial generosity, and we have witnessed churches and agencies that would never have cooperated previously working together to save lives. Millions of people around the world are sacrificing their income by staying home to protect people they do not know. God is truly at work.

Christopher Cheney documented that virus outbreaks in the recent past have posed challenges, but the novel coronavirus has an uncommon potential to wreak havoc. The swine flu pandemic hit the United States in 2009 and 2010 with about 12,500 deaths and an estimated 60.8 million cases, according to the CDC. Additionally, during the 2014–2016 Ebola outbreak, eleven people were treated for the viral disease in the United States with two deaths. Cheney noted that the Imperial College COVID-19 Response Team had declared the novel coronavirus as the most serious public health threat from a respiratory virus since the 1918 Spanish flu pandemic.

He cited Ericsson who explained that the major difference is the poor response to COVID-19 testing. He enumerated that the testing for swine flu was efficient and rapid, which helped a great deal in keeping it under control and flattening the epidemiologic curve. Testing was done to recognize the swine flu, and there were treatments. Testing was rapidly developed to recognize when the virus was becoming resistant to one reagent so we could switch to another reagent, but we have nothing like this now to control the COVID-19 epidemic.

Furthermore, he buttressed that we do not have recognized treatment for COVID-19 presently that is recognized and actively in use. We only have an experimental agent, but it is only for hospitalized patients who are in dire need of a rescue medication. Ericsson enumerated further that a key lesson studied from swine flu is that we need to have a plan in place that we can rapidly adapt mostly a plan that must be flexible enough to deal with the new realities of whatever develops. He stated that out of many challenges of new viruses that had shown forth in the recent past, there has never been the one that is potentially as dangerous as COVID-19.

He also corroborated that once we could recognize suspected people who were entering the country, just as any traveler who had Ebola symptoms, they would be jumped on immediately, isolated, and tested. Another lesson obtained from the Ebola virus was that it is necessary to quickly develop vaccines, unlike the novel coronavirus vaccine which is still underway. He stressed that there must be plans for off-site assessment of people if there is ever going to be a surge of disease such as Ebola. This would mean not evaluating many people in the hospital just as tents are set up outside hospitals. In comparison with Ebola, COVID-19, which is not symptomatic in a large segment of patients, results in sending many people home without admitting them into the hospital. He said we have to think through during Ebola because of the possibility of necessitating off-site facilities in the event of a pandemic.[91]

Makini Brice and Richard Cowan conveyed that the leading United States infectious disease expert, Anthony Fauci, had again warned Congress on May 11 that a premature lifting of lockdowns could lead to additional outbreaks of the deadly coronavirus, which has killed more than 134,000 Americans as of the time of writing this book and has brought the economy to its knees. Fauci also urged states to follow health experts' recommendations and to wait for signs, including a declining number of new infections, before reopening. He noted a slowing in the growth of cases in hotspots such as New York as of May 11, even as other areas of the country were seeing spikes.

Brice and Cowan added that some states already have begun reopening their economies, and others have announced plans to faze that out during the summer months, even as opinion polls shows most Americans are concerned about reopening too soon.[92]

---

[91] Christopher Cheney, "Coronavirus: Infectious Disease Expert Shares Lessons Learned from Other Recent Outbreaks," 2020, Accessed on May 14, 2020, https://www.healthleadersmedia.com/clinical-care/coronavirus-infectious-disease-expert-shares-lessons-learned-other-recent-outbreaks.

[92] Makini Brice and Richard Cowan, "Fauci Tells Congress US Coronavirus Outbreak Not Yet Under Control," *Financial Post*, 2020, Accessed on May 11, 2020, https://business.financialpost.com/pmn/business-pmn/fauci-tells-congress-u-s-coronavirus-outbreak-not-yet-under-control.

Alejandro De La Garza enumerated that during the coronavirus era, a host of epidemiological terms have entered common public use, such as the now-ubiquitous "social distancing," and the newly politicized "flatten the curve." Garza explained that as states and local governments seek a way out of lockdowns that have brought their economies to a near-standstill, "contact tracing" has made its way into everyday conversation, and he explains how contact tracing can help society battle the COVID-19 epidemic. Accordingly, he explained that "contact tracing" is a little like detective work where trained staff interview people who have been diagnosed with a contagious disease to figure out who they may have recently been in contact with, and they will now go and tell these people they may have been exposed to COVID-19 and then encourage them to quarantine themselves to prevent spreading the disease any further. This is just like a public health work and part investigation.

Furthermore, he buttressed that contact tracing was used during the 2014 Ebola virus outbreak and in the SARS outbreak in 2003. Also, it has been used to combat sexually transmitted infections and other communicable diseases like tuberculosis. As COVID-19 has gone global, countries like South Korea and New Zealand have aggressively used contact tracing in an attempt to control outbreaks.

Health care workers will inform all contacts and give them instructions on symptoms to look for or direct them to self-isolate. Garza reinforced that contact tracing could be a very timely and laborious process which ranges from interviewing infectious patients and reaching out to dozens of contacts. With a virus like COVID-19, which spreads through the air, things can get complicated quickly. Contact tracers might end up trying to find those who sat near an infected individual on a plane or a bus, even if the sick person never met them. This is a radically different task from "contact tracing" with a sexually transmitted infection like HIV, which tends to involve a much shorter, more well-defined list of contacts for investigators. Health care workers may also have trouble getting in touch with contacts if phone records are not up-to-date or if an infected patient is already too sick to help identify their recent contacts.

Garza stated that contact tracing COVID-19 infections has proven particularly difficult as some infected people do not show any symptoms, and the period of time between getting infected and becoming infectious appears to be relatively short. But still, at the height of a pandemic, contact tracing can be useful within smaller community settings, such as in health care facilities or nursing homes. Many countries that are battling the coronavirus have used the combination of old-school "contact tracing" techniques and more technologically sophisticated methods.

Gaza informed that there is a joint effort between Apple and Google to add software to smartphones that would aid in contact tracing, and the Google's CEO also emphasized that using it is optional and that there is no personally identifiable information coming to the tech companies as part of the initiative.[93]

Recent findings from both Yale and Melbourne researchers amplify the call for immediate validation and implementation of saliva sampling for SARS-CoV-2. Researchers are working around the clock, innovating ways to improve the COVID-19 testing process, and recently, a group of researchers from Yale University presented findings that suggest that one improvement could be made right at the beginning of the testing process in the choice of the sample to be tested. Although the current gold standard is to use samples collected from nasopharyngeal swabs (NPS), the group found that using saliva for SARS-CoV-2 detection is more sensitive and consistent than using a nasopharyngeal swab. They assert that saliva should be considered as a reliable sample type to improve COVID-19 testing, although available SARS-CoV-2 detection tests had suffered from multiple challenges including low sensitivity and reliance on swabs.[94]

---

[93] Alejandro De La Garza, "What Is Contact Tracing? Here's How IT Could Be Used to Help Fight Coronavirus," *Time*, 2020, Accessed May 9, 2020, https://time.com/5825140/what-is-contact-tracing-coronavirus/.

[94] "SARS-COV-2 Detection in Saliva Samples Is Sensitive and Consistent," *Genetic Engineering & Biotechnology News*, 2020, Accessed April 28, 2020, https://www.genengnews.com/news/sars-cov-2-detection-in-saliva-samples-is-sensitive-and-consistent/.

Churches and faith-based organizations remains the light to our communities and the world at large, especially in these dark times because the church is like a city set upon a hill (Matt. 5:14). The government and faith-based churches have learned to work together in order to slow the spread of the coronavirus. Now the best practice is for churches to conduct their worship remotely and follow minimum health protocols. We are called to love the Lord with all our heart, soul, and mind and to love our neighbors as ourselves (Matt. 22:37), even to love one another as Christ loved us (John 13:34). Daniel 2:21 elucidates, "And he changeth the times and the seasons: he removeth kings, and setteth up kings: he giveth wisdom unto the wise, and knowledge to them that know understanding."

According to Bulbulia, et al., they stated that virus and religion is not about a transmission of religious ideas which some have described as using epidemiological model but the role of religious practices in spreading SARS-COV-2, the virus responsible for the COVID-19 pandemic. They corroborated this with South Korea's experience who as of the end of the first week of March 2020 almost have two-thirds of coronavirus infections (nearly 5,000 cases) traced back to "Patient 31," an individual who worshipped at Shincheonji Church of Jesus in Daegu. The church had insisted on in-person meetings, banning health masks, praying while touching others, and refusing to turn over its membership list to health officials. Routinely accused by mainline Protestant Christian denominations of being a secretive sect, now it is being blamed for contributing to the local epidemic of COVID-19. It didn't help that the church's leader eighty-eight-year old Mr. Lee Man-hee explained the epidemic as the Evil One fighting back against the rapid growth of the church he founded. Koreans are outraged and urging the government to prosecute Mr. Lee for murder due to gross willful negligence.

They also specified that some pastors of churches in Trinidad in the West Indies disagreed with government health officials. The pastors were continuing to hold in-person services on the basis that a failure to attend worship in person is evidence of a lack of faith. Bulbulia, et al., noted that collective worship is an effective mechanism for accelerating the spread of COVID-19. However, they

observed that though recalcitrant religious congregations are accelerating viral transmission, it is notable that most religious groups are
innovating in response to opposing demands of collective worship
and social distancing. For example, religious communities all over
the world are conducting online services, stretching the world's data
bandwidth at certain times of the week to stream live videos of suit-
ably modified rituals, sermons, and prayers.[95]

Many religious communities are also disseminating practical
health information and offering urgent financial help in the wake
of rapidly degrading economic conditions. The behaviors of problematic churches are attracting the media's attention, but in many
regions of the world, religious communities are more beneficial than
harmful. While it is impossible at present to sum over the global
diversity of religious communities, the fact that so many religious
communities are active in the fight against COVID-19 is a vivid
reminder that concept "religion" does not carve human social behaviors neatly at any joint. For this reason, the question of whether religion is contributing to the global COVID-19 health crisis is poorly
formulated.

They also implicated that though religious groups do not line
up neatly on one or another side of the global pandemic response,
religious community-making tends to be an intensifier of response,
strengthening resolve, and motivating action. They concluded that
standard epidemiological models of viral spread don't take into
account human factors such as religious ideologies and values. Human
beings are complex, and the way religion weaves itself through the
lattice of human life is incredibly intricate. Surfacing such human
value factors is a public obligation.

Just as health officials try to explain their recommendations, so
experts in the scientific study of religion need to surface religion-abet-
ted value judgments that impact behaviors relevant to viral spread.
Experts need to explain where religion is causing problems and find

---

[95] Bulbulia, et al., "Religion and the COVID-19 Pandemic," *Religion, Brain &
Behavior*, 10:2, 2020, Accessed April 28, 2020, https://doi.org/10.1080/21535
99X.2020.1749339, 115–117

creative ways to communicate alternative ways of thinking.[96] We must not stand against God's Word in our quest for zeal (Rom. 10:2). Our zeal must not be without the revelation knowledge of God.

Paul states in Romans 13:1–5:

> Let every soul be subject unto the higher powers. For there is no power but of God: the powers that be are ordained of God. Whosoever therefore resisteth the power, resisteth the ordinance of God: and they that resist shall receive to themselves damnation. For rulers are not a terror to good works, but to the evil. Wilt thou then not be afraid of the power? do that which is good, and thou shalt have praise of the same: For he is the minister of God to thee for good. But if thou do that which is evil, be afraid; for he beareth not the sword in vain: for he is the minister of God, a revenger to execute wrath upon him that doeth evil. Wherefore ye must needs be subject, not only for wrath, but also for conscience sake.

While it is needful to follow the state guidelines which is the authority set up by God for every nation as long as it does not contradict God's Word, Jesus Christ, the resurrection and life, still watches over all. It is because of us He neither sleeps nor slumbers. He is working on our behalf to perfecting all that which concerns us. He is relentlessly interceding for the believers as our High Priest after the order of Melchizedek (Rom. 8:34; Heb. 5:10, 6:20). Remember, He upholds all things by the Word of His power. He has engravened us in the palms of His hands, and our walls are continually before Him (Isa. 49:16). There is nothing too hard for Our God (Jer. 32:17, 27)

God is still in the business of healing all forms of sickness and disease, including all plagues, raising the dead, making the lame walk, giving eyes to the blind, and making the deaf hear. He is a moun-

---

[96] Ibid.

tain mover; He calms the storm of life, and He is a waymaker. He opens up the Red Sea, He walks on water, He walks out of the grave triumphantly, and He ever lives to intercede for us. He knows your name, He knows the number of the hairs on your head, He knows your need, and He is always there for you 24/7. You can count and depend on Him, and He will answer you. *He* is the same yesterday, today, and forever. He can never change (Mal. 3:15; Heb. 13:8).

Peradventure you are feeling down or thinking that all hope is gone as you read this book or you are alone in quarantine, maybe you are surrounded by walls of trouble or you have been forsaken by family and friends; you might even be thinking there is no way out of this myriad of sorrows of losing precious loved ones and troubles. Read through my personal true-life chronicles about how Jesus—the resurrection and the life, the only one that can cancel all appointment with death and hell—showed up in my case. I can vividly tell you that He is never late. He is always on time and He is always on point.

Remember the Scriptures state in Revelation 12:11, "And they overcame him by the blood of the Lamb, and by the word of their testimony; and they loved not their lives unto the death."

And David declares in Psalms 119:46, "I will speak of thy testimonies also before kings and will not be ashamed."

Chronicles of True-Life Experiences
Deliverance from the Flood of Death

In October 1979, my family and I had just finished our nightly prayer devotions, and we went to bed. We are a family of seven, and every one of us kept our Bibles on the dining table where we gathered daily for family prayers. Suddenly, around 10.30 p.m., there was a very heavy thunderstorm and rainstorm, which lasted for about twelve hours. All the houses in the community where I lived had high security bricked fences and gates. The heavy rain caused a great flood that resulted in the loss of lives and properties that year.

Surprisingly, the adjacent fence collapsed into my father's house fence, which also crumpled into our exit door and thus created a water canal from all of the neighbor's houses into our house. The water began to flow into our house. By this time, the electricity had already been out. I had my mother crying that the water had begun to rise inside our house, and then my father went into everyone's rooms to wake us up to for all gather in one room. My father tried to open the exit doors so we could quickly get out of the house. At the same time, he kept calling our names in the dark one after the other to be sure we were all safe. We kept responding to our names, and we were all glad that our dad was also alive.

He was walking through the whole house to see how we could exit, but we were already in the middle of water. He instructed us to all climb the heavy iron burglary proof bars built over all the windows of the house until we reach the ceiling and that we should hold on tight since he could not really see anyone in the dark. As of this time, the water had almost risen to the ceiling.

We had prayed intensely, and right within me, I thought the whole scenario was a dream. I was also thinking we had prayed a night before, so why would God allow this to happen and let this flood drown the whole family? My father had called unto the neighbors to help with a loud noise, but unfortunately, there was no response. We later found out in the morning that the neighbors drowned in the flood. Since all hope to be saved was gone, and the flood of water had reached my father's neck, he also decided to climb the iron cast bars and called our names again. He said that he knew God could not destroy the entire family and that one way or the other, deliverance would come. However, the deliverance had to come in about five minutes' time, or else we would all be drowned by the flood.

Suddenly, my father prayed by giving thanks to God, declaring Him faithful to a thousand generations. He told the Lord that we were all sinners both by nature and commission and that we had all made Jesus Christ as Lord and Savior. However, for the sake of my three-week-old brother who had not sinned, though he is a sinner by nature, God should deliver the entire family. With tears, he told the Lord he was completely out of wisdom and that he did not know what else to do, and immediately, he said in Jesus Christ's name.

Suddenly, a strong force blew off the entire wall adjacent to the wall that had the window where we held on to the iron cast. The entire wall fell toward the outside of the house.

All the water inside the house and the water rushing in from the back of the house that was coming from the neighbors now had a channel to flow, and the flood of water was subdued. I have always wondered, what if the entire house collapsed on us? The wall could have fallen inside, the electricity could have been turned on, and we all could have been electrocuted, or the flood could have driven all of us away; but the Almighty God made a way for us where there was no way.

Later in the morning, when we returned to the house to pick up valuables and personals that remained, we realized everything had been carried away by the flood, including the floor carpets, but to our utter amazement, all of the our Bibles and call-to-worship bell that were placed at the center of the dining table were all on the floor. However, the dining table, stove, couches, refrigerator, and carpet had been carried away by the flood. Indeed, when the enemy comes in like a flood, the Spirit of God will lift up a standard against him (Isa. 59:19).

The Lord spared my life and my entire family. God cancelled every appointment we had with death, and I was able to witness that firsthand as a child. The Scripture declares in Revelation 12:15–16:

> And the serpent cast out of his mouth water as a flood after the woman, that he might cause her to be carried away of the flood. And the earth helped the woman, and the earth opened her mouth, and swallowed up the flood which the dragon cast out of his mouth.

Deliverance from the Wicked One

My father once told me that I was the expression of Paul described in Romans 8:29–30, which says:

> For whom he did foreknow, he also did predestinate to be conformed to the image of his Son, that he might be the firstborn among many brethren. Moreover, whom he did predestinate, them he also called: and whom he called, them he also justified: and whom he justified, them he also glorified.

According to him, when I was about eighteen months old, my parents had a housemaid whom they were thinking of dismissing due to her incompetence. The very day she was to leave, she placed me on the balcony of a two-story building and left the house. However, my father had been instructed by the Holy Spirit to leave work early in order to quickly dismiss the housemaid. To his utter amazement, he saw me far off, holding the rail of the balcony. He began to pray silently to God that I should not have eye contact with him, which would definitely trigger the release of my hands from the balcony railings and thus fall headfirst from the two-story building. He immediately hurried up the stairs to rescue me.

After my dad furnished me with the story, I remembered the words of David, the sweet Psalmist of Israel in Psalm 124:5–8:

> Then the proud waters had gone over our soul. Blessed be the Lord, who hath not given us as a prey to their teeth. Our soul is escaped as a bird out of the snare of the fowlers: the snare is broken, and we are escaped. Our help is in the name of the Lord, who made heaven and earth.

It is imperative to know that the same spirit that raised Jesus Christ from the dead dwells in us and that eternal life will disgrace eternal death and sustain our biological lives. Jesus declares in John 10:28–29:

> And I give unto them eternal life; and they shall never perish, neither shall any man pluck them out of my hand. My Father, which gave them me, is greater than all; and no man is able to pluck them out of my Father's hand.

Deliverance from Deadly Poison

I had gone to minister somewhere in Europe. It was a conglomerate of churches meeting for a one-week prophetic and miracle service. Before the meeting, there were prayers, intercessions, thanksgiving, worship, and fasting to prepare. On the first day of the meeting, the hospitality department brought dinner. I decided to take a quick shower before I ate the food, but the Holy Spirit witnessed in my heart that I must not touch the food. I ended up eating a honey oat bar for dinner.

Meanwhile, the food was presented and packaged in sealed coolers and tightly covered. But the noise of the forced opening of the coolers woke me up early in the morning, and the solid food inside had turned to liquid dripping off from the cooler unto the desk where it was placed. I was flabbergasted at the sight knowing that could have been taking place inside my stomach. Apparently, the food was contaminated, but the voice of the Lord made the difference.

David declares in Psalm 29:3–10:

> The voice of the Lord is upon the waters: the God of glory thundereth: the Lord is upon many waters. The voice of the Lord is powerful; the voice of the Lord is full of majesty. The voice of the Lord breaketh the cedars; yea, the Lord breaketh the cedars of Lebanon. He maketh them

also to skip like a calf; Lebanon and Sirion like a young unicorn. The voice of the Lord divideth the flames of fire. The voice of the Lord shaketh the wilderness; the Lord shaketh the wilderness of Kadesh. The voice of the Lord maketh the hinds to calve, and discovereth the forests: and in his temple doth every one speak of his glory. The Lord sitteth upon the flood; yea, the Lord sitteth King forever.

Deliverance from High Voltage Electric Shock

I was about eleven years old when I came across a high voltage electric cable that fell down from power lines due to a heavy wind on the path where I was walking to play football and do some exercise. Unknowingly, I thought I could just twist part of it to make a jump rope for my exercise.

Suddenly, as I held the cable with wet sweaty hands, I was electrocuted, and immediately, I somersaulted and landed on the floor, unconscious. Still on the floor, I was looking up to see if anyone was around to rescue me, but thank you Jesus Christ, the Son of God, who lifted me, and I did not sustain any injury.

Young children have always been prone to high voltage shock caused by mischievous exploration and exposure at work, and certainly, electric shock occurs whenever an individual comes into contact with an electrical energy source, thereby releasing electrical energy to flow through the portion of the body, causing shocks.

Complete Dedication to God

It is a blessing to be joined to the bone of your bone and flesh of your flesh during your life journey for the fulfilment of God's divine kingdom and purpose here on the earth. God revealed my wife to me when I was nineteen years old. The primary function of the Holy

Spirit is to show us things to come, and the secret of the Lord is with the righteous. While it is the glory of God to conceal a matter, the honor of kings is to search it out. The Lord revealed everything about my wife, before I met her, and children even before they came out my loins. I waited patiently, prayed prayers of thanksgiving for ten solid years, before I finally met my beloved wife.

Shortly after the birth of our first child, I was offered a six-figure job, which the Lord did not approve of me to take, but I accepted the offer for a short period of time to support the family and ministry. Graciously, the Lord used my wife to remind me of the Lord's mandate upon my life and the instruction for my destiny. Immediately, I tendered my letter of resignation on the first day of work. I bless God because I was not disobedient to the heavenly vision for my life.

There was another incident that occurred while I was lecturing at another institution. The Lord revealed to me that my time was up at the job. During this period, my wife was interceding fervently for me daily, asking the Lord for mercy and grace. One day while I was lecturing, a very hot air from nowhere came upon me, and suddenly, I collapsed. However, before the paramedics arrived, I was back on my feet because of the intercession of my wife. By God's divine will and timing, she was praying the same time the incident occurred because the Lord instructed her to do so without her knowing the details.

During a mission trip to Kuwait and parts of the Middle East and Mediterranean countries, the Lord revealed through my wife that we should take the Gospel to Iraq since its border is with Kuwait. We made this trip during the Iraq war. While the team and I were in Iraq, we were faced with countless traps of death and destruction, but thanks be to God who used the ceaseless prayers of my wife to that place.

Prior to September 11, 2001, the Lord revealed to me through a vision of two planes entering a high-rise building. Neither did I grasp the full understanding nor the intent and purpose of the vision. However, my wife and I prayed the prayer of agreement, and the Lord instructed me to postpone all mission trips. On September 11, 2001, while I was lecturing some group of students, I saw the terrific event on the news. Immediately, I burst into tears because that was exactly what the Lord showed me four days before.

Solomon dedicated the temple to the Lord for the Lord's use according to 1 Kings 8:63, "And Solomon offered a sacrifice of peace offerings, which he offered unto the Lord, two and twenty thousand oxen, and a hundred and twenty thousand sheep. So, the king and all the children of Israel dedicated the house of the Lord."

I am that house, the temple of the living God, dedicated to the Lord, and through the intercession of a dedicated wife, the Lord delivered me from the paws of the lion. David declares in Psalms 4:3, "But know that the Lord hath set apart him that is godly for himself: the Lord will hear when I call unto him."

Miraculous Supply of Gasoline

During my final year in the university, I traveled out of town for a conference that I was led to attend. The distance was about 220 miles away from my campus, and I was driving at an average of seventy-five miles per hour. I was accompanied by a friend who happened to be my assistant and a student of the same university. We arrived at the venue tardy and did not remember to fill the gas tank that was already on empty. I went ahead to facilitate the conference, which ended at 11:00 p.m. that night. I did not intend going back to school because it was already late, even though I had to do a final preparation for an exam at 6:00 p.m. the next day.

After inquiring from the Lord on what to do, just as King David will always acknowledge the Lord in all his ways (Prov. 3:3–4), the Lord instructed me to travel back to school (Ps. 32:8). After an incessant trial of looking for gas to fill the tank, I went back to the Lord, and He told me to go back to school, and I asked Him, "Lord, how do I get gas to fill the gas tank because the drive is 220 miles away?"

And the Lord instructed me to just be driving and never to look at the dashboard but to continuously keep my eyes off until I get back to the school campus. As of this time, there were no available gas stations open to buy the gas on the way. To make it worse, that road was usually bombarded with armed robbers, and it was just too dangerous to travel at that time of the night. However, I am very sure I heard the Lord, and I obeyed His voice and started praying in the Holy Spirit without looking at the dashboard until I arrived in front of my dormitory at the campus.

God's Word attested in 1 John 4:16–18:

> God is love; and he that dwelleth in love dwelleth in God, and God in him. Herein is our love made perfect, that we may have boldness in the day of judgment: because as he is, so are we in this world. There is no fear in love; but perfect love casteth out fear: because fear hath torment. He that feareth is not made perfect in love.

When I looked at the dashboard, the car suddenly stopped. My friend and I burst in laughter and began to give God all the glory for miraculously supplying the car with gas. This might be unbelievable for many people, but my response was from the Scripture, which says in Romans 3:3–4:

> For what if some did not believe? shall their unbelief make the faith of God without effect? God forbid yea, let God be true, but every man a liar; as it is written, that thou mightest be justi- fied in thy sayings, and mightest overcome when thou art judged.

God: The Waymaker

After holding a series of prayer meetings and Bible studies with some of our brethren and indigenous missionaries serving at one of the most restricted nations in the world with high levels of persecu- tion index, we decided to have Bible study and prayers at a secret place on a school campus in the Middle East along the Mediterranean.

We did not realize that some "religious police" had been monitoring and watching all of our evangelistic activities, but we successfully finished the meeting. Right after the meeting, on our way to the car park, we encountered six religious police pursuing us. Our team kept walking faster to get to the car park, and when we looked back, we noticed that the police were still following us systematically.

We were praying silently in the Holy Spirit to keep the spirit of fear away from us, and we entered a departmental building surrounded by a wall. Suddenly, we saw a door in the wall that led to the other side, and we thought it was built in the wall for exit or egress. We opened the door and saw our car on the parking lot and were moving toward the car, but when we looked back, we did not see both the door in the wall and the religious police again. The Lord safeguarded our lives because we put our trust in Him.

It is written in 1 Corinthian 10:13:

> There hath no temptation taken you but such as is common to man: but God is faithful, who will not suffer you to be tempted above that ye are able; but will with the temptation also make a way to escape, that ye may be able to bear it.

Angelina Theodorou documented that as of 2012, at least seventeen nations (9 percent worldwide) have police that enforce religious norms according to a new Pew Research analysis of 2012 data. Theodorou stated that these actions are particularly common in the Middle East and North Africa, where roughly one-third of countries (35 percent) have police enforcing religious norms.

She specified that in Vietnam, the government's religious security police continued to monitor "extremist" religious groups, detaining and interrogating suspected Dega Protestants or Ha Mon Catholics. Also, in Malaysia, state Islamic religious enforcement officers and police carried out raids to enforce Sharia law against indecent dress, banned publications, alcohol consumption, and *khalwat* (close proximity to a member of the opposite sex). Additionally, in sub-Saharan Africa, Theodorou noted two countries in the region, Nigeria and Somalia, that have religious police. In Nigeria, the Hisbah (religious police) are largely funded and supported by governments in several states where they enforce their interpretation of Sharia law. Theodorou indicated that as of 2012, religious police forces were not present in any country in Europe or the Americas.[97]

Serve Your Generation and Generations Beyond

The Word of God declares in Acts 13:22, 30, 35–37:

> [A]nd said, I have found David the son of Jesse, a man after mine own heart, which shall fulfil all my will.
> But God raised him from the dead...thou shalt not suffer thine Holy One to see corruption.
> [A]fter he had served his own generation by the will of God.
> [H]e whom God raised again saw no corruption.

My parent always takes us (children) to spend part of our summer holiday with my grandmother. I was told my grandfather was married to my grandmother, but also, there were concubines. One of them lived at the family house.

My grandmother (blessed memory) who was responsible for my spiritual upbringing, an elder at the Baptist church, and also a prophetess at a fast-growing Pentecostal Church informed me that God Almighty had anointed and ordained me to be His servant to the nations before I entered my mother's womb and that the enemy plotted to terminate that purpose. This task will remain impossible

---

[97] Angelina Theodorou, "Religious Police Found in Nearly One-in-Ten Countries Worldwide." Pew Research Center, *Fact Tank News in the Numbers*, 2014, Accessed May 19, 2020, https://www.pewresearch.org/fact-tank/2014/03/19/religious-police-found-in-nearly-one-in-ten-countries-worldwide/.

for the enemy because the Scriptures declare in Ecclesiastes 3:14 that, "I know that, whatsoever God doeth, it shall be forever: nothing can be put to it, nor any thing taken from it: and God doeth it, that men should fear before him."

My grandmother usually engaged in several days of fasting and prayer based on the previous revelation of an impending danger against me. She also instructed me to get involved in a regular once a week prayer and every first day of the month and warned me be to behave myself wisely.

On the first day of July in 1980, I was observing an ordinance of fasting and continuous silent prayer as instructed by my grandmother. Immediately after school assembly, I had a strange nudge to get out of the class and walk out of the gate and cross to the other side because someone was waiting for me.

Instruction had begun, and the classroom teacher had already done the roll call. I was already at my seat in the classroom, and no student for whatever reason was permitted to leave the class, talk less of walking out of the school except with the teacher's permission. It was practically impossible to walk out of the classroom because of the school security and the strict school system. There were serious penalties for any student found loitering around the school premises and not seated in the classroom, receiving instruction.

I stood up without taking permission from the teacher, walked out of the class, and opened the heavy iron gate. While all this was happening, none of the teachers or security stopped me to inquire from me where I was going. The gateman did not even stop me while I was opening the gate. As I crossed over the highway that was in front of the school, after looking at the left side and the opposite right side and looking at the left side again, there being no oncoming vehicles, suddenly I was hit hard, and that was it.

The next thing was I heard the sound of several marching sounds like army boots. I could hear them marching in their heavy boots, and one said to me, "Let him go. He will not die but live to declare the glory of God in the land of the living." The person continued to say, "I have need of him, and I will use him to serve his generation and generations to come. I will work through him and perfect everything that concerns him. Through him, many shall be redeemed and come to know, serve, and love me. He is a light unto the nations of the earth."

The next time I came out of that experience, I found myself at the hospital on a stretcher, and as I opened my eyes and came back to life, I saw my mother and many other people weeping. I did not know what had happened, and the first word that came out of my mouth was, "Give me a mirror so I can look at myself and be sure this is real." I kept shouting and pleading that I needed a mirror to be sure this was real. My grandmother had already hinted to me that this accident was coming and that I needed to fast and pray as usual.

My mother told me that I was knocked down by a fast speeding bus that dragged me on the bitumen concrete highway for about 220 feet. The bumper of the car was damaged, the front windscreen broken, and I had bruises all over my body and face, but miraculously, none of my bones were broken—no fracture or dislocation.

I am so full of tears of joy and appreciation as I write this book, knowing fully well that only God must have delivered me from death. The Scripture declares in Psalms 34:20, "He keepeth all his bones: not one of them is broken."

The Lord performed His wonders in my life to the extent that I did not even have any surgery apart from staying at the hospital at the recovery room for examination for about a week. Neither did I receive any blood transfusion after losing quite some blood. I testify to the praise and the glory of God that I am a living miracle, and not a jot out of God's Word for my life or any reader of this book shall go unfulfilled. The Bible declares in John 16:33, "These things I have spoken unto you, that in me ye might have peace. In the world ye shall have tribulation: but be of good cheer; I have overcome the world."

We can be challenged as children of God by the enemy, but we are not permitted to be defeated because of the indwelling Holy Spirit of God that is at work in us.

Unstoppable Vision

When I was about eight years old, I was drawn to playing the piano. Since my parents couldn't afford to buy me one nor get me a private teacher, I had to join the church's choir to learn the basics of music and also learn how to play a piano. I was auditioned to sing the tenor part. I would come to choir practice early enough during choir practice so I could learn how to play piano from the musical skills taught in choir.

However, there was this man who was one of the church's pianists. He would always beat me anytime he saw me practicing on the piano. He would take me inside and flog me and instruct me never to place my hands on the piano again, despite the fact that the piano was free for anyone interested. He physically abused me for about four years. He wanted to destroy my passion and zeal toward music and playing piano. I cannot count how many times he beat me to the point of wounding me. He told me that if I ever told my parents, they would double the beating because he would tell them I wanted to damage the church's piano, and this made me more afraid to the point where I could not inform my parents about this abuse.

Actually, in those times in Africa, parents would beat you more without any inquiry if they should be informed that their child wanted to damage the church's piano.

While I was defiantly learning by hearing how to play the church's piano, I had discovered some basic skills, and I would go earlier at the time this man was not there, preferably before the choir rehearsals to practice despite the almighty beating and flogging. If this man saw me, I would pay the price of being dragged into a corner and be severely beaten with a stick.

Nonetheless, after four years of secret abuse for practicing to play piano with my church's piano freely, meant for beginners and leaners, the church's high school was celebrating Christmas cantata service at the church's premises, and it was this same man that was supposed to play the piano for them, but he did not show up. I happened to be at the church, and I voluntarily offered to play for the high school with my very little piano skills. I thought I could not make it but because I was on the spotlight. I did my best with God being on my side. During the two-hour program, I sensed the hand of God upon me, just like David, the sweet Psalmist of Israel. I played most of the songs from my head without reading the musical notes because these were songs that I was already used to during rehearsal.

I never thought I could receive a very loud applause and recognition after the event. I wasn't looking for one. I was too excited to be called upon to play. To me, I was doing myself a big favor of passionately fulfilling my dream. I wasn't also expecting to receive a little scholarship given to me by the church's high school toward my college education.

Surprisingly, the man that used to physically abuse me arrived at the time I was called out for recognition and the award. Apparently, he had been held back by traffic. After that experience, he never stopped me from practicing on the church's piano.

Thankfully, during my first year in college, my parents were able to buy be a small keyboard, and I was able to polish my piano skills with a few of my friends. I thank God for healing me from the wounds and fear of playing piano because sometimes, whenever I play, even on my own keyboard, I always think that someone will drag me into a corner or a room to physically abuse me. This was a significant miracle and testimony for me.

Of a truth, no one (except yourself when you quit) can stop you from fulfilling your God-given dream if you follow it with passion. You are unstoppable. David, the sweet Palmist of Israel, was unstoppable by the ferocious lion, bear, Goliath, Saul, and his own personal error. You are unstoppable by the power of the Holy Spirit that is in you. Christ is in you, the hope of glory.

It was written of Jesus Christ in Acts 2:22–24:

> Ye men of Israel, hear these words; Jesus of Nazareth, a man approved of God among you by miracles and wonders and signs, which God did by him in the midst of you, as ye yourselves also know. Him, being delivered by the determinate counsel and foreknowledge of God, ye have

taken, and by wicked hands have crucified and slain. Whom God hath raised up, having loosed the pains of death: because it was not possible that he should be holden of it.

Dream Big—Our God Is Able

There are men and women presently who are not born again but are "wiser in their generation" than the children of light. While some of these men might not be the best example to follow because they have not yet professed Jesus Christ as their Lord and Savior, their utterance in regard to what their passion and what drives their magnanimity could be noted. Observe that the Bible connoted that these men are wiser "in their generation," but in this present generation, the Lord is raising a chosen generation, children of light (1 Pet. 2:9) whose wisdom will blast off and surpass the wisdom of the men of this world. The Word of God declares in Psalm 17:14, "[M]en of the world, which have their portion in this life, and whose belly thou fillest with thy hid treasure: they are full of children and leave the rest of their substance to their babes."

Regarding the limited mundane activities of this world, Jesus declares in Luke 16:8 and 20:34, "[F]or the children of this world are in their generation wiser than the children of light... And Jesus answering said unto them, the children of this world marry, and are given in marriage."

Dr. Ben Carson stated, "I struggled academically throughout elementary school yet became the best neurosurgeon in the world in 1987." That is to say that the difficulties you are facing could be an indication that you are on the verge to succeeding in life, so never quit from the race.

Oprah Winfrey lamented, "I was raped at the age of nine, yet I am one of the most influential women in the world." You cannot allow the hurt of the past to hinder your glorious future. You must learn to forget things that are behind and press forward to what is ahead of you (Phil. 3:13). He told me to say to you, the righteous, that it shall be well with you (Isa. 3:10).

Bill Gates remarked, "I didn't even complete my university education but became the world's richest man." Though education is needful, it cannot necessarily make you rich. Education is designed to polish your life so you can be rich. You obtain needful knowledge that will help increase your skillset and help you understand the world better so as to know how to interact with it.

Tyler Perry, an American actor, writer, producer, and director whose net worth is more than a billion USD according to Forbes, affirmed, "It doesn't matter if a million people tell you what you can't do or if ten million tell you no. If you get one yes from God that's all you need. God gives everyone a lane, and no one can beat you on your lane. Just stay focused on Him and what you are supposed to do. And everything will be all right. Rather than focus on your critics, focus on the people who are impacted by your work."

The Scriptures expounded Romans 9:15–16, "For he saith to Moses, I will have mercy on whom I will have mercy, and I will have compassion on whom I will have compassion. So, then it is not of him that willeth, nor of him that runneth, but of God that sheweth mercy."

God does not just have the "final say" in our lives. He also has the "only say."

Joyce Meyer pronounced, "I was sexually, mentally, emotionally, and verbally abused by my father as far back as I can remember until I left home at the age of eighteen, yet I am one of the most influential preachers in the world." This is to make everyone understand that we serve a God of restoration, and you can still recover your dignity in life and be all that God wants you to be.

Cristiano Ronaldo stated, "I told my father that we would be very rich, but he couldn't believe me. I made it a reality." You will have what you say if truly you believe it. There is so much power in your words. The Bible says, "Death and life are in the power of the tongue: and they that love it shall eat the fruit thereof" (Prov. 18:21).

Lionel Messi affirmed, "I used to serve tea at a shop to support my football training and still became one of the world's best footballers." Believe in your God-given dream, and never let anyone hinder you. The dream of God for your life, though it tarries, wait for it, for it will not, and it will surely come (Hab. 2:3).

Steve Jobs indicated, "I used to sleep on the floor in my friends' rooms, returning coke bottles for food, money, and getting weekly free meals at a local temple. I later on founded the Apple Company." Just because you are little today or being ridiculed does not mean your tomorrow shall be small. Your tomorrow shall be great. The Bible declares in Job 8:7, "Though thy beginning was small, yet thy latter end should greatly increase."

The former British PM, Tony Blair, said, "My teachers used to call me a failure, but I became a prime minister." Never allow someone else's opinion of you to define who you are or limit what you are predestined to become in life.

Bishop David Oyedepo specified, "I started Living Faith Church from a lawn tennis court with three members only and preached prosperity. Many of my friends criticized me, but today, we have the largest church auditorium in the world and two world-class universities." It does not matter how many people back you up. Do not lose God's backing. God will only back up that which originates from His Word.

Isaiah 29:11–12 declares:

> And the vision of all is become unto you as the words of a book that is sealed, which men deliver to one that is learned, saying, Read this, I pray thee: and he saith, I cannot; for it is sealed: And the book is delivered to him that is not learned, saying, Read this, I pray thee: and he saith, I am not learned.

Nelson Mandela specified, "I was in prison for twenty-seven years and still became president." This is to let everyone know that with God, all things are possible, and all things are possible to them that believe (Mark 9:23, 10:27). God did not only have the final say in your life but the only say.

Mike Adenuga stated, "I drove a taxi to finance my university education, but today, I'm a billionaire." For all of us, the redeemed, we only have one position in life, and that is "above only." Topmost of the top (Deut. 28:13).

Harland Sanders, Founder of KFC, said, "I was on the verge of suicide when an idea of opening a restaurant hit me after I retired as a cook in the navy." To say it is too late is a language of failures. God is ever ready with you whenever you are ready to believe Him. Your own day can be today.

Aliko Dangote said, "I worked for my uncle since I was a small boy. People looked down on me. I later on took a loan from my uncle to open a tiny shop. I worked hard to make ends meet. Now I am the richest man in Africa." God is the designer of your life. It will take being enlightened by the Spirit of God to follow the path of God for your life. Every child of God must follow God's path for their life. The Scriptures declare in Romans 8:14, "For as many as are led by the Spirit of God, they are the sons of God."

Barack Hussein Obama stipulated, "I am a son of a Black immigrant from Kenya. I graduated from Harvard and later on became a senator in Chicago. I was also the president of the most powerful nation on Earth." As God's children, we are chosen for greatness.

Think about what God said about us in Ephesians 1:4, "According as he hath chosen us in him before the foundation of the world, that we should be holy and without blame before him in love."

God, our wise master builder and heavenly potter, has designed us to take the lead in every affair of life, and it does not matter your background, race, or where you come from. What does matter is whether you believe it or you do not.

Dr. Akinwumi Adesina, the president of the African Development Bank, affirms, "Many of you might not know that I came from a poor background, and while I was studying for my master's at Purdue University, there was a day during a very cold winter without sweater, jacket, or gloves that all I had left with me was twenty-five cents. I prayed to God and said, 'God, you have to do a miracle for me today.' God gave me an assistantship, and he supernaturally provided me a hundred dollars and other assistant-ships during my PhD, and I wouldn't be what I am today without a world-class education I received at this top-rated world-class university." The book of Hebrews 7:25 substantiates, "Wherefore he is able also to save them to the uttermost that come unto God by him, seeing he ever liveth to make intercession for them."

There is an unstoppable grace God will lavish on those who follow Him humbly, and He will always show up in our lives whenever we reach the dead end, having done all to do but still standing, though not knowing what to do again. He always knows what to do, and He will never leave us nor forsake us.

Strive Masiyiwa indicated, "The opportunity is in the problem. The moment I see a problem, I immediately begin to think about the opportunities that can be created by trying to solve it. You can find opportunities if you are looking for them. God will do nothing, except you pray. And you have to be clear what you want." Strive is a London-based Zimbabwean billionaire businessman and philanthropist who is the founder and executive chairman of the international technology group Econet Global. The Word declares in Romans 8:37, "Nay, in all these things we are more than conquerors through him that loved us."

Folorunsho Alakija, the richest Black woman in Africa, boldly declares, "I never went to a university and I am proud to say so because I don't think I have done too badly. I told much of my life as I could to encourage people, to encourage others to get to where they should be, where they want to be. People should not just look at people who are on top. They should go and study how they got there and the challenges they had to face as they were climbing the ladder. I once dared to dream and I could succeed, then you can." The Word of God answers in Philippians 4:13, "I can do all things through Christ which strengtheneth me."

Let's come off it; if we believe ten, we will receive. We are to believe all that God has for us, and God is to perform what we believe. We are not to pay for what we desire from God's Word but to believe, follow, and obey God's instructions to possessing them, and so is eternal life.

Arnold Schwarzenegger lamented, "I traveled to America in search of financial independence when I was fifteen years old. I became the world's strongest man seven times and Mr. Universe. I then got my economics degree. Then I became one of Hollywood's best actors before I was voted twice as Governor of California." The Lord had said of man in Genesis 11:6, "And the Lord said, Behold, the people is one, and they have all one language; and this they begin to do: and now nothing will be restrained from them, which they have imagined to do."

It is high time we begin to cast down wicked imaginations against our destinies and begin to receive God's thought for our lives.

The Lord declares to us in Jeremiah 29:11, "For I know the thoughts that I think toward you, saith the Lord, thoughts of peace, and not of evil, to give you an expected end."

We, God's children, who are of the highest order of dominion must begin to think and imagine His Word comes to pass in our lives, looking at the invisible (2 Cor. 4:18; Heb. 11:2, 12:2), and calling those things which be not as though they were (Rom. 4:17). The scripture says, "For as a man think, so is he" (Prov. 23:7). Therefore, let us begin to think on God's thoughts for our lives. The Scriptures infer in Philippians 4:8:

> Finally, brethren, whatsoever things are true, whatsoever things are honest, whatsoever things are just, whatsoever things are pure, whatsoever things are lovely, whatsoever things are of good report; if there be any virtue, and if there be any praise, think on these things.

When you think about Elon Musk who said, "I'm talking about moving there," the "there" in this statement is Mars. According to Tom Huddleston Jr., Elon Musk is never one to shy away from setting ambitious goals. He is a billionaire whose most ambitious goal is about going to Mars. Huddleston indicated that for Musk, personally, a successful mission would be something of a culmination of his efforts to build a viable private space company. He founded

SpaceX in 2002 (two years before he joined the electric car company, Tesla) with the goal of eventually building more affordable spacecraft that would make it possible to one day reach and colonize Mars. He had also said in the past that he plans to send an unmanned SpaceX rocket to Mars, carrying only cargo, by 2022. It does remain to be seen how feasible that plan actually is, much less Musk's plan for a second mission that would transport humans to the Red Planet by 2024.

Huddleston cited Jim Cantrell who announced that Musk's focus with SpaceX has always been more about eventually reaching Mars than on making money. Cantrell indicates, "Elon really doesn't care about the money. He wants to go to Mars." SpaceX has also raised nearly $1.7 billion from investors since the beginning of 2019, giving the company a valuation of around $36 billion, and still that valuation has not changed billionaire Musk's goal of putting humans on Mars. Huddleston stated that Musk wants to send a million people to Mars by 2050.[98]

Born to Overcome

As a child of God, we have inherited His divine nature which can never be answerable to defeat and unfulfillment. God, who is also our Father, can never fail. It is impossible to our God to fail. No viral attack is too powerful to numb our God. God does not and can never know failure, and as God's own children that were born by the incorruptible Word of God (1 Pet. 1:4, 23), we are careers of His divine nature. No matter the challenges, we are destined to overcome. It is written in 1 John 5:4, "For whatsoever is born of God overcometh the world: and this is the victory that overcometh the world, even our faith."

---

[98] Tom Huddleston Jr., "Why SpaceX's Historic Manned NASA Flight Is Important for Elon Musk's Mars Ambitions," *Make It*, CNBC, 2020, Accessed May 27, 2020, https://www.cnbc.com/2020/05/27/what-spacexs-historic-nasa-flight-means-for-elon-musks-mars-goals.html.

None of God's children possesses a DNA that is meant for failure and defeat but for great exploits in victory. Therefore, there is no fight, however fierce, no skirmish, however tough, that you cannot overcome in life. You can walk triumphantly over all life's battles as long as you abide in God and know Him intimately. Your level of exploits in life becomes unlimited.

There is no limit to the victory that God will manifest through over Satan, our adversary anytime, anywhere, and anyhow. God is highly committed to your divine accomplishment. We are the apple of God's eye, and God is out against anybody and anything that is against you. God's written word declares in Isaiah 49:25–26:

> But thus, saith the Lord, Even the captives of the mighty shall be taken away, and the prey of the terrible shall be delivered: for I will contend with him that contendeth with thee, and I will save thy children. And I will feed them that oppress thee with their own flesh; and they shall be drunken with their own blood, as with sweet wine: and all flesh shall know that I the Lord am thy Saviour and thy Redeemer, the mighty One of Jacob.

The Lord will not allow you to be tossed around by anybody, whether a group, government, or authority. You are a very important and sensitive subject in God's agenda.

Your life and destiny are forbidden zones to the adversaries based on the veracity and integrity of His Word. The Bible declares in Psalm 106:8–10:

> Nevertheless, he saved them for his name's sake, that he might make his mighty power to be known. He rebuked the Red sea also, and it was dried up: so, he led them through the depths, as through the wilderness. And he saved them from

the hand of him that hated them and redeemed
them from the hand of the enemy.

God will not tolerate your being messed up or treated anyhow. Those who attempt to do you harm will pay dearly for it with their lives. He will do anything to protect and preserve us. Those who will take advantage of you and go free cannot succeed. You are not permitted to be defeated as a child of God. Even if you cannot make sense of the outcome of the battle, be rest assured that by the help of the Holy Spirit, you will always overcome. He is the greater one that is in you. He is at work in you right now. He is greater than all your concerns and will humiliate every attack of the enemy against your glorious destiny. The Scriptures allude in Genesis 12:3, "And I will bless them that bless thee, and curse him that curseth thee: and in thee shall all families of the earth be blessed."

As the seed of Abraham, those who bless you are blessed, and those who curse you are cursed (Gal. 3:29, 4:28).

CHAPTER 6

Terminating the Spirit of Fear

This is a mighty weapon in the hands of our adversary. The Bible admonishes us not to fear despite a thousand falling at our side and ten thousand at our right side, but the plague shall not come near us (Ps. 91:10–12). However, COVID-19 has brought so much fear to many people in the world, which is why God's people must be filled with faith that comes by hearing, believing, and acting on God's Word. We are not to give the devil any place, not even the spirit of fear. This can only happen when we are filled with the Word of God (Rom. 10:17; Eph. 4:27; James 1:22). The Bible clarifies in 2 Corinthians 4:13, "We having the same spirit of faith, according as it is written, I believed, and therefore have I spoken; we also believe, and therefore speak."

Acts 6:5, 11:24 described Stephen and Barnabas thus:

> And the saying pleased the whole multitude: and they chose Stephen, a man full of faith and of the Holy Ghost.
> For he was a good man, and full of the Holy Ghost and of faith: and much people was added unto the Lord.

Jacek Debiec explained that the pandemic of fear is unfolding alongside the pandemic of the coronavirus. He corroborated that due to the global reach and instantaneous nature of modern media, fear contagion spreads faster than the dangerous invisible coronavirus. He added that watching or hearing someone else that is afraid spreads fear without necessarily even knowing what caused the other person's fear. He stressed that fear contagion is an evolutionarily old phenomenon that researchers observe in many animal species. It can serve as a valuable survival function. He substantiated that in a herd of antelopes pasturing in the sunny African savanna, when one of them senses a stalking lion, all of the antelopes will momentarily freeze, which will quickly set off an alarm call that makes them all run away from the predator, and in the blink of an eye, other antelopes follow suit.

Debiec stated that brains are hardwired to respond to threats in the environment such as sight, smell, or sound cues that signal the presence of the predator that automatically triggers the first antelope's survival response, which is first immobility, and then escape. The amygdala, a structure buried deep within the side of the head in the brain's temporal lobe, is key for responding to threats which receives sensory information and quickly detects stimuli associated with danger. Afterward, the amygdala will now forward the signal to other brain areas, including the hypothalamus and brain stem areas to further coordinate specific defense responses.

According to Debiec, the outcome of all of these is commonly known as fright, freeze, flight, or fight. In the same vein, human beings share the same automatic unconscious behaviors with other animal species, which explains the direct fear the antelope feels when sniffing or spotting a lion nearby. However, fear contagion goes one step further when the antelopes automatically run for their lives, following one frightened group member. He indicated that their escape was not directly initiated by the lion's attack but by the behavior of their terrified group member, which is momentarily freezing, sounding the alarm, and running away, and the group as a whole will pick up on the terror of the individual and acted accordingly. Likewise, as other animals, people are also sensitive to panic or fear expressed by other humans. Human beings are exquisitely tuned to detect other people's survival reactions.

Debiec presented experimental studies that have identified a brain structure called the anterior cingulate cortex (ACC) as fundamental for this ability. This surrounds the bundle of fibers that connect the left and right hemisphere of the brain, and so when you watch another person express fear, your ACC lights up. He noted that studies in animals confirmed that the message about another's fear travels from the ACC to amygdala where the defense responses are set off, and it makes sense why an automatic unconscious fear contagion would have evolved in social animals that can help prevent the demise of an entire group bound by kinship, protecting all their shared genes so they can be passed on to future generations. He stipulated that studies had shown that social transmission of fear is more robust between animals, including humans, that are related or belong to the same group as compared to between strangers. Nevertheless, fear contagion is an effective way of transmitting defense responses not only between members of the same group or species but also across species.

Fear contagion happens automatically and unconsciously, making it hard to really control a phenomenon that explains mass panic attacks that occur during music concerts, sports events, or other public gatherings. Once fear is triggered in the crowd through someone who supposedly thought he heard a gunshot, there is then no time or opportunity to verify the source of terror, but fear travels from one to the next, infecting each individual as it goes, and where everyone starts running for their lives in mass panic, it always leads to tragedy. Fear contagion does not require direct physical contact with others, but media distributing terrifying images and information can effectively spread fear. It will be more productive when information about danger and safety is clearly provided with straightforward instructions on what to do because whenever one is under significant stress, it is harder to process details and nuances.[99]

---

[99] Jacek Debiec, "Fear Can Spread from Person to Person Faster Than the Coronavirus." Michigan Medicine Department of Psychiatry, The Conservation under Creative Commons License (2020) https://medicine.umich.edu/dept/psychiatry/news/archive/202005/fear-can-spread-person-person-faster-coronavirus (accessed December 22nd, 2020).

Fearful news makes money today and brings death, and whenever the spirit of death smells fear, it will come upon its host. Fear is a doorway to death. Hebrews 2:14–15 declares:

> Forasmuch then as the children are partakers
> of flesh and blood, he also himself likewise took
> part of the same; that through death he might
> destroy him that had the power of death, that is,
> the devil; and deliver them who through fear of
> death were all their lifetime subject to bondage.

The scripture identifies fear as a spirit (2 Tim. 1:7), which is more than someone being afraid of some bad thing. Fear is demonically inspired. Fear is a scary demon that oppresses the mind. Fear makes people make wrong choices and also opens the door for depression. Some will shut everyone out of their lives because of the spirit of fear. Some are rich and handsome but will not be able to live a fulfilled life because of a fearful spirit. Whenever you are afraid, trust in the Holy Spirit to help you cast out the spirit of fear (Ps. 56:3).

Life carries elements of risk, and we need faith to overcome the risk. Psalm 23:4 states, "Yea, though I walk through the valley of the shadow of death, I will fear no evil: for thou art with me; thy rod and thy staff they comfort me."

God cannot be with you and see you put to shame, sickness, disease, and suffer death. Many are trapped inside the jail of the fear of death where the enemy is waiting for them. Some have an inferiority complex, jealousy, and an inability to release pain from the past because of fear. According to Proverbs 29:25, "The fear of man bringeth a snare: but whoso putteth his trust in the Lord shall be safe."

A snare is an instrument that is used to trap or entangle birds and mammals. It makes the prey to be impeded, limited, or in difficulties. We need the spirit of faith to disperse the spirit of fear.

Job lost his ten children and wealth to fear. Those who are afraid carry the spirit of death along with them. This is different from the healthy fear of God, which is respect for God, and being aware of the penalty we will face when we disobey Him. Job 3:25 laments, "For the thing which I greatly feared is come upon me, and that which I was afraid of is come unto me."

Job was praying for and not with his children and safeguarding his businesses. Possibly, he was afraid he was going to lose them. Whatever you cannot let go will leave you because you have no power to hold on to anything. Only God can keep everything for you. Job was an upright and righteous man, but the devil smelled fear around him, and that led to the death of his children and loss of his properties. You must load yourself with God's Word and always come to the throne of grace to obtain mercy and find grace to help in times of need (Heb. 4:16).

How many hours do we spend on social media and many other things that distract us from God's Word? Many things have over-crowded our lives. We have been cluttered with the cares and anxieties of the world and distractions of this age and the pleasures and delight and false glamor and deceitfulness of riches and the craving and passionate desire for other things that have been allowed to creep in and choke and suffocate God's Word in our lives (Mark 4:19 AMP). The gospel of John 12:24–25 states:

> Verily, verily, I say unto you, except a corn of wheat fall into the ground and die, it abideth alone: but if it dies, it bringeth forth much fruit. He that loveth his life shall lose it; and he that hateth his life in this world shall keep it unto life eternal.

The Bible admonishes that there is no fear in love, for perfect love casts out all fear. All fear means "all fear," including the fear of death, and whosoever fears is not made perfect in love. Our love for God and for one another must be perfected because fear has torment (1 John. 4:17–18).

Many years ago, when John G. Lake was ministering in South Africa, his faith in God's eternal life saved his life in an unprecedented way during the bubonic plague that struck the country.

He was exposed to the plague day after day, he and another minister. They had been laying hands and praying for those suffering from the disease. They had also helped bury the bodies of the dead. Before long, the medical doctors working at the hospital asked John Lake what made it impossible for him not to contract the disease. John Lake response was to go with them into the medical lab where he instructed the doctors to take the samples of the plague and place them under a microscope and verify that they were alive and moving, and then place the same germs on his hand and look at them under the microscope again. The germs died instantly upon contact with his hand. The eternal life of God that was exuding from John Lake's spirit into his flesh instantly killed the germs.

Lake had such faith in the power of the divine life that even the bubonic plague could not exterminate him nor touch him because when it did, God's power flowed within him and immobilized it in his tracks. This same power could be made available to us if we would believe in God's resurrection power. Johanes Susanto declares, "Although working hard by faith to help sick people, Lake, all of his family, and his assistant never caught the plague. This amazed many people and doctors, especially when a medical laboratory test proved that deadly plague germs died instantly in his hands, proving Lake's conviction of divine healing and health by the Holy Spirit in Christ."[100]

Terminating Achan, the Troubler of Israel

An appointment with death can be made on your behalf, such as in the case of Achan who made an appointment with death on behalf of his children when he took the accursed thing. Korah, Dathan, Abiram, and Gehazi are other examples (Num. 16; 2 Kings 5:27).

---

[100] Johanes L. Susanto, "A Practical Theology Evaluation of the Divine Healing Ministries of Smith Wigglesworth and John G. Lake: A Continuationist Reformed Perspective," Dissertation submitted for the Doctor of Theology, University of South Africa 55, 2007, Accessed May 19, 2020, http://citeseerx.ist.psu.edu/viewdoc/download?doi=10.1.1.921.7297&rep=rep1&type=pdf.

Joshua 7:1, 24–25 declares:

> But the children of Israel committed a trespass in the accursed thing: for Achan, the son of Carmi, the son of Zabdi, the son of Zerah, of the tribe of Judah, took of the accursed thing: and the anger of the Lord was kindled against the children of Israel.
>
> And Joshua, and all Israel with him, took Achan the son of Zerah, and the silver, and the garment, and the wedge of gold, and his sons, and his daughters, and his oxen, and his asses, and his sheep, and his tent, and all that he had: and they brought them unto the valley of Achor. And Joshua said, why hast thou troubled us? the Lord shall trouble thee this day. And all Israel stoned him with stones, and burned them with fire, after they had stoned them with stones.

Terminating Nabal, the Fool

Christ took our place on the cross of Calvary and died for us. We are not supposed to be snared again by death nor allow the spirit of death to hang around us. David was anointed king that had no appointment in the palace. To God, David was king, but to the people, Paul was king. God's approval was upon David, and there could not be two kings in Israel. Are you anointed, but not appointed, then wait for your time? Abigail was married to Nabal (whose name means fool), and David sent his servant to ask Nabal for the supply of food which was of the "training to reigning" season in the life of David.

Nabal recognized David as a runaway rebellious servant of Saul and declined his request, and David, out of anger, wanted to kill him. You can find this kind of character inside Saul, and there is a Saul in David that needed to be destroyed before David assumed the throne so Israel would not have another Saul on the throne in the person of David. Abigail knew of the plan of David to exterminate every male that belong to Nabal, but Abigail, with her godly character, intervened and averted being destroyed with Nabal in the order of Ananias and Sapphira (1 Sam. 25:18–39; Acts 5:1–11). You too can escape death by teaming up with Christ. Remember, the fool had said in his heart there is no God, and the fool also said take it easy, eat, drink, and be merry (Ps. 14:1; Luke 12:15–22)

The aftermath effect of coronavirus will still be here for several decades, but how it works together for the good of those who love the Lord must be what we are after. Obviously, no one prays for this horrific event to be enacted on the planet, but God knows best. Jean Twenge had been researching generational differences and cultural trends, which fundamentally is how cultural events impact people, and has stipulated that the coronavirus outbreak is quite bigger than 9/11 and might also be bigger than the Great Recession. She also stated that the coronavirus outbreak could become the biggest and most impactful cultural event of our lifetime.

Twenge postulated that neither 9/11 nor the Great Recession so profoundly altered as many aspects of day-to-day life in such a short period of time the way the coronavirus has affected schools, work, travel, entertainment, and shopping. She added that 9/11 and the recession do not really have direct impact on so many people around the world. But coronavirus outbreak and our reactions to it will intersect with the trends of the past and also have an impact on the futures of many people, especially the generation of those who were born after 1995.

Twenge specified that the coronavirus is already having deep psychological effects on many people, bringing in anxiety, fear, and worry. Also, fewer or zero social interactions and anxiety may turn into depression. This is because social interaction with peers is paramount for young people, and with schools closed, working at home encouraged, and larger gatherings canceled, that could end for now. However, texting, social media, and video chat can help fill the void, although these virtual communications are still not as good as face-to-face contact.

To an already vulnerable generation, this situation might not be pleasant because between 2011 and 2018, and based on the most recent data available, the rate of depression, self-harm, and suicide did soar among teens, and 2020 might well make things even worse, especially if mental health resources are more difficult to obtain as the pandemic worsens.[101]

Terminating Letters of Death

Paul declared that we our open letters written by the Spirit of God not on tablets of stone but on tablets of human hearts. We are known and read by everyone (2 Cor. 2–3). Literarily, we must be the fifth gospel. Men might not have the time to read the Gospels of Matthew, Mark, Luke, and John, but they can read the events of our lives as the fifth gospel. Everyone is called to be conformed to the image of Jesus Christ. All of us are carriers of letters, and when you are born again, you ought to become a carrier of God's Word.

Jezebel was good at writing letters of conspiracy that led to death. She wrote a death letter to kill Naboth. You must reject every letter of destruction from COVID-19 and other future pandemics. Paul was carrying a letter of death and, on the road to Damascus after his encounter with the Lord Jesus Christ of Nazareth, took the letter of death away from him and exchanged it for the letter of life (Acts 9:3). His letter of life to the Church at Corinth reads in 1 Corinthians 15:51–55:

> Behold, I shew you a mystery; We shall not all sleep, but we shall all be changed, in a moment, in the twinkling of an eye, at the last trump: for the trumpet shall sound, and the dead shall be raised incorruptible, and we shall be

---

[101] Jean Twenge, "The Coronavirus Could be Generation Z's 9/11," *The Conversation, Academic Rigor Journalistic Flair,* 2020, Accessed May 17, 2020, https://theconversation.com/the-coronavirus-could-be-generation-zs-9-11-133740.

changed. For this corruptible must put on incorruption, and this mortal must put on immortality. So, when this corruptible shall have put on incorruption, and this mortal shall have put on immortality, then shall be brought to pass the saying that is written, Death is swallowed up in victory. O death, where is thy sting? O grave, where is thy victory?

What is read in the life of many people might be letters of divorce (Deut. 24:1; Isa. 50:1; Jer. 3:8; Mark 10:4), barrenness, and misfortune. You could exchange any letter or any lifestyle for a letter of life. Jeremiah 22:30 indicates, "Thus saith the Lord, write ye this man childless, a man that shall not prosper in his days: for no man of his seed shall prosper, sitting upon the throne of David, and ruling any more in Judah."

Uriah was a Hittite warrior in King David's army. The meaning of his name was "Yahweh is my light" He had become a worshipper of Yahweh and had married a Hebrew wife, Bathsheba (daughter of oath). David committed adultery with Bathsheba while Uriah was engaged in warfare, and that led to Bathsheba becoming pregnant. David had Uriah recalled to Jerusalem and to his wife in order to hide what had transpired. Uriah, however, felt that he was bound by the consecration of a soldier and refused to be with his wife, which would have been a cover-up for David's sin. David, in desperation, wrote Joab instructions by a letter of death, unknowingly carried by Uriah, which was a command to brilliantly have Uriah murdered, and these instructions were carried out (2 Sam. 11:2–27). Job declares in Job 13:26, "For thou writest bitter things against me, and makest me to possess the iniquities of my youth."

Terminating Death Sentence

Hezekiah was sick unto death, which means a terminal sickness, and the Lord, through Prophet Isaiah, told him to set his house in order and that he would die. But Hezekiah cried unto the Lord, and before Prophet Isaiah left the king's court, the Lord spoke to him to tell Hezekiah that he would not die, but rather an extra fifteen years shall be added unto his life. It's very interesting that there are sins committed unto death which the Bible commended us not to pray about (Isa. 38:1–5). This also reveals to us that when our sins are forgiven, then it is easier for the Lord to uproot any sickness or malady in our lives. Jesus reiterated in Matthew 9:5, "For whether is easier, to say, thy sins be forgiven thee; or to say, Arise, and walk?"

The "sin unto death" referred to in 1 John 5:16–17, which we are not to pray about, literarily means living a habitual life of sin like Esau until one can never respond to mercy and grace that brings repentance.

> "When a Christian sin and he or she already have a preconceived notion that they will repent later in the future or always thinking that God will forgive them because God is a merciful God, it's like someone standing on a dangerous terrain. God is merciful, there is no doubt about it, however, if the individual continues to wallow in sin and God continue to forgive and have mercy, that can make the individual to develop a hardened heart and be trapped in sin, which leads to death. Whenever a Christian sin, the realization of that sin ought to lead to godly sorrow that produces repentance. We cannot continue in sin and expect God's grace to abound and most definitely, God is not willing that any perish but that all come to repentance. "The Lord is not slack concerning his promise, as some men count slackness; but is longsuffering to us-ward, not willing that any should perish, but that all should come to repentance." (2 Pet. 3:9)

When one sins unto death, God is done with the individual and will never reel in the person again. We must be aware of not sinning day after day against God's mercy and grace. It was written of Esau in Hebrews 12:16–17:

> Lest there be any fornicator, or profane person, as Esau, who for one morsel of meat sold his birthright. For ye know how that afterward, when he would have inherited the blessing, he was rejected: for he found no place of repentance, though he sought it carefully with tears.

God's desire for his children is never death by demonic eviction through cancer, calamity, sickness, or sorrow but a deliberate departure that takes place when God tells the person to leave the earth by giving us glimpses of glory and our heavenly reward. As God's redeemed sons and daughters, we have already died the death through being crucified with Christ to the flesh and carnal lifestyle (Gal. 2:20). Paul said in 1 Corinthian 15:31, "I die daily," and thus he must resurrect daily (Phil. 3:10), and when we depart this earth, it must be a divine departure.

When your time comes to take off, for those who will not be here when Jesus Christ returns for the saints in the air, you decide you will never exit through sickness. And if the adversary places any infirmity or sickness on you, you get healed first and then head for heaven when you and your Lord Jesus are ready. The Bible declares about Abraham in Genesis 25:8, "Then Abraham gave up the ghost, and died in a good old age, an old man, and full of years; and was gathered to his people."

A pandemic of any kind must bow to the resurrection power and the powerful name of Jesus Christ, for unto the Lord every knee must bow (Rom. 14:11; Phil. 2:10) and we must continuously dwell in the secret place of the Most High (Ps. 91:1) as we run into His name, which is as a strong tower (Prov. 18:10). Although the rapid spread of COVID-19 around the world has caused more than 580,000 deaths and has infected more than about five million people as of July 2020,[102] Stephanie Parker noted that there had not been a continent where COVID-19—started in December 2019—had not been confirmed, except Antarctica. She indicated that the United States has the most COVID-19 cases in the world. The swift spread has been attributed to delay response to such a highly contagious disease that has never been seen before and other factors.

Parker cited Stacker's timeline composition of the COVID-19 pandemic from its first mention by Dr. Li Wenliang in Wuhan, China, to better understand what has happened and what might follow and how the situation changes daily. She concluded that the virus keeps spreading and that the surest way to flatten the curve is to keep people apart through social distancing because COVID-19 is a highly contagious virus that has become a global health crisis.[103] The stories of those who has lost loved ones during the COVID-19 pandemic are captivating across the United States and the entire world.

Katherine Rosman of *The New York Times* reported about the tragic death of couples across the United States. According to her, "The cruelty is darker when both partners die, often within a few days of each other. It's the coronavirus version of dying of a broken heart, but the cause of death isn't a metaphor but a pandemic."[104]

George Johnson rationalized that when the clock struck midnight on January 1, 2020, no one thought the world would be in the midst of a humanitarian crisis just a few months later. He buttressed that the New Year's resolutions had turned into prayers for survival, just as COVID-19 has done damage to many lives worldwide with thousands of deaths. He postulated that for many people around the world living with HIV, the restrictions that we are experiencing because of the coronavirus are nothing new. He noted that this is not

---

[102] John Hopkins University and Medicine, "Coronavirus Resource Center," Accessed May 7, 2020, https://coronavirus.jhu.edu/map.html.

[103] Stephanie Parker, "From Wuhan to New York City: A Timeline of COVID-19's Spread," *Stacker*, 2020, Accessed April 30, 2020, https://thestacker.com/stories/4039/wuhan-new-york-city-timeline-covid-19s-spread.

[104] Katherine Rosman, "After a Lifetime Together, Coronavirus Takes Them Both," *The New York Times*, 2020, Accessed May 2, 2020, https://www.nytimes.com/2020/05/02/us/coronavirus-couples.html.

the first time government inaction resulted in the spread of a deadly disease, just as in the case of the HIV epidemic known since 1981 was ignored by the United States until 1984 when it was known throughout the world. He concluded that the same delay in tackling COVID-19 has led to history repeating itself with deadly consequences for the underserved populations.[105]

It is the revelation knowledge of God's Word that can only be an effective and offensive weapon that no COVID-19 and any other future pandemics can withstand. The Bible calls it the sword of the Spirit. Ephesians 6:17 states, "And take the helmet of salvation, and the sword of the Spirit, which is the Word of God." God's Word will destroy every work of the enemy. It has the inert omnipotence ability to tear down the strongholds of unseen viruses and carnal thoughts of wicked men and unregenerate souls. It can be dispatched to heal cancers, destruction, and all diseases (Ps. 107:20). With it, you rebuke every spiritual, soulish, and physical attack of the enemy.

God's Word is a weapon of mass destruction that will cause you to win in every battle, every contest, and every challenge. So the answer to any destruction or problem is the knowledge of God's Word and obedience of the same. When we give God's Word first place and final authority in every area of our lives, we will begin to witness the victorious and triumphant power of God in our lives and in our nation like never before.

Terminating Man's Impossibilities by God's Possibilities

We want to bless the name of the Lord for every commonsense attempt and scientific approach of the government to flatten the curve of the COVID-19 pandemic. Ella, et al., enumerated that the actual number of people diagnosed all around the globe is even much

---

[105] George M. Johnson, "For People Living with HIV, the Coronavirus Pandemic Feels Familiar," Accessed April 22, 2020, https://www.msn.com/en-us/health/medical/for-people-living-with-hiv-the-coronavirus-pandemic-feels-familiar/ar-BB12UF6e?li=BBnb7Kz&ocid=mailsignout.

higher due to testing shortages that have led to many unreported cases and suspicions that some governments are hiding the scope of their nations' outbreaks. There are now more than 13.5 million people who have tested positive for the coronavirus around the world according to data from Johns Hopkins University. They specify that Air France is the latest airline to require passengers to wear face masks on flights, an effective policy that began in early May. They will also be checking passengers' body temperatures with a noncontact infrared thermometer. Delta, American, United, Frontier, and JetBlue previously announced they would require passengers to wear face coverings. Ella, et al., stated that Remdesivir, the drug donated and developed by Gilead, will be used to treat patients with COVID-19, according to the HHS.[106]

According to Nectar Gan, authorities in Chinese are using technology to track who is likely to be healthy and who poses a risk. Gan stressed that residents have been assigned a color-coded QR code on their phones and that color correlates to what they are able to do. He substantiated that although the lockdown has been lifted in Wuhan, residents still need to produce a green QR code to leave their compounds, and for those returning to work, they also need to produce a letter from their employer. Even to get into places such as restaurants, people need to show that QR code, and only people with a green code will gain entry.

Gan explained that if one's code is yellow or red, it means the individual has been flagged for some reason. Maybe the person had been on a plane with a person infected with coronavirus which will automatically flag the individual, and their code might even change color. He pointed out that those with a yellow or red code might be asked to self-isolate or even have to go into state quarantine. Gan stated that the whole thing relies on big data, and that means local governments have a database of people's travel history, their health

---

[106] Ella, et al, "Coronavirus Live Updates: More than 2,500 New Cases in Florida Since Reopening May 11, 2020," *ABC News*, 2020, Accessed May 9, 2020, https://abcnews.go.com/US/coronavirus-live-updates-global-covid-19-death-toll/story?id=70592970.

history, and whether they have been in close contact with anyone who has coronavirus.[107]

According to Justin, et al., they informed that finding a treatment for COVID-19, the respiratory disease caused by the coronavirus, could move the world closer to easing lockdown measures put in place to help slow its spread. They added that in the United States, the government's top infectious-disease expert had said that early results of a closely watched clinical trial offered "quite good news" regarding a potential COVID-19 therapy made by the biotechnology company Gilead Science Inc. They also cited Gilead who indicated that it had become aware of results from the NIAID trial showing its experimental drug, Remdesivir, helped patients recover more quickly than standard care, suggesting it could become the first effective treatment for an illness that has turned modern life inside out. The National Institute of Allergy and Infectious Diseases' (NIAID) trial enrolled more than a thousand patients internationally and compared the Remdesivir treatment alongside supportive care with a placebo. Patients who got the drug recovered in an average of eleven days while those who get a placebo recovered in fifteen days. The results were highly significant in terms of the time to recovery.

The United States Food and Drug Administration made an arrangement with Gilead to make the medicine available quickly. Originally developed to treat other novel viruses, Remdesivir has placed Gilead at the head of the race to develop a treatment for COVID-19. The drug, which has also been tested on Ebola, is not approved for use anywhere in the world. However, Gilead's study and the NIAID trial could signal a profound shift in the race to get the novel coronavirus under control. The availability of a treatment would allow the world to start reopening economies as well as offer

---

[107] Nectar Gan, "How China Is Using Color-coded QR Codes to Control the Spread of Coronavirus," *CNN Coronavirus News*, 2020, Accessed April 20, 2020, https://www.cnn.com/world/live-news/coronavirus-pandemic-04-08-20/h_a8055bb5065e8c22d68ae98de8afa7b2.

psychological relief to billions of people who have been self-isolating and fatigued to hide from the virus.[108]

According to Drew Andrew and Jennifer Jacobs, the Trump administration has organized a Manhattan Project-style effort to drastically cut the time needed to develop a coronavirus vaccine with a goal of making enough doses for most Americans by the end of 2020. The operation was termed "Operation Warp Speed." The program pulled together private pharmaceutical companies, government agencies, and the military to try to cut the development time for a vaccine by as much as eight months. The project's goal was designed to have 300 million doses of vaccine available by January 2021.

Andrew and Jacobs informed that vaccine development is typically slow and high risk; however, the project's goal is to cut out the slow part. Operation Warp Speed will use government resources to quickly test the world's most promising experimental vaccines in animals, then launch coordinated human clinical trials to winnow down the candidates. Also, the best prospective vaccines would go into wider trials at the same time mass production ramps up.

They also announced one of the world's most promising vaccine candidates developed by a team at Oxford University in London. Scientists at the US National Institutes of Health inoculated six rhesus macaques with the Oxford vaccine and then exposed them to the coronavirus, according to *The New York Times*. The result was that all six were healthy more than four weeks later. The researchers proceeded to test their vaccine in a thousand patients and also planned to expand to stage two and three clinical trials that will involve about five thousand more people.

The Bill & Melinda Gates Foundation in the United States shifted much of its research effort to the coronavirus virus. Vaccines are one of the most effective tools against viral disease as they can prevent people from becoming sick at all. Typically, they are a short-

---

[108] Justin, et.al, "Prognosis: Fauci Calls Data from Gilead Virus-Drug Trial 'Good News,'" *Bloomberg*, 2020, Accessed April 30, 2020, https://www.bloomberg.com/news/articles/2020-04-29/gilead-remdesivir-trial-for-covid-19-has-met-primary-endpoint.

cut to the immunity that most people acquire after they get sick by viruses and recover. During the illness, the immune system produces antibodies that it can subsequently use to fight off later exposure to the same pathogen. Vaccines use a live weakened virus, a dead one, or pieces of the pathogen to trick the body into building defenses without having to get sick.[109]

According to Georgia Simcox of MailOnline, Ghebreyesus stressed that most countries are still in the early strategies of their epidemics while some that were early affected by this pandemic are beginning to witness a resurgence of cases. He also cited WHO emergencies expert, Mike Ryan, who warned against opening up global travel too quickly which, according to him, would require a very careful risk management. Ghebreyesus substantiates, "Make no mistake. We have a long way to go. This virus will be with us for a long time."[110]

Is this the end of coronavirus? Or will there be a major second wave of coronavirus? This is a question that has been pulsating in the hearts of many people. There is always the risk of a potential resurgence or second wave of COVID-19 as stated by Peter Beaumont in *The Guardian*. He claimed that epidemics of infectious diseases behave in different ways, but the 1918 influenza pandemic is regarded as key example of a pandemic that occurred in multiple waves with the latter more severe than the first. He explained that other flu pandemics, including those in 1957 and 1968, had multiple waves. Case in point, the 2009 H1N1 influenza which was a pandemic started in April and was followed in the US and temperate northern hemisphere by a second wave in the autumn. However, Beaumont clarified that

---

[109] Drew Armstrong and Jennifer Jacobs, "Trump's 'Operation Warp Speed' Aims to Rush Coronavirus Vaccine," *Bloomberg*, 2020, Accessed April 30, 2020, https://www.bloomberg.com/news/articles/2020-04-29/trump-s-operation-warp-speed-aims-to-rush-coronavirus-vaccine.

[110] Georgia Simcox, "WHO Warns Coronavirus Will Be with Us for a Long Time and Says Most of the World's Population Remains at Risk from Catching the Disease." MailOnline, 2020, Accessed April 22, 2020, https://www.dailymail.co.uk/news/article-8246431/WHO-warns-coronavirus-long-time-worlds-population-risk.html.

how and why multiple wave outbreaks occur and how subsequent waves of infection can be prevented has become a staple of epidemiological modelling studies and pandemic preparation, which have looked at everything from social behavior and health policy to vaccination and the buildup of community immunity, also known as herd immunity. He also emphasized that conventional wisdom among scientists suggests second waves of resistant infections occur after the capacity for treatment and isolation becomes exhausted realistically, when the social and political consensus supporting lockdowns is being overtaken by public frustration, which triggered protests in the US and elsewhere and the urgent need to reopen economies.

Furthermore, he highlighted that the threat will only decline when susceptibility of the population to the disease falls below a certain threshold or when widespread vaccination becomes available. Beaumont cited Justin Lessler, an associate professor of epidemiology at Johns Hopkins University, who stated that epidemics are like fires that rage uncontrollably when fuel is plentiful, smolders slowly when fuel is scarce, but no one knows how much fuel is still available for this coronavirus. He stresses:

> Epidemiologists call this intensity the "force of infection," and the fuel that drives it is the population's susceptibility to the pathogen. As repeated waves of the epidemic reduce susceptibility…they also reduce the force of infection, lowering the risk of illness even among those with no immunity.[111]

WHO Chief, Tedros Ghebreyesus, warns "the worst is yet ahead of us…let's prevent this tragedy. It's a virus that many people still don't understand."[112]

---

[111] Peter Beaumont, "Will There Be a Second Wave of Coronavirus?" *The Guardian's Development Desk,* 2020, Accessed April 22, 2020, https://www.theguardian.com/world/2020/apr/20/will-there-be-second-wave-of-coronavirus-.

[112] Tedros A. Ghebreyesus, "The Worst is Yet Ahead of US" *The Telegraph*, 2020, Accessed April 22, 2020, https://www.youtube.com/watch?v=yboX5UeMWdI.

Emma Graham-Harrison cited WHO on immunity passports issuance to people who have recovered from COVID-19 because there is yet no evidence that they will be protected from a second infection, and also that the idea of issuing some form of certificates to people who have been sick with the virus on the assumption they would be immune to reinfection has been gaining ground in many places, including the UK as authorities cast around for ways out of socially and economically devastating lockdowns. He stressed that WHO warned in a scientific briefing that "there is currently no evidence that people who have recovered from COVID-19 and have antibodies are protected from a second infection."

Instead, the certificates could pose a health risk by providing unjustified assurances of protection to individuals and their communities. WHO stated, "at this point in the pandemic, there is not enough evidence about the effectiveness of antibody-mediated immunity to guarantee the accuracy of an 'immunity passport' or 'risk-free certificate...'" WHO added that people who assume that they are immune to a second infection because they have received a positive test result may ignore public health advice and that the use of such certificates may therefore increase the risks of continued transmission.[113]

According to Kathleeen Dohemy, Pfizer had launched a Phase 1/2 clinical trial for a vaccine for COVID-19, and it collaborated with an immunotherapy company, BioNTech, to test four different vaccine candidates at once. Pfizer expects to produce millions of vaccine doses in 2020.

She added that the platform under study is similar to the one used by Moderna, which hopes to begin a Phase 2 study by the summer of 2020. These types of vaccines use messenger RNA to convey genetic information to the body's cells. Once mRNA in a vaccine is in the cell, the cells can translate this genetic information to create

---

[113] Emma Graham-Harrison, "WHO Warns Against Coronavirus Immunity Passports," *The Guardian*, 2020, Accessed April 27, 2020, https://www.theguardian.com/world/2020/apr/25/who-warns-against-coronavirus-immunity-passports

an immune response, and because the companies are evaluating four different mRNA candidates at once, they can shift gears quickly if one does not work, but as of early May, according to Fast Cures, a center of the Milken Institute, 123 vaccines for COVID-19 are still under study in various phases of development.[114]

Eric Schmitt, et al., explicated that one of the hallmarks of the United States military relies in its ability to project power around the world, often under the banner of slogans intended to strike fear in its adversaries: "Ready to fight tonight" for US troops in South Korea, "America's 911" for the Marine Corps expeditionary units at sea, And the list goes on. However, the foe now is the novel coronavirus that has really struck deep and has affected more than 1,200 military personnel and their family members. Schmitt, et al., noted that US warships typically spend months at sea monitoring the activities of adversaries. The ships assigned to the Pacific Fleet patrol the South China Sea, the East China Sea and areas in between, sometimes undertaking the so-called freedom of navigation operations that bring them close to disputed islands in the area. The goal of these voyages is to drive home to China that the United States does not recognize Beijing's claims of ownership.

Nevertheless, the virus has proven far more damaging than any recent encounters with traditional adversaries and has exposed a vulnerability of a force often referred to as the world's policeman because all the focus on the battles in Afghanistan, Iraq, Syria, Yemen, and the power conflict with China and Russia has exerted a crippling effect on an American aircraft carrier in days. Schmitt, et al., stated that for the military, the core issue is that as the virus spreads, it becomes increasingly difficult to carry on with training and missions.[115]

---

[114] Kathleen Dohemy, "Pfizer Starts Clinical Trials of COVID-19 Vaccine," WebMD, 2020, Accessed May 12, 2020, https://www.webmd.com/lung/news/20200507/pfizer-starts-clinical-trials-of-covid-19-vaccine.

[115] Eric Schmitt, et al., "Prepare for War or Fight Coronavirus: US Military Battles Competing Instincts," *The New York Times* 2020, Accessed May 21, 2020, https://www.nytimes.com/2020/04/01/us/politics/coronavirus-aircraft-carrier-roosevelt.html?action=click&module=RelatedLinks&pgtype=Article.

Man may try, and he is trying, but only God can help. Except the Lord builds the house, the builders are laboring in vain, and except the Lord watches the city, the watchmen are doing so in vain. Jesus Christ is the stone which the builder has refused, and He has become the chief cornerstone (Ps. 118:22, 127:1). The Gospel according to Mark 10:27 and 9:23 declares, "And Jesus looking upon them saith, with men it is impossible, but not with God: for with God all things are possible. Jesus said unto him, If thou canst believe, all things are possible to him that believeth."

And so there is a correlation with God who only can handle that which is impossible to man and man who believe that God can do so. Man, because of his limitation, cannot handle impossible things, but that is where God steps in. That is where divinity takes over humanity and faith in His Word transcends us to that same realm of divinity. Has it not been written that God has made us to sit together with Him in the heavenly places far above every principality and power and every name, including COVID-19 and any other future pandemic (Eph. 1:16–23, 2:6–7, 4:10)?

Terminating Death by Standing between the Living and the Dead

Who could cancel the dream of death that the baker had in the same prison with Joseph? Only Jesus Christ through his spiritual weapon of mass destruction (Gen. 40:16–22). He redeemed the thief on the right side at Golgotha when he said to him, "Today you shall be with me in paradise" (Luke 23:43). Who else can deliver Jonathan from perishing with Saul? He was to walk and suffer with David in the woods after escaping the destructive javelin of his father, Saul, but for the comfort of the palace. He was to be the second on the throne with David instead of Joab. David asked, "How are the mighty fallen" (2 Sam. 1:19, 25, 27)? Jonathan, before his death, laments in 1 Samuel 23:17, "And he said unto him, Fear not: for the hand of Saul my father shall not find thee; and thou shalt be king over Israel, and I shall be next unto thee; and that also Saul my father knoweth."

Jonathan departed from Saul into the congregation of the dead after he visited David in the woods, but instead of continuing with him to suffer for a while (1 Pet. 5:10), he went back to the palace. The Bible says in 1 Samuel 23:18, "And they two made a covenant before the LORD: and David abode in the wood, and Jonathan went to his house."

I perceive someone reading this book needs to rush out of the congregation of the dead and begin to dwell among the congregation of the living. The Word of God declares in Proverbs 21:19, "The man that wandereth out of the way of understanding shall remain in the congregation of the dead."

Who else can stand between the living and the dead except our only High Priest after the order of Melchizedek whose name is Jesus Christ (Heb. 5:10, 6:20), the only one that has the spiritual weapons of mass destruction that have annihilated every virus and pandemic if we appropriate the same? The Bible declares in Numbers 16:47–49:

> And Aaron took as Moses commanded, and ran into the midst of the congregation; and, behold, the plague was begun among the people: and he put on incense, and made an atonement for the people. And he stood between the dead and the living; and the plague was stayed. Now they that died in the plague were fourteen thousand and seven hundred, beside them that died about the matter of Korah.

Faith in God's Word is likened to a shield of faith that will quench every fiery dart of the enemy, including COVID-19, just as the Word of God declares in Ephesians 6:16, "Above all, taking the shield of faith, wherewith ye shall be able to quench all the fiery darts of the wicked."

Man can only roll away the stone to Lazarus' tomb. The remains are already stinking after four days, but man has no power to raise

Lazarus. And hence the command of Jesus Christ at the tomb of Lazarus, "Take ye away the stone" (John 11:39). Man had helped to take away the stone of COVID-19 and other pandemics that this world has ever encountered, but it is time for us to now let the Lord know that we have done, our part, and only God can do the impossible. When we acknowledge God as the only one who can call forth Lazarus, who can make the vaccine effective, who can stop future pandemics, and who can destroy every second or a third wave of coronavirus, that is the time He will show up to eradicate all of these with His spiritual weapon of mass destruction.

The Gospel according to Mark accounted in Mark 16:1–3, regarding who will help the women push away the stone that was used to seal Jesus's tomb:

> And when the sabbath was past, Mary Magdalene, and Mary the mother of James, and Salome, had bought sweet spices, that they might come and anoint him. And very early in the morning the first day of the week, they came unto the sepulchre at the rising of the sun. And they said among themselves, who shall roll us away the stone from the door of the sepulchre?

Who can annul the covenant of death entered into by Judas Iscariot through the love of money? Who can hinder the covenant of death entered into by Ananias and Sapphira when they both lied against the Holy Ghost in the newly established Church of Jesus Christ where the Holy Spirit is the Director and Chief Executive Officer? We are called to be part of the body of the living church because our God is a living God and not the God of the dead. First Timothy 3:15 asserts, "But if I tarry long, that thou mayest know how thou oughtest to behave thyself in the house of God, which is the church of the living God, the pillar and ground of the truth." We serve the God of the living and not the dead (Matt. 22:32).

Who can break the curse that Jacob passed upon Rachel, unknowingly, when Rachel sat on the idol of her father? Jacob declares in Gen. 31:32, "With whomsoever thou findest thy gods, let him not live: before our brethren discern, thou, what is thine with me, and take it to thee. For Jacob knew not that Rachel had stolen them."

How many idols are you sitting upon? How many idols are the nations of the earth sitting upon and won't let go? Later in life, Rachel had to weep for her children (Jer. 31:15; Matt 2:18) when Herod massacred them during the infant days of Jesus Christ. But God reassured Rachel and every wailing woman (Jer. 9:20) that had lost precious ones to refrain from weeping and dry the tears on their eyes. The Lord said your work shall be rewarded because there is hope in thine end and that your children will come again to their border (Jer. 31:16–17).

Who can stop COVID-19 and other pandemics that attack a man while sleeping on a bed? The Bible declares in 2 Samuel 4:5–11:

> And the sons of Rimmon the Beerothite, Rechab and Baanah, went, and came about the heat of the day to the house of Ishbosheth, who lay on a bed at noon. And they came thither into the midst of the house, as though they would have fetched wheat; and they smote him under the fifth rib: and Rechab and Baanah his brother escaped.

Who else can annul the conspiracy against Amon, the king of Israel, in his own house where he was slain (2 Kings 21:23–24)? Who else can stop Hazael (a type of COVID-19) from suffocating Benhadad, the king of Syria in his own house (2 Kings 8:7–15)? Who else can stop the edict of Elijah against Ahaziah who had contacted Beelzebub, the god of Ekron, regarding his disease? Second Kings 1:4 declares, "Now therefore thus saith the Lord, thou shalt not come down from that bed on which thou art gone up, but shalt surely die. And Elijah departed."

Who else can annul the death sentence against the rich fool that trusts in his own wealth? Jesus Christ laments in the parable of Luke

12:20, "Thou fool, this night thy soul shall be required of thee: then whose shall those things be, which thou hast provided?"

Jezebel vowed to cut off the head of Elijah who had slain the four hundred and fifty prophets of Baal at brook Kishon (1 Kings 18:19). The four hundred prophets of groves or Asherah never showed up at mount Carmel. Elijah went to heaven in a whirlwind (2 Kings 2:1), but John the Baptist will soon come in the spirit and power of Elijah to prepare the way of the Lord (Luke 1:17), and he truly came (Matt. 17:10–12). Jezebel also came in the spirit of Herodias who later had sworn to cut off the head of John the Baptist (Matt. 14:1–10; Rev. 2:20). Who else would have stopped the death of John the Baptist? Nobody else but Jesus Christ. *If* John the Baptist had decreased his ministry to zero and followed Jesus Christ, he would have been protected under the protective arm of Jesus Christ just as one of his disciples and never would have been dead through offenses (Luke 17:1).

Who else would have annulled the death of Apostle James that Jesus prophesied to when his mother came to Jesus to secure a position for him and his brother on the right and left side of Jesu Christ? The Bible declares in in Matthew 20:21–23:

> And he said unto her, what wilt thou? She saith unto him, Grant that these my two sons may sit, the one on thy right hand, and the other on the left, in thy kingdom. But Jesus answered and said, Ye know not what ye ask. Are ye able to drink of the cup that I shall drink of, and to be baptized with the baptism that I am baptized with? They say unto him, we are able. And he saith unto them, Ye shall drink indeed of my cup, and be baptized with the baptism that I am baptized with: but to sit on my right hand, and on my left, is not mine to give, but it shall be given to them for whom it is prepared of my Father.

Who else halted the death of Peter when he was incarcerated in prison by Herod and getting ready to be slaughtered just like he did to Apostle James, the brother of John, as recorded in Acts 12:1–17? It was nobody else but Jesus Christ who had prayed for Peter. The Bible asserts in Luke 22:31–32:

> And the Lord said, Simon, Simon, behold, Satan hath desired to have you, that he may sift you as wheat. But I have prayed for thee, that thy faith fails not: and when thou art converted, strengthen thy brethren.

Obviously, the church had prayed for Peter, but their prayer was not in faith because when Peter was released, they did not even believe he would be released. Their whole praying principle at the church was wonderful, but God will only respond to faith, for it is impossible to please God without faith, and only the prayer of faith can save the sick (Heb. 11:6; James 5:14–15).

Who else can stop the projection of death into your future but Jesus Christ? Esau said within himself as recorded in Genesis 27:41, "And Esau hated Jacob because of the blessing wherewith his father blessed him: and Esau said in his heart, The days of mourning for my father are at hand; then will I slay my brother Jacob."

Who else can stop every satanic conspiracy of death against you? Ahithophel conspired with David's son and others to kill David (2 Sam. 15:12, 31). More than forty men conspired together to kill Paul (Acts 23:12–13). Only God could have altered their plans through his spiritual weapon of mass destruction, just like He did for Israel when they were held captive by Pharaoh in Egypt.

He delivered Jehoshaphat from destruction when the Moabites, Ammonites, and other nations came to destroy him and his nation (2 Chron. 20). God used His massive spiritual weapon of mass destruction on Jehoshaphat's enemy.

Terminating Every Appointment
with Death with God's Word

What you don't say, you will never see. "He shall have whatsoever he saith" (Mark 11:23). The book of Proverbs 18:21 declares, "Death and life are in the power of the tongue: and they that love it shall eat the fruit thereof." The Lord responded to the murmurings and complaints of the children of Israel by saying, "As truly as I live, saith the Lord, as ye have spoken in mine ears, so will I do to you (Num. 14:28).

Psalms 91:2 pronounces, "I will say of the Lord, He is my refuge and my fortress: my God; in him will I trust." I will say the Lord means to terminate all appointment with death; you have to say it. A man can either kill himself by the wrong use of his tongue or establish his heritage of living a very long and satisfying life by using his tongue rightly.

The Lord destroyed thousands of people in the wilderness just because of what they said. Their corpses fell in the wilderness at the rate of a hundred to two hundred per day dying, like flies as they suffered the wages of the sin of unbelief. This was far from what they had anticipated. The book of Numbers records their journey, their failure, and the demise of that Exodus generation that wanders in the wilderness en route to the promised land. An eleven-day journey turned into forty years of wilderness camping and high death tolls because of their fearful description of the promised land. The Amplified version of Deuteronomy 1:2 states:

> It is [only] eleven days' journey from Horeb (Mount Sinai) by way of Mount Seir to Kadesh-barnea [on Canaan's border; yet Israel wandered in the wilderness for forty years before crossing the border and entering Canaan, the promised land].

As you confess God's Word, be aware that repeated refusal to trust God can lead to being removed from the forefront of God's purposes for our lives (Num. 14:22–24). Trials should be expected but cuddled with joy (James 1:2–4). It is impossible to please God without faith, and it is impossible to have faith without trials. God uses trials for our spiritual development (1 Cor. 10:13). Murmuring and complaining highly offends God because He has revealed to His children that He loves and cares for them. Yet, God is faithful even when we are not. He just cannot deny Himself (2 Tim. 2:12). He will accomplish His desires and fulfill His promises regardless of the unbelief of others. Romans 3:3–4 declares, "For what if some did not believe? shall their unbelief make the faith of God without effect? God forbid."

CHAPTER 7

Releasing Spiritual Weapon of Mass Destruction to Terminate COVID-19 and Future Pandemics

There are some serious pestilences prevalent in our days. We are living in the days that Jesus prophesied will come in Luke 21:11, 13, 18–19:

> And great earthquakes shall be in divers places, and famines, and pestilences; and fearful sights and great signs shall there be from heaven.
>
> And it shall turn to you for a testimony.
>
> But there shall not an hair of your head perish. In your patience possess ye your souls.

In this chapter, we will be identifying some of the enemy's weapons of mass destruction, including COVID-19, and how to intercept and destroy them with a counter spiritual weapon of mass destruction. We must remember that the scripture admonishes in Revelation 13:10, "He that leadeth into captivity shall go into captivity: he that killeth with the sword must be killed with the sword. Here is the patience and the faith of the saints."

Understanding God's Weapon of Mass Destruction

Richard Mesic enumerated that the attractiveness of both ballistic missiles and weapons of mass destruction (WMD) to various actors throughout the world pose a serious threat to US security and that these weapons and delivery systems are popular in part because they are highly visible symbols of military prowess, and as such, provide significant influence on regional balances of power, even among friends and allies. He highlighted that such weapons give the appearance of being unstoppable, even by active defenses. Mesic detailed that unlike a ballistic missile that is armed solely with conventional high explosives that is inefficient and expensive, a WMD is a bearing missile used for coercion or in extreme circumstances with valuable warheads that have enhanced potentials. A WMD might be chemical, biological, or nuclear. The most usable are chemical agents but the easiest to counter, while biological agents that may be least suitable for ballistic missile delivery are the most difficult to counter; and nuclear weapons are the most expensive and challenging but are the least likely (one hopes) to be used.

He explained that biological weapons are sometimes referred to as the "poor man's nuclear weapons" both because of their potential, pound-for-pound, to inflict human casualties on a scale comparable to nuclear weapons and because their cost could be less than the cost of even modest nuclear arsenals by a factor of ten or more, and they are of increasing concern to national security policymakers and warfighters. He also warned that the threat a WMD poses may be a forcing function for revolutionary changes and causes a warranted and much broader consideration of WMD and their implications in the overall strategic context.

Biological weapons put awesome destructive potential within the reach of many states, and using them would entail awesome operational and political risks. He also enumerated that the potential effectiveness of modern lethal and nonlethal chemical agents, in purely clinical terms, is well understood, although their strategic and tactical military potential in the very dynamic and complex battlefields of the future is more uncertain. and chemical weapons also have a negative image relative to more "humane" and discriminating instruments of warfare.

Mesic added that the relatively crude approximately fifteen-kiloton implosion and gun-type atomic weapons dropped on Hiroshima and Nagasaki ended World War II but introduced the world to the awesome power and effects of nuclear fission devices. He explained that in a relatively short time, the development of thermonuclear weapons ("H-bombs") did rewrite the book on destructive potential with modern weapons producing the power equivalent of about a thousand tons of high explosives per pound of warhead (a 2,000,000 to 1 increase in efficiency over high explosives).

Mesic revealed the characteristics of biological weapons to be unconventional as they only affect living organisms, such as anthrax that can kill humans and never harm a tank. They also take a relatively long time before their effects are observed. They are largely antipersonnel, not antimateriel, that produce a delayed effect (kicking in minutes to hours to days or even weeks after exposure). This release may or may not be associated with observable phenomena (such as flybys of a hostile aircraft or a bomb, artillery, or missile attack). Once dispersed, the agent cloud is generally invisible. People in its path will not see it coming and will not notice when the cloud engulfs them, but effective treatment is possible with adequate warnings of an attack.

Mesic explained that chemical agents can be delivered by a variety of means, and a small amount can cover a large (but "controllable") area, and a very effective defense is possible with adequate warning. However, nuclear weapons can produce antipersonnel and or antimateriel effects, and the effects are devastating, prompt, and long-term. He substantiated that the principal characteristic of nuclear weapons in the proliferation context is that very few are likely to be available because the critical nuclear materials (plutonium and/or highly enriched uranium) required to fabricate these weapons are difficult and expensive to make. He buttressed that several actions, operationally, including preventive strikes on WMD facilities, preemptive strikes on WMD stocks and delivery means, active defenses—such as airborne laser (ABL), Theater High-Altitude Area

Defense (THAAD), and Patriot missiles—and passive defense measures—such as nuclear hardening, inoculations, antibiotics, warning systems, masks, and collective shelters—can be taken, and of all these, the most important are passive defense measures.[116]

However, with the succinct understanding of these physical weapons of mass destruction (WMD),that can do significant harm and damage on a large scale, none has proven to deal with COVID-19, but there is nothing like the use of spiritual weapons of mass destruction (SWMD) that are more powerful, massive, profuse, direct at hitting its target, exhaustive, overwhelming, and very effective. SWMD will not only defuse but also humiliate every other weapon. No virus can stand it, not even coronavirus and any other known pandemics. This spiritual weapon of mass destruction is called "Weapon of Mass Revelation Knowledge of God's Word."

Isaiah 5:3 and Hosea 4:6 state:

> Therefore my people are gone into captivity, because they have no knowledge: and their honourable men are famished, and their multitude dried up with thirst.
> My people are destroyed for lack of knowledge.

Jesus Christ announces against the gates of hell (including all coronaviruses, endemics, or pandemics) in Matthew 16:18, "And I say also unto thee, That thou art Peter, and upon this rock I will build my church; and the gates of hell shall not prevail against it."

---

[116] Richard F. Mesic, eds. Jeremy Shapiro and Zalmay Khalilzad, *Countering Weapons of Mass Destruction and Ballistic Missiles, Strategic Appraisal: United States Air and Space Power in the 21ˢᵗ Century* (RAND Corporation, CA: Santa Monica, VA: Arlington, PA: Pittsburg, 2002), 283–342.

Countermeasures Weapons against COVID-19 Missiles

The associated press had detailed that there have been some new flareups in Rome and South Korea, and the fear of a second wave of contagion underscored the dilemma authorities faced as they tried to reopen their economies. Italian authorities were worried that people were getting too friendly at cocktail hour during the country's first weekend of eased restrictions.

They documented responses around the world, especially in the US and other hard-hit countries that are wrestling with how to ease curbs on business and public activity without causing the virus surging back. They cited Governor Andrew Cuomo who reported that three children had died in New York state from a possible complication of the coronavirus involving swollen blood vessels and heart problems and that at least seventy-three children in New York had been diagnosed with symptoms similar to Kawasaki disease, which is a rare inflammatory condition and toxic shock syndrome. However, there has not been proof that the mysterious syndrome is caused by the virus.

They noted that health authorities in the United States are watching for a second wave, roughly two weeks after states began a gradual reopening, with the state of Georgia largely leading the way. The governments of different countries warn that controls will be reimposed if the public fails to follow social-distancing guidelines.[117]

COVID-19 and other pandemics are fiery darts shot from the enemy. Their defense system is only the shield of faith. Ephesians 6:16 states, "Above all, taking the shield of faith, wherewith ye shall be able to quench all the fiery darts of the wicked." David deployed ballistic missile defense systems against a particular plague that was destroying Israel's populace when the devil moved David to count

---

[117] "Reopenings Bring New Cases in South Korea, Virus Fears in Italy," COVID-19 Pandemic WGN9, *The Associated Press*, 2020, Accessed May 9, 2020, https://wgntv.com/news/coronavirus/reopenings-bring-new-cases-in-s-korea-virus-fears-in-italy/.

Israel after God had warned that such an act should not be practiced among His people.

First Chronicles 21:1, 7, 26–28 states:

> And Satan stood up against Israel, and provoked David to number Israel.
>
> And God was displeased with this thing; therefore he smote Israel
>
> [S]o the Lord sent pestilence upon Israel: and there fell of Israel seventy thousand men.
>
> And David built there an altar unto the Lord, and offered burnt offerings and peace offerings, and called upon the Lord; and he answered him from heaven by fire upon the altar of burnt offering. And the Lord commanded the angel; and he put up his sword again into the sheath thereof. At that time when David saw that the Lord had answered him in the threshing floor of Ornan the Jebusite, then he sacrificed there.

God, who is the righteous Judge, had permitted the census to be taken with the design that this sin of David would make room for Him to punish Israel for other sins. This is because when God has a plan in mind, He sometimes uses Satan and his demons as an instrument to work out His own will and purpose, such as when God allowed a lying spirit to fill the mouth of Ahab's prophet who in turn would prophesy that Ahab should go to battle, which would lead to his death. Satan was also an instrument for Job's persecution, but at the end of it all, he walked in double blessings (Job 1–2, 42). David's countermeasure missiles deployed against that plague that had destroyed almost seventy thousand people was complete dedication through genuine repentance and an outcry for mercy to God and giving sacrificial offerings unto God.

G. Lewis and T. Postol stated that the United States is in the midst of an ambitious effort to build and deploy a wide range of ballistic missile defense systems. They noted that proponents of the systems have argued that they will be effective against a host of current and postulated threats from ballistic missiles, but in reality, success or failure of this will depend not only on the technology used in defenses but also on the tactics and technologies used in missile attacks.

Lewis and Postol illustrated that resourceful and determined attackers always seek to stress a defense beyond its limits, and they can do this by altering their weapons' characteristics with tactics or devices known as countermeasures, such as maneuvers, decoys, and infrared and radar stealth, which hinder or prevent the defense from identifying or hitting their incoming missiles. They clarified that the ability of a defense to adapt to and deal with countermeasures is the ultimate test of its combat worthiness.[118]

Bill Powell indicated that it had been a bedrock belief of US policy for forty years that it was possible to bring the People's Republic of China smoothly into the family of nations, and now, one of the architects of that policy was finally acknowledging the obvious. According to Powell, the coronavirus global pandemic has brought relations between Beijing and Washington to its lowest point since China reopened to the world in 1978, and any chance that the pandemic might spur Washington and Beijing to set differences aside and work together on treatments and other aspects of the pandemic—such as how exactly it started—is long gone.

But the aftermath of the Wuhan outbreak more closely resembles the building of the Berlin Wall in 1961 than either Pearl Harbor or 9/11. What follows will not be a sharp burst of savage conflict but a global scramble to shape the new order rising from the rubble of old. Furthermore, he explained that as with the wall, the forces that led to the dispute over the Wuhan outbreak were unleashed years before the events that made history. And the change they represent is likely irreversible, no matter who sits in the White House, and that notion has fully settled in here.

---

[118] G. N. Lewis, T. A. Postol, "Future Challenges to Ballistic Missile Defense," *IEEE Spectrum*, 34:9, 1997:60.

He enumerated that 66 percent of Americans now have a negative view of China, according to a recent Pew Research poll. Likewise, in China, state-owned media and a government-controlled Internet has beaten up nationalism and anti-Americanism to levels unseen since the US accidentally bombed Beijing's embassy in Belgrade during the Balkan wars in 1999. He explained that the world's two most powerful nations are now competing in military and cyber warfare. Similarly, the competition to dominate the key technologies of the twenty-first century is also intensifying, the kind of rivalry that has not been witnessed since the Soviet Union collapsed in 1991. China's pursuit of preeminence across a wide range of technologies in areas like quantum computing and artificial intelligence is central to the economic clash with the US, but China also has significant military components.

He added that since the 1990s, when Chinese military planners were stunned by the US lightning victory in the first Iraq war, they have consistently focused their efforts on developing war-fighting capabilities relevant to their immediate strategic goals while creating the ability to one day leapfrog US military technologies, and quantum computing is an example.

Powell cited David Kilcullen, who wrote that our enemies have caught up or overtaken us in critical technologies or have expanded their concept of war beyond the narrow boundaries within which our traditional approach can be brought to bear already adapted, and unless we too adapt, our decline is only a matter of time.

China is not yet a "peer power" as US national defense analysts put it. But the steadily aggressive pursuit of quantum technologies and a wide array of others that also have dual-use applications increasingly convince Pentagon planners that Beijing will one day be one. The year 2049 will mark the Chinese Communist Party's hundredth anniversary of taking power in Beijing, and that is the year Chinese propaganda outlets have said China will see the completion of its rise to the dominant power on earth.

The most significant difference in the emerging geopolitical standoff between Washington and Beijing is obvious: China is economically powerful and deeply integrated with both the developed and developing worlds. Powell cited Rosemary Gibson, who remarked that if China shut the door on exports of medicines and their key ingredients and raw material, US hospitals, military hospitals, and clinics would cease to function within months if not days. Powell emphasized that in the wake of the pandemic, the US is suffering a defeat that should be unthinkable, and it is losing the propaganda war, particularly in the developing world. He proposes that right now, Washington and its allies should focus more on how to cope effectively with a powerful rival with the mission being wage the twenty-first century's Cold War while ensuring it never turns hot.[119]

Holiness: A Spiritual Weapon of Mass Destruction

Holiness is the foundation of releasing spiritual weapons of mass destruction on COVID-10 and any other pandemic. It's not a coincidence that we have been told to clean our hands during this pandemic. The Bible declares in James 4:8, "Draw nigh to God, and he will draw nigh to you. Cleanse your hands, ye sinners; and purify your hearts, ye double minded."

According to a Penn Medicine article, frequently cleaning and disinfecting the home is very essential for keeping every member of the family safe and healthy. While person-to-person transmission of COVID-19 poses a much greater risk than transmission via surfaces, the Centers for Disease Control (CDC) has recommended cleaning and disinfecting high-touch surfaces at least once a day, even if no one leaves the house since items and people that come into the house could lead to the possibility of exposure. The novel coronavirus can remain in the air for up to three hours and live on surfaces such as

---

[119] Bill Powell, "America Is in a New Cold War, and this Time, the Communists Might Win," *Newsweek Magazine*, 2020, Accessed May 21, 2020, https://www.newsweek.com/2020/06/05/america-new-cold-war-this-time-communists-might-win-1504447.html?utm_source=WhatCountsEmail&utm_medium=RAND%20Policy%20Currents+AEM:%20%20Email%20Address%20NOT%20LIKE%20DOTMIL&utm_campaign=AEM:631600804.

cardboard for up to twenty-four hours and plastic and stainless steel for up to three days.

There is a difference between cleaning a surface which can simply remove dirt and particles, but disinfecting kills viruses and bacteria. The article suggested the most important items to disinfect every day, which are cupboard and drawer knobs/pulls, faucets, kitchen and bathroom counters, toilets (especially the seat and handle), refrigerators, dishwashers, oven and microwave handles, remote controls and game controllers, cell phones, tablets and other mobile devices, computers, keyboards and mice, doorknobs/handles, table surfaces, staircase railings, and light switches or switch plates. Furthermore, the article buttressed that no matter what you do, the best way to lower the risk of contracting COVID-19 or passing it to someone else is to wash the hands more frequently. The CDC recommends a vigorous twenty-second scrub with soap and water that extends beyond the hands to the wrists, between the fingers, and under the fingernails.[120]

Second Timothy 2:19, 21 declares:

> Nevertheless the foundation of God standeth sure, having this seal, The Lord knoweth them that are his. And, let everyone that nameth the name of Christ departs from iniquity.
>
> If a man therefore purge himself from these, he shall be a vessel unto honour, sanctified, and meet for the master's use, and prepared unto every good work.

Whenever holiness is in place, there will be miracles, signs, and wonders in our lives. The power of mighty signs and wonders can only flow in the life of a holy vessel. Gehazi's destiny was to catch double, even triple the portion of the grace of God upon Elisha, but he lost it because sin was found in him. Although signs and wonders

---

[120] Penn Medicine, "How to Clean and Disinfect Your Home Against COVID-19," *Health and Wellness*, 2020, Accessed May 26, 2020, https://www.pennmedicine.org/updates/blogs/health-and-wellness/2020/april/cleaning-against-covid.

are the heritage of God's children, it will take a life of holiness for it to be delivered into our lives. The Bible details in Hebrews 12:14, "Follow peace with all men, and holiness, without which no man shall see the Lord."

God has called us unto holiness and not unto uncleanliness (1 Thess. 4:7). All the promises of God can only be delivered to us on the platform of holiness. The promises of God to his children can only be delivered to us with holiness. God our Father will never allow evil to befall his children. Even when we are challenged, he will always make a way of escape for us.

Second Corinthians 6:14–18, 7:1 state:

> Be ye not unequally yoked together with unbelievers: for what fellowship hath righteousness with unrighteousness? and what communion hath light with darkness? And what concord hath Christ with Belial? or what part hath he that believeth with an infidel? And what agreement hath the temple of God with idols? for ye are the temple of the living God; as God hath said, I will dwell in them, and walk in them; and I will be their God, and they shall be my people. Wherefore come out from among them, and be ye separate, saith the Lord, and touch not the unclean thing; and I will receive you. And will be a Father unto you, and ye shall be my sons and daughters, saith the Lord Almighty.
>
> Having therefore these promises, dearly beloved, let us cleanse ourselves from all filthiness of the flesh and spirit, perfecting holiness in the fear of God.

Demons always scatter and bow to Jesus Christ because they recognize him as the Holy one of God. Mark 1:24 states, "Saying, let us alone; what have we to do with thee, thou Jesus of Nazareth? art thou come to destroy us? I know thee who thou art, the Holy One of God."

All the hosts of heaven are not crying, "Faithful, faithful, faithful" to our God; neither are they hollering out, "Mighty, mighty, mighty," although our God is faithful and mighty. All they cry is, "Holy, Holy, Holy, Lord God Almighty, who was, who is and who is to come" (Rev. 4:8).

Holiness, which is the practice or the doing of righteousness or a righteous deed, must come forth out of the church so as to exalt our nations. Proverbs 14:34 indicates that "righteousness exalteth a nation: but sin is a reproach to any people." And if righteousness can exalt a nation out of COVID-19, how much more would it exalt a family or an individual out of all pandemics of this life? Jesus declared in John 8:46, "Which of you convinceth me of sin?" *He* has the boldness to ask this question because He was a man of absolute holiness, a sanctified vessel, and as a result, He enjoyed supernatural manifestations throughout His life here on earth. He said in John 14:21, "He that hath my commandments, and keepeth them, he it is that loveth me: and he that loveth me shall be loved of my Father, and I will love him, and will manifest myself to him."

We have to keep God's commandment of holiness to discharge our God-given spiritual weapon of mass destruction against COVID-19 and another future pandemics. If you are not a lover of holiness, you can never be a candidate of God's power. When we walk in holiness, we will be like our God with whom there is no impossibility. First Peter 1:15–16 commands, "But as he which hath called you is holy, so be ye holy in all manner of conversation; Because it is written, Be ye holy; for I am holy."

When we walk in God's holiness, we gain direct access to God's divine revelation, and revelation provokes revolutions. When you live in a habitual life of sin, you are limited to information from the Word of God, and you will have no access to His revelations.

Apostle John, in his letter, decries in 1 John 3:5–9:

> And ye know that he was manifested to take
> away our sins; and in him is no sin. Whosoever

abideth in him sinneth not: whosoever sinneth hath not seen him, neither known him. Little children let no man deceive you: he that doeth righteousness is righteous, even as he is righteous. He that committeth sin is of the devil; for the devil sinneth from the beginning. For this purpose, the Son of God was manifested, that he might destroy the works of the devil. Whosoever is born of God doth not commit sin; for his seed remaineth in him: and he cannot sin, because he is born of God.

When we walk in God's divine holiness, we carry God's manifest presence, and everything had to clear off the way when God's presence is there. God's manifest presence guarantees an all-round breakthrough. The Bible says in Psalms 97:3–5, 114:7:

A fire goeth before him, and burneth up his enemies' round about. His lightnings enlightened the world: the earth saw, and trembled. The hills melted like wax at the presence of the Lord, at the presence of the Lord of the whole earth.

Tremble, thou earth, at the presence of the Lord, at the presence of the God of Jacob.

There is no way a man can carry God's presence without holiness. We must all strive to stay pure and clean. David states in Psalms 24:3–5:

Who shall ascend into the hill of the Lord? Or who shall stand in his holy place? He that hath clean hands, and a pure heart; who hath not lifted up his soul unto vanity, nor sworn deceitfully. He shall receive the blessing from the Lord, and righteousness from the God of his salvation.

The Name of Jesus Christ of Nazareth: A Spiritual Weapon of Mass Destruction

Names are very important in biblical Christianity. God had to change the names many of his children, such as Abram, which means exalted father, to Abraham, which means father of a multitude (Gen. 17:5). God also changed the name Sarai, which meant princess, to Sarah, which means mother of nations so as to match her glorious future (Gen. 17:15–16). When God changed a person's name and gave him a new name, it was usually to establish a new identity.

God changed the name of some of His disciples to match their assignments. James and John, the sons of Zebedee, were surnamed Boarneges, which means the sons of thunder. Simon was renamed Cephas, which means the stone. Peter was identified as an unstable character, but because of the commission given to him, he needed the stability of a stone to operate in that office. Apostle Paul was formerly known as Saul of Tarsus, but everything became new for him on his road to Damascus, including his name, so as to carry out his assignment effectively.

Isaiah 9:6 describes the power that is in the name of Jesus:

> For unto us a child is born, unto us a son is given: and the government shall be upon his shoulder: and his name shall be called Wonderful, Counsellor, The mighty God, The everlasting Father, The Prince of Peace.

The name of Jesus is full of wonders, the type that will destroy COVID-19 and every demonic hoard. He gave us all the authority to use His name (Mark 16:17–18).

Jesus declares in John 14:13, "Whatsoever ye ask in my name, that will I do." Nothing shall be impossible to those who know the power that is in the name of Jesus.

Acts 3:6 states, "Then Peter said, Silver and gold have I none; but such as I have give I thee: In the name of Jesus Christ of Nazareth rise up and walk." The name of Jesus Christ has counsels that will reveal to you the right path to follow in life and the wrong path to avoid. Counsel is an integral part of wisdom, and we all need wisdom to manifest as the sons of God.

The name of Jesus Christ releases might. We have the strength of God in the place of weakness, and confidence comes in the place of frustration. Furthermore, the name of Jesus Christ of Nazareth releases the supernatural power of God that launches us into the world of the supernatural. When the name of Jesus is invoked, it compels peace, which is the requirement for the supernatural to flow. Exodus 14:14 declares, "The Lord shall fight for you, and ye shall hold your peace."

The name of Jesus is the only authentic solution to the problem of sin. Acts 4:12 announces, "Neither is there salvation in any other: for there is none other name under heaven given among men, whereby we must be saved." Obedience earned for Jesus, the most exalted name in heaven, on earth, or under the earth.

Everything answers to that name—death, grace, every sin, poverty, failure, novel coronavirus or COVID-19, H1N1, HIV, bareness, poverty.

Owens Jarus detailed the twenty worst plagues and epidemics that have ravaged humanity throughout its existence, often changing the course of history and, at times, signaling the end of entire civilizations:[121] Spanish fever; Circa 3000 BC; Plague of Athens: 430 BC; Antonine Plague: AD 165–180; Plague of Cyprian: AD 250–271; Plague of Justinian: AD 541–542; The Black Death: 1346–1353; Cocoliztli epidemic: 1545–1548; American Plagues: sixteenth century; Great Plague of London: 1665–1666; Great Plague of Marseille: 1720–1723; Russian plague: 1770–1772; Philadelphia yellow fever epidemic: 1793; Flu pandemic: 1889–1890; American polio epidemic: 1916; Spanish Flu: 1918–1920; Asian Flu: 1957–1958; AIDS pandemic and epidemic: 1981–present day; H1N1 Swine Flu

---

[121] Owens Jarus, "20 Worst Epidemics and Pandemics in History," *Life Science, All About History*, 2020, Accessed May 26, 2020, https://www.livescience.com/worst-epidemics-and-pandemics-in-history.html.

pandemic: 2009–2010; West African Ebola epidemic: 2014–2016; Zika Virus epidemic: 2015–present day.

Whatever has a name is compelled to bow at the name of Jesus, which means at the mention of the name of Jesus Christ of Nazareth, all heavenly forces are set to ensure the purpose to which that name was mentioned in faith. All of these aforementioned names must bow to the name of Jesus Christ when we invoke that name in faith. For at the name of Jesus Christ of Nazareth, every force of opposition in all the realms of existence surrenders.

You can use the name to establish your victory over every challenge of COVID-19 or for a financial turnaround. You can use the name of Jesus Christ to restore peace in your life, marriage, and family. You can use the name of Jesus Christ to destroy every habitual life of sin and, therefore, manifest the nature and the character of Jesus Christ. The name of Jesus contains within itself the power and the authority to which every other situation and circumstances bow.

You can walk in total triumph in this life when you have faith in the name of Jesus Christ of Nazareth. Philippians 2:9–11, declares:

> Wherefore God also hath highly exalted him, and given him a name which is above every name: That at the name of Jesus every knee should bow, of things in heaven, and things in earth, and things under the earth; And that every tongue should confess that Jesus Christ is Lord, to the glory of God the Father.

Prayer: A Spiritual Weapon of Mass Destruction

There is a type of prayer that avails much, which provokes the release of signs and wonders. This means there are prayers that avail little or do not avail. The prayer that avails much releases tremendous earth-rending power, which is dynamic in its working.

James 5:17–18 declares:

> Elias was a man subject to like passions as we are, and he prayed earnestly that it might not rain: and it rained not on the earth by the space of three years and six months. And he prayed again, and the heaven gave rain, and the earth brought forth her fruit.

The amplified version of James 5:16 states:

> Therefore, confess your sins to one another [your false steps, your offenses], and pray for one another, that you may be healed and restored. The heartfelt and persistent prayer of a righteous man (believer) can accomplish much [when put into action and made effective by God—it is dynamic and can have tremendous power].

This kind of prayer releases spiritual weapon of mass destruction upon every invading power of hell, such as COVID-19. This is not a religious gibbering kind of prayer but a kind of prayer of faith that involves your heart, which will without doubt attract heaven's attention. James 5:15 proclaims, "And the prayer of faith shall save the sick, and the Lord shall raise him up; and if he has committed sins, they shall be forgiven him."

Hannah prayed a heartfelt prayer as she poured out her heart to the Lord, and that changed the trajectory of her destiny (1 Sam. 1:11–15, 19). Hezekiah prayed to the Lord, and his prayer caught heaven's attention. His prayer connects to the Throne of God, and the answer was dispatched without any hinderance (Isa. 38:1–6). Elijah, whose ministry was backed with profound signs and wonders, was a refence point for an effective and fervent prayer. The God that answers by fire shows up with miracles (1 Kings 18:36–37).

Jesus Christ, our Lord and Savior, raised Lazarus from the dead through a heartfelt prayer (John 11:41). It was not a cat and dog discussion but a deep-seated connection with the throne of heaven. Once you position your heart aright and you are praying according to God's will, which is His Word, you will never miss your target in prayer. This prayer is the prayer of faith, and hence, without faith, it is impossible to please God. The tears of the blind men did not move Jesus to act on their behalf (Matt. 9:27–29) but their faith. We all need the instrument of faith in prayers to work miracles.

We must understand that faith is a substance that is tangible and can be handled. It is not a figment of man's imagination nor a phycological state of mind. Faith is the cheapest way for our continuous victory, and it is also the ticket to the life of the miraculous. For every genuine child of God, faith has become your seal of authority in the battle of life.

First John 5:4 states, "For whatsoever is born of God overcometh the world: and this is the victory that overcometh the world, even our faith."

Holy Communion: A Spiritual Weapon of Mass Destruction

The Gospel of John 5:51–57 pronounces:

> I am the living bread which came down from heaven: if any man eat of this bread, he shall live forever: and the bread that I will give is my flesh, which I will give for the life of the world. The Jews therefore strove among themselves, saying, How can this man give us his flesh to eat? Then Jesus said unto them, Verily, verily, I say unto you, except ye eat the flesh of the Son of man, and drink his blood, ye have no life in you. Whoso eateth my flesh, and drinketh my blood, hath eternal life; and I will raise him up at the last day. For my flesh is meat indeed, and my blood is drink indeed. He that eateth my flesh,

and drinketh my blood, dwelleth in me, and I in him. As the living Father hath sent me, and I live by the Father: so he that eateth me, even he shall live by me.

The life of the flesh is in the blood of Jesus Christ, and you receive God's eternal life anytime you partake of the communion table. The very life of God, Zoe, is injected into your bodies, and you are in union with Jesus Christ, the head of the church. He is the vine (John 15:1, 5), and we are the branches, so that whatever flows in Jesus (the vine) begins to flow in us (the branch). When you partake of the communion (the flesh and the blood of Jesus), eternal life swallows up human life, which is susceptible to demonic oppressions. Jesus said in John 6:55, "For my flesh is meat indeed, and my blood is drink indeed."

This is like the rod of Moses in the hands of Aaron that turned to a snake and swallowed up the rod turned to snakes that belonged to Jannes and Jambres, the Egyptian magicians (Ex. 7:12). Whenever you partake of the Lord's table, death is swallowed up in victory. Sickness, disease, depression, and weakness is swallowed up by God's eternal life. It is a powerful spiritual weapon of destruction against every attack of the enemy, including all viruses and pandemics.

Isaiah 25:8 declares, "He (Jesus) will swallow up death in victory; and the Lord God will wipe away tears from off all faces; and the rebuke of his people shall he take away from off all the earth: for the Lord hath spoken it."

There is no medicine that can be compared with the flesh and blood of Jesus Christ. It has no side effect. It is your miracle meal for your sustenance here on this earth. It is a special meal to acquire strength for your life's journey here on earth. Jesus said in John 6:53, "Except ye eat the flesh of the Son of man, and drink his blood, ye have no life in you."

God had provided for Adam the tree of life in the Garden of Eden that will make them to live forever. If only they had eaten the tree of life, they would not have experienced sickness and disease. God never made provisions for man's healing at creation because He never intended that man should ever be sick. He only gave man what to eat. It was after man was corrupted and dethroned that Satan's wicked rule and oppression began. That was why God sent Jesus Christ, His only begotten Son, who in turn feeds us with His own flesh and blood to rejuvenate our bodily systems.

The communion table is a provision from the office of the heavenly Surgeon General Jesus Christ of Nazareth. He is the Great Physician, the Balm of Gilead. The very life of God is embedded in the communion. Acts 2:46 corroborates, "And they, continuing daily with one accord in the temple, and breaking bread from house to house, did eat their meat with gladness and singleness of heart."

You must have ultimate faith in the communion table as it contains everything you will ever need for our healing. It will make you live like Jesus lived here on earth. You become as strong as stone because Jesus is the one working out all things for you, and you will operate in the stature of the divine. John 6:57 states, "As the living Father hath sent me, and I live by the Father: so he that eateth me, even he shall live by me."

Nothing compares in value to the healing virtue that is found in the flesh and blood of Jesus. You become spiritually indestructible, and sickness will no longer overcome you or attack you. By continually partaking of the communion, you can no longer be humiliated or molested by sickness and disease. This is because the communion takes care of everything that weakens you and mocks your redemptive testimony. That does not mean we should ignore our medical providers, but it does mean only God can make the medicine work. Jeremiah 30:13, 46:11 declare:

> There is none to plead thy cause, that thou mayest be bound up: thou hast no healing medicines.
>
> Go up into Gilead, and take balm, O virgin, the daughter of Egypt: in vain shalt thou use many medicines; for thou shalt not be cured.

We take biblical initiatives of praying over our medicines before we use them, trusting the Lord to make it to work and not cause any side effect, for whatsoever is not of faith is sin (Rom. 14:23). Jesus said in John 6:48, 50, "I am that bread of life…which cometh down from heaven, that a man may eat thereof, and not die."

Jesus announces in 1 Corinthians 11:23–31 that as often as you observe this ordinance, you remember Him and not our past sins, limitations, or infirmities.

> For I have received of the Lord that which also I delivered unto you, that the Lord Jesus the same night in which he was betrayed took bread: And when he had given thanks, he brake it, and said, Take, eat: this is my body, which is broken for you: this do in remembrance of me. After the same manner also he took the cup, when he had supped, saying, this cup is the new testament in my blood: this do ye, as oft as ye drink it, in remembrance of me. For as often as ye eat this bread, and drink this cup, ye do shew the Lord's death till he come. Wherefore whosoever shall eat this bread, and drink this cup of the Lord, unworthily, shall be guilty of the body and blood of the Lord. But let a man examine himself, and so let him eat of that bread, and drink of that cup. For he that eateth and drinketh unworthily, eateth and drinketh damnation to himself, not discerning the Lord's body. For this cause many are weak and sickly among you, and many sleep. For if we would judge ourselves, we should not be judged.

Those who refuse to discern the Lord's body and blood as the source of eternal life; those who ignore and disregard it; those who eat it in sin; those who refuse to surrender their lives to Jesus Christ in sincerity and truth and then eat this miracle meal eat damnation instead of justification to themselves, and so it is very vital for you to examine yourself before eating it and be sure you are in a right relationship with the Lord. You must surrender your life to Jesus Christ and be in tune with Him rather than totally avoid the communion and continue to live in sin. It is wrong to walk out on Holy communion, just like Judas, and afterward, he hung himself on the tree just a few hours before Jesus's perfect hanging on the cross, taking away all of our sins and curses. We must learn to judge ourselves so we will not be judged (1 Cor. 11:31).

Remember that eternal life is free, church entrance is free, salvation is free, the love of God is free, heaven is free—provided you are genuinely saved—and the breath of God through His Word is free, and although all these cost Jesus Christ His very own life, men still have to choose to pay for the things that destroy us and that will ultimately lead us to hell. We always think of birthdays, Valentine's day, Father's Day, Mother's Day, Children's day, Labor Day, Memorial Day, Martin Luther King's Day, Teacher's Day, Christmas Day, Independence Day, Boxing Day, Easter Sunday, Saint Patrick's Day—but only few remember the Judgment Day. Is it going to be a day of celebration or condemnation for you?

The Bible adds in John 3:19–21:

> And this is the condemnation, that light is come into the world, and men loved darkness rather than light, because their deeds were evil. For everyone that doeth evil hateth the light, neither cometh to the light, lest his deeds should be reproved. But he that doeth truth cometh to the light, that his deeds may be made manifest, that they are wrought in God.

Choose eternal life that resides inside the communion as you make yourself right with God that you and yours may live during any pandemics or satanic attacks (Deut. 30:19). Do not forget that the Bible declares that for this reason, many are weak, sick, and many even die (1 Cor. 11:30). The children of Israel ate manna in the wilderness for their wilderness sustenance. The Bible declared in Psalms 105:37 that there was not one feeble person among them: "He brought them forth also with silver and gold: and there was not one feeble person among their tribes."

The communion infuses God's kind of life into your bloodstream, bones, marrow, mind, and spirit-man. As you take the communion, whatever is contrary to eternal life inside your system will be destroyed. This is an end-time mystery and the wisdom of the Almighty God for the triumph of the saints, the Church of Jesus Christ to survive in this demon-infested and wicked world. Observe the words and actions of Jesus Christ at the communion table from Matthew 26:26–28:

> And as they were eating, Jesus took bread, and blessed it, and brake it, and gave it to the disciples, and said, Take, eat; this is my body. And he took the cup, and gave thanks, and gave it to them, saying, Drink ye all of it. For this is my blood of the new testament, which is shed for many for the remission of sins.

Praise: A Turbocharged Spiritual Weapon of Mass Destruction

Praise is the most destructive spiritual weapon of mass destruction. It opens all doors for any captive held back by any force of darkness. Nothing in the power of hell can resist or intercept it. It has multiplication power, which ushers the skilled user into an unlimited realm of walking in the supernatural. Jesus gave thanks over five loaves and two fish, and it was multiplied to feed five thousand, and twelve baskets of the remnant were gathered (John 6:11–13). There's something powerful about praising God and thanking Him for fulfilling His promises in your life, even when you are still waiting to see them coming to pass (Ps. 65:1–2). It is like putting a turbocharger on your faith, and it pushes you forward more quickly into the place where, like Abraham, you are fully persuaded that what God has promised, He is able to perform (Rom. 4:16–21).

There is a fountain you connect to in thanksgiving and praise that ensures your continuous triumph over life's circumstances. The Bible declares in Psalms 67:5–7:

> Let the people praise thee, O God; let all the people praise thee. Then shall the earth yield her increase; and God, even our own God, shall bless us. God shall bless us; and all the ends of the earth shall fear him.

The power in praise is released as you praise God in and for whatever circumstances you find yourself in. First Thessalonians 5:18 states, "In everything give thanks: for this is the will of God in Christ Jesus concerning you."

Praise that is the will of God must first be done before you can obtain the promise of signs and wonders. Hebrews 10:35–36 admonishes, "Cast not away therefore your confidence, which hath great recompence of reward. For ye have need of patience, that, after ye have done the will of God, ye might receive the promise." No matter what is happening in your world, praise God, and you will obtain the promise.

Praise brought Lazarus out of the grave because God inhabited the praise of His people. Those who live a praiseful life are carriers of His presence. David declares in Psalm 22:3, "But thou art holy, O thou that inhabitest the praises of Israel."

It is time for us to bring God down into our situations and circumstances. Angels will always respond to our prayers, and they could be hindered as in the case of Daniel (Dan. 10:13, 20) or even made dumb as in the case of Zacharias (Luke 1:19–20), but when we praise, God comes down by Himself as in the case of Paul and Silas (Acts 16:25–29).

When Peter was in jail, prayer was made for him without ceasing, and God sent an angel (Acts 12:7). The angel of the Lord opened the prison doors of the apostles as well in Acts 5:19.

When the children of Israel came out of Egypt, God was their sanctuary. The sea saw them and fled, Jordan was driven back, and the mountains skipped like rams, the little hills like young lambs. It was God's presence through praise that took them through and gave them victory over their enemies.

Exodus 15:1, 20, and 21 declare:

> Then sang Moses and the children of Israel this song unto the Lord, and spake, saying, I will sing unto the Lord, for he hath triumphed gloriously: the horse and his rider hath he thrown into the sea.
>
> And Miriam the prophetess, the sister of Aaron, took a timbrel in her hand; and all the women went out after her with timbrels and with dances. And Miriam answered them, Sing ye to the Lord, for he hath triumphed gloriously; the horse and his rider hath he thrown into the sea.

Praise will give us ultimate victory over all enemies. As for Paul and Silas, it was written that all the prison doors were opened when God stepped in through an earthquake, and everyone's chains fell off (Acts 16:26).

In 2 Chronicles 20, King Jehoshaphat stepped back and allowed God to go ahead of him in battle. They began to sing praises in the middle of their own coronavirus, so to speak, and God took their place in battle. He became their spiritual vaccine again their destroyer. Praise will always compel our God to take over our battles. It is a covenant technique.

After all, Jesus turned water into wine (John 2:6–19) as the one who is ever greater than all chemists. He was born without normal conception to prove that He is greater than the biologist and gynecologist (Isa. 7:14; Luke 1:26–37). As greater than all physicists, He walked on water that He made to beat down the law of buoyancy (Matt. 14:29). He disapproved the law of gravity when He ascended into heaven (Mark 16:19). As greater than all economists, He disapproved the law of diminishing return by feeding five thousand two fish and five loaves of bread and another four thousand with seven loaves and few fish (Matt. 14:19, 15:29–39; John 6:13). As the only physician who heals all, He cured the sick and the blind without administering a single dose of medication with side effect (Matt. 15:30; Mark 1:34).

His story is the greatest history ever, and so He is the beginning and the end (John 1:1–5; Rev. 22:13, 21:6). As the leader of the universe and governor of all the nations of the earth, He is called Wonderful, Counselor, the Mighty God, Everlasting Father, the Prince of Peace, and the government shall be upon His shoulders (Isa. 9:6–7). To have a relationship with God, our Father, He is the only way to the Father who declares that no one can come to the Father except through Him (John 14:4–6).

He is the Greatest Man in History that matters. Jesus had no servant, and yet they called Him Master. He had no degree, and yet they called Him Teacher. He had no medicine, yet they called Him Healer and physician. He had no army, yet kings feared Him. He won no military battles, yet He conquered the whole world and has made us more than conqueror and has the universe under His control. He committed no crime, yet they crucified Him. He was buried in a tomb, yet He lives forevermore.

You do not have to be strong to succeed; just be obedient to praising God and start using this spiritual weapon of mass destruction that works any day and anywhere in any given situation and circumstance. There is no mountain that God's presence that comes down through praise cannot fix. There is no body of water—may it be the Red Sea, River Jordan, River Euphrates—that He cannot dry to make a way for you. Praise is our ultimate access to His presence. When God steps down, no demon can stop Him or stand in His way. No COVID-19 can resist our God.

Praise pleases God and gives no room for murmuring or complaining that complicates matters (Num. 11:1). Being thankless is one of the hallmarks of the last days (2 Tim. 3:2). That you have breath, you are to praise the Lord. Not that you have money or houses or vehicles but inasmuch as you have the breath of life in your lungs, you are to praise the Lord (Ps. 150:6). Gratitude will cause God's presence to cocoon you. You will be living in the bubble of His shekinah glory. You will be living a life of the miraculous.

Praise always pleases God, and when God is pleased, He will release into your life everything that pleases you from His Word. Praise makes the supernatural to become natural in your life. Every obstacle will give way for anyone that lives a life of praise. It's a mighty spiritual weapon of mass destruction against COVID-19 or any other force of wickedness in your life.

David, the sweet Psalmist of Israel, the man of war that never lost a battle, who slayed the lion, bear, and Goliath, who sought for the presence of God by bringing the Ark of God to Jerusalem and pitching a tent for it, who praised the Lord with and, in the dance (Ps. 149:3, 150:4), declared in Psalms 34:1–3, 69:30–31:

> I will bless the Lord at all times: his praise shall continually be in my mouth. My soul shall make her boast in the Lord: the humble shall hear thereof and be glad. O magnify the Lord with me and let us exalt his name together.
>
> I will praise the name of God with a song and will magnify him with thanksgiving. This also shall please the Lord better than an ox or bullock that hath horns and hoofs.

Would you begin to act like David who was girded with linen ephod but danced before the Lord with all his might, regardless of what was going on around him (2 Sam. 6:14)? Your victory and ultimate triumph are guaranteed over every opposition of life, including COVID-19 as you use this spiritual weapon of mass destruction that no enemy in heaven on earth and under the earth can withstand.

Praise is a potent weapon in spiritual warfare. It brings you into the hurt-free zone of life because the Almighty takes over the battle, making you a relaxed overcomer. It's time to get your musical instruments and tambourine to begin to praise our God. Psalm 149:3–4 states, "Let them praise his name in the dance: let them sing praises unto him with the timbrel and harp. For the LORD taketh pleasure in his people: he will beautify the meek with salvation."

David did not care about what people would say whenever he danced before the Lord, his God, and every enemy mocking him was terribly judged (2 Sam. 6:14, 20–23). When you use praise for warfare, it is more than being emotionally carried away but bringing down the enemy citadel and confidence through praise.

Psalm 68:1–4 indicates:

> Let God arise, let his enemies be scattered: let them also that hate him flee before him. As smoke is driven away, so drive them away: as wax melteth before the fire, so let the wicked perish at the presence of God. But let the righteous be glad; let them rejoice before God: yea, let them exceedingly rejoice. Sing unto God, sing praises to his name: extol him that rideth upon the heavens by his name Jah, and rejoice before him.

Praise is a God-given weapon for humiliating our adversary. None of your enemies can escape God's judgment. It is safe when you enter the realms of high hosanna praises. The higher your praises, the stronger His presence, and the more fearful will His acts in your midst be. The story of Matthew 21:8–16 denotes that when we praise God, He will invade our temple, which is our body (2 Cor. 6:16) and drive out whatever sickness or disease that might be buying or selling:

> And a very great multitude spread their garments in the way; others cut down branches from the trees, and strawed them in the way. And the multitudes that went before, and that followed, cried, saying, Hosanna to the son of David: Blessed is he that cometh in the name of the Lord; Hosanna in the highest. And when he was come into Jerusalem, all the city was moved,

> saying, Who is this? And the multitude said, This is Jesus the prophet of Nazareth of Galilee. And Jesus went into the temple of God, and cast out all them that sold and bought in the temple, and overthrew the tables of the moneychangers, and the seats of them that sold doves. And said unto them, It is written, My house shall be called the house of prayer; but ye have made it a den of thieves. And the blind and the lame came to him in the temple; and he healed them. And when the chief priests and scribes saw the wonderful things that he did, and the children crying in the temple, and saying, Hosanna to the son of David; they were sore displeased, And said unto him, Hearest thou what these say? And Jesus saith unto them, Yea; have ye never read, Out of the mouth of babes and sucklings thou hast perfected praise?

You have to turn the presence of God loose on your behalf with your high hosanna praise. Engage in target praise warfare. Perhaps there is an issue in your life that seems to have resisted prayer and disregarded fasting; it has no choice but to bow to praise. Every wall of Jericho will come crashing down as you engage praise in battle. Joshua 6:20 states:

> So the people shouted when the priests blew with the trumpets: and it came to pass, when the people heard the sound of the trumpet, and the people shouted with a great shout, that the wall fell down flat, so that the people went up into the city, every man straight before him, and they took the city.

The only thing that will refuse to bow to God will be the only thing that will refuse to bow to the power of sincere high hosanna praise, and nothing can dare God, whether visible or invisible, created or not yet created. This is because praise provokes divine presence, which in turn delivers the fearful acts of God in your life. Let somebody make a joyful noise unto the *Lord* (Ps. 100:1).

Rebuking COVID-19 Contrary Winds: A Spiritual Weapon of Mass Destruction

Storms are customary in the lives of every redeemed child of God, and the earlier we embrace this truth, the better. Storms of life are part and parcel of our redemptive package. You don't need to commit sin to experience life's troubles. Remember, Jesus never sinned, yet the storms attempted to destroy Him. The storms of life have access to anyone. The Scriptures allude in James 1:2–4:

> My brethren, count it all joy when ye fall into divers temptations. Knowing this, that the trying of your faith worketh patience. But let patience have her perfect work, that ye may be perfect and entire, wanting nothing.

The storms of life raged against Jesus's ship, and on other occasions, He faced diverse trials and temptations. If the storms attempted Jesus, who then will they not attempt? If Jesus had to face storms, what makes you think you will not face the storms of life? You cannot get to the next grade in school without examination. Before God can ever place you in any position, He will first prove you to determine what stuff you are made of. Just as no student is ever promoted in school without first sitting for and passing examinations, likewise, no child of God ever moves forward without facing challenges.

Like the children of Israel, there will be the Egyptian taskmasters to contend with, apart from the divinely arranged Red Sea, the Jordan River, and the walls of Jericho on your way to your Canaan. Though Joseph knew he was going to be king, he still had to pass through slavery and imprisonment to arrive at the top. We must understand that these storms are not designed to destroy or overwhelm us, but they are there to promote us. The storms are not meant to tear you apart but to enthrone you.

Most of all, thanks be to God that every storm has an answer. No change is intractable, and there are several ways of solving every problem, if only you will maintain the right stance. It is what we see exemplified in the life of Jesus in Mark 4:38. The storm was raging vehemently against the ship Jesus was in, causing it to be filled with water and begin to sink. But in the midst of this contrary situation, Jesus was asleep on a pillow in the hinter part of the ship. Jesus was asleep on a pillow in the midst of a very tempestuous storm. That speaks of perfect rest, and it is a demonstration of unadulterated faith.

Mark 4:39 states, "And he arose, and rebuked the wind, and said unto the sea, Peace, be still. And the wind ceased, and there was a great calm."

You can challenge every storm of your life. It is time to rebuke that contrary wind blowing around you. There is no storm that does not have ears and a mind to understand and recognize the authority behind the voice that is speaking by the Word of God. Observe from the scripture above that Jesus did not rebuke the devil here. He basically challenged the storm. He spoke directly to the root cause of the problem, and it obeyed, because storms are not hard of hearing. Business failure is not deaf; barrenness has ears to hear; COVID-19 and its second wave also has ears, and so does every storm of life, including all forms of influenza. It is time to rebuke every wind that is contrary to God's will for your life.

Jesus did not stop at rebuking the wind; He also declared the peace of God and the peace that He is. He is the prince of peace, and there could not be anything contrary to peace around Him. We are to address the contrary issues, situations, and circumstances of our lives, such as the novel coronavirus that has eaten deep into the lives of several people and nations. The power of life and death is in your tongue (Prov. 18:21). It's time to address that embarrassing situation right now. Declare whatever you desire that is in line with the Word of God. It is time to challenge your challenges. The storms you cannot address will not submit to you. Look at every storm and say, "You are too small to overcome me, because the Greater One lives in me."

You have the same authority as Jesus because He said greater works than these shall we do also (John 14:12). Therefore, arise like Jesus did and wield your scepter of authority by rebuking the winds and speaking peace to the turbulence around you.

Anastasis:
Resurrecting into Jesus Christ

According to *Strong's Concordance NT* (386), the word *anastasis* is defined as a standing up, a raising up, or rising. It is used in resurrection or a rising again. Christ's physical resurrection is the foundation of Christianity, which also guarantees the future resurrection of all believers (John 6:39, 40, 44).

Anastasis refers to the physical bodily resurrection of Christ and people (both of the redeemed and the unredeemed). In the Gospel of John 11:25, the Lord Jesus, in effect, said, "I AM presently the resurrection and the life;" not "I am going to be and he that believe in me, though he were dead, yet shall he live" (John 11:25). Paul substantiated in 1 Corinthians 15, 12–13, 19:

> Now if Christ be preached that he rose from the dead, how say some among you that there is no resurrection of the dead? But if there be no resurrection of the dead, then is Christ not risen.
> If in this life only we have hope in Christ, we are of all men most miserable.

Martha did not believe that the resurrection power of the Lord Jesus could be made manifest before the last day when she said in John 11:24, regarding her dead brother, Lazarus, "Martha saith unto him, I know that he shall rise again in the resurrection at the last day." It is amazing to see that the Lord Jesus called Himself the resurrection before He was resurrected in faith, calling the things which be not as though they are (Rom. 4.17). This is the same thing He said to Moses at the burning bush, "I AM THAT I AM" (Ex. 3.14). Just as the "I AM" is the light of the world, the bread of life, the vine, the way, the truth, the life, the good shepherd, and many other things, so also is He "the resurrection and the life."

The resurrection power that can raise the dead is available in Christ *now* and not just on the resurrection day in the future. However, this does not mean we can be resurrected and glorified now, but it does mean a pre-glorification resurrection experience is available *now* in this life before the grand event of the resurrection and glorification of our physical bodies.

Paul confirms this in Philippians 3:10–11 from the Amplified Version of the Bible:

> [For my determined purpose is] that I may know Him [that I may progressively become more deeply and intimately acquainted with Him, perceiving and recognizing and understanding the wonders of His Person more strongly and more clearly], and that I may in that same way come to know the power outflowing from His resurrection [which it exerts over believers], and that I may so share His sufferings as to be continually transformed [in spirit into His likeness even] to His death, [in the hope] that if possible I may attain to the [spiritual and moral] resurrection [that lifts me] out from among the dead [even while in the body].

He also mentioned this in 2 Corinthians 4:10–11, 5:4:

> Always bearing about in the body the dying of the Lord Jesus hat the life also of Jesus might be made manifest in our body. For we which live

are always delivered unto death for Jesus's sake, that the life also of Jesus might be made manifest in our mortal flesh.

For we that are in this tabernacle do groan, being burdened: not for that we would be unclothed, but clothed upon, that mortality might be swallowed up of life.

The news of death during the COVID-19 pandemic is everywhere. Surprisingly, many people now know COVID-19 or coronavirus more than Jesus Christ because of the fangs of death attach to it. However, God has a plan that resides in his resurrection and life.

Yan, et al., reported that the victims of coronavirus have represented some of the best of humanity. From an ER doctor who risked his life trying to save others to a grandmother and refugee who worked tirelessly to provide a better life for her children. Even as the number of deaths reach such a grim milestone, Americans are at odds over whether it's necessary to keep taking protective measures, including wearing a face-covering.[122]

The Associated Press (AP) described Washington in the fraught freighted number of American moments, which is a round one brimming with zeroes—100,000—a hundred thousand. A thousand hundred. Five thousand score. More than eight thousand dozen all are dead in the last week of May 2020 when America's official coronavirus death toll reaches six digits. One hundred thousand lives wiped out by a disease unknown to science a half a year ago.

According to *AP*, the numerous comparisons for this staggering numbers are places like the beaver stadium, seen often on the television as the home to Penn State football and one of the country's largest sports venues that could hold about 106,572 people when full. Also, the 2018 estimated population of South Bend, Indiana,

---

[122] Yan, et al., "Coronavirus Has Killed More than 100,000 People Across the US," *CNN Health*, Accessed May 28, 2020, https://www.cnn.com/2020/05/27/health/us-coronavirus-wednesday/index.html.

was 101,860, and about 100,000 people visit the Statue of Liberty every ten days.

The report also stated that gun violence killed more than 37,000 people a year on average between 2014 and 2018 in the United States, and 9/11 took exactly 2,996 lives, a figure that the US coronavirus tally passed in early April, and adding to the complexity is how different coronavirus deaths are from a mass shooting or a cataclysmic natural disaster to 9/11. Unlike all of these, the COVID-19 saga unfolds gradually over time, growing steadily more severe, and resists the time-tested American appetite for loud and immediate storylines. Furthermore, *AP* stated that in the fourteenth century, the Black Death ravaged humanity, taking many millions, although no one knows exactly how many died, but today, when the dead are counted, some coherence is reached, and the thinking is that if the virus cannot be stopped, at least it can be quantified by human effort that is far more palatable than a society where we cannot establish who is no longer among us.[123]

Rhys Blakely authors that virus hunters had spent five years tracking down their quarry, a colony of horseshoe bats teeming with an ominous collection of coronavirus strains. He enumerated that in a single cave in the Chinese province of Yunnan, a team of researchers had found inside these small mammals all the genetic building blocks of SARS, which is a virus closely related to COVID-19 that killed nearly eight-hundred people in 2003 while causing economic mayhem across Asia.

Blakely stressed that the researchers had warned that all the elements were in place as they presented their findings two years ago for a new SARS-like disease to skip again from animals to humans. And as the world reels from the worst pandemic in a century, scientists are calling for new systems that react to these kinds of warnings and have

---

[123] COVID-19 Pandemic VOA News, "American Virus Deaths at 100,000: What Does a Number Mean?" *The Associated Press*, 2020, Accessed May 28, 2020, https://www.voanews.com/covid-19-pandemic/american-virus-deaths-100000-what-does-number-mean.

investigated that we need new tools to track the emergence of exotic new pathogens and a battery of new antiviral drugs to treat them.

He cited Vincent Racaniello who believe that we need to gather better intelligence on our formidable microbial foes. He states, "The first thing people need to understand is that every virus that you can think of that infects people, polio, measles, herpes, chickenpox, they all came from animals," and he might also have added influenza, Ebola, and HIV/AIDS. He supported the creation of a new global atlas of zoonotic pathogens, a catalogue of the bugs that exist in other species that have the potential to spill over into the human population, and he also purports that researchers would use it, in part, to develop "plug and play" vaccine technologies that could rapidly be modified to counter new threats. He stated that bats are an obvious starting point because they are abundant, accounting for a fifth of all mammals. They thrive across a vast range of habitats; individuals often cover large distances, and they harbor an extraordinary range of viruses.

Additionally, he substantiated that the pandemic preparedness and vaccine research center, a collaboration with the drugmaker, AstraZeneca, aims to become a global sentry. It will evaluate techniques for screening blood transfusions around the world to search for the genetic signatures of ominous novel pathogens, and it will seek to galvanize research into antiviral treatments and diagnostics. Furthermore, Blakely noted that it also plans to monitor for signs of unusual illnesses across Africa, Asia, and the Indian subcontinent, and it will look at tracking zoonoses, diseases that can be transmitted to humans from animals. SARS and COVID-19 are thought to have leapt from bats to humans via intermediary "amplifier" species.

Moreover, he elucidated that mice also carry the dangerous hantaviruses; dromedary camels harbor MERS, another coronavirus that kills a third of the humans it infects; HIV/AIDS, which has killed thirty-two million people since 1981, came from chimpanzees; and the growing human population will still brush up against more novel microbes as we clear wild areas.

Blakely cited Racaniello who claimed that there are millions and millions of dogs in China who might be the next source of influenza pandemic, and he added that influenzas are particularly tricky customers, largely because of how two entirely separate strains can swap genetic material if they cross paths in a single host. He explained that once in the lungs of a mammal, an avian strain can "reassort" or mix genes with any human influenza viruses that are also present, which can ultimately lead to an entirely new viral strain, capable of sustained human-to-human transmission, and if this virus has not circulated before, the entire global population will be susceptible.

Racaniello advocated that a dog would be infected with two different influenza viruses, one human and another from the feces of a bird makes a new virus, which then makes the jump to the pet's owners, and it takes off. Additionally, he clarified that the cataloguing of animal viruses is to build weapons against them, and one focus could be on so-called pan-viral treatments, medicines that have the potential to be effective against a range of pathogens. He also stressed that the main obstacle to the development of an effective coronavirus treatment has been a lack of funds and that investment is instead skewed toward treatments for chronic diseases such as diabetes, which tend to be taken daily and for a lifetime.

Blakely confirmed that the contours of the post-lockdown world are unknown, but scientific consensus is rock-solid on one point: COVID-19 will not be the last virus to sweep the planet because over the past three hundred years, there have been ten influenza pandemics and avian flu outbreaks that have bubbled away, and just as we have now seen three coronaviruses in three successive decades—SARS in 2003, MERS in 2012, and COVID-19 in 2019—bigger cities, global travel, intensive animal farming, and a rising human population will have to increase vulnerability.

Blakely declared in the words of the science writer David Quammen the label "zoonosis," the term for an animal infection transmissible to humans, is already "a word of the future, destined for heavy use in the twenty-first century."[124]

---

[124] Rhys Blakely, "After COVID-19, How We Can Prepare for a New Pandemic. Better Monitoring and More Investment in Drugs Could Prevent Another Global Disaster" The TIMES (2020) https://www.thetimes.co.uk/edition/news/after-covid-19-how-we-can-prepare-for-a-new-pandemic-zg8pdfkm7 (accessed May 13, 2020).

Kim Hjelmgaard cited Fadela Chaib, the WHO spokesman who indicated that coronavirus came from an animal and not manipulated or produced in a laboratory as alleged. Chaib clarifies, "It is probable, likely, that the virus is of animal origin." This is contrary to the theory that suggests the virus could be man-made and linked to a Chinese biowarfare program or that the virus is naturally occurring from a bat but accidentally escaped the Wuhan Institute of Virology research facility in China due to poor safety protocols. This research facility has been historically studying coronaviruses in bats, and it's in proximity to where some of the infections were first diagnosed, and China reported a lax safety record in its labs. She explained that there still remained some outstanding questions over how precisely the coronavirus jumped the species barrier to humans, noting that an intermediate animal host could be the most likely explanation. She added that coronavirus, which causes the disease COVID-19, most probably has its ecological reservoir in bats.[125]

Anastasis: God's Eternal Life Reservoir

Consider the reservoir of life that was in men that lived before the flood that destroyed the world of Noah but at the same time lifted up the ark of Noah.

The Bible accounts in Genesis 5:4, 11, 14, 17, 20, 21–24, 27:

> And all the days of Seth were nine hundred and twelve years: and he died.
> And all the days of Enos were nine hundred and five years: and he died.
> And all the days of Cainan were nine hundred and ten years: and he died.

---

[125] Kim Hjelmgaard, "WHO Says Coronavirus Came from an Animal and Was Not Made in a Lab" *USA TODAY* (2020), https://www.usatoday.com/story/news/world/2020/04/21/coronavirus-who-says-evidence-shows-covid-19-not-made-lab/2995236001/ (Accessed April 22, 2020).

And all the days of Mahalaleel were eight hundred ninety and five years: and he died.

And all the days of Jared were nine hundred sixty and two years: and he died.

And Enoch lived sixty and five years, and begat Methuselah. And Enoch walked with God after he begat Methuselah three hundred years, and begat sons and daughters. And all the days of Enoch were three hundred sixty and five years. And Enoch walked with God: and he was not; for God took him.

And all the days of Methuselah were nine hundred sixty and nine years: and he died.

Only the great-great-grandson of Adam Mahalalel lived 895 years and died a little younger than the others. Also, Enoch walked with God and was taken up by God after living for 365 years. All of these people lived almost a millennium, which is like living from 1020 to 2020. The reservoir of the life of God in these people kept them going and granted them longevity. They subdued every agent of deaths, including viruses and plagues, and fulfilled their days. The scripture buttresses in Romans 6:23, "For the wages of sin is death; but the gift of God is eternal life through Jesus Christ our Lord." Sin brought death to humanity, including the COVID-19 invasion, but the gift of God is eternal life.

It is time to receive and embrace this gift of God which is eternal life. The life span limit in Psalm 90 is not referring to the New Testament saint. The only people that the seventy- or eighty-year limit was given to were the rebellious wilderness-wandering Israelites who refused to go into the promised land, and God set that limit because the Word has gone out of His mouth in Numbers 14:22–23.

In this regard, God's people must reset their expectations of lifetimes to be the original intention of God which was one hundred and twenty years. You must not allow that which is not from the beginning. Genesis 6:3 declares, "And the Lord said, 'My spirit shall not always strive with man, for that he also is flesh: yet his days shall be an hundred and twenty years.'"

Jesus declares in Matthew 19:8, "He saith unto them, Moses because of the hardness of your hearts suffered you to put away your wives: but from the beginning it was not so."

This is the reason why you should adjust your sight and choose that which is from the beginning, which is at least one hundred and twenty years. This is not living in a nursing home weak, fragile, sick, and senescing but living life to the fullest for one hundred and twenty years. Moses made it so to that age with full vitality intact. This is attainable by faith.

Matthew 16:26 and Mark 9:23 state, "But Jesus beheld them, and said unto them, with men this is impossible; but with God all things are possible... Jesus said unto him, If thou canst believe, all things are possible to him that believeth."

It's time to turn to God's Word. It's time to stop watching as the world turns. The scriptures alluded in Romans 8:11, "If the spirit of him that raised up Jesus from the dead dwells in you, he that raised up Christ from the dead shall also quicken your mortal bodies by his sprit that dwelleth on you." This means the Spirit of God that dwells in you will "restore vigor," "stimulate to revive" or "restore life to" or "become more active."

Jesus notifies us that the event of His Second Coming will be like the events that surrounded the days of Noah. Jesus states in Matthew 24:37, 39, "But as the days of Noah were, so shall also the coming of the Son of man be... And knew not until the flood came, and took them all away; so shall also the coming of the Son of man be." This means if the Lord turns the life span of men to be one hundred and twenty as He did in the days of Noah, similarly, the provision has been made in our days, just like it was in Noah's days. Our merciful God will not send the flood to the earth until the last possible moment. He waited until there was only one God-fearing family left on the earth that He could depend on. He postponed judgment until just one man, Noah, stood between the annihilation of the human race and future generations.

Just like in the days of Noah, the only safe place against the flood of pandemics and all other sicknesses and disease on this planet is in the ark, and God made sure Noah and his family were in it. Noah satisfactorily died at the age of nine hundred and fifty years (Gen. 9:28–29), and men still lived past the age of one hundred and twenty after Noah's flood.

The Bible accounted in Genesis 11:10–15:

> These are the generations of Shem: Shem was a hundred years old, and begat Arphaxad two years after the flood. And Shem lived after he begat Arphaxad five hundred years, and begat sons and daughters. And Arphaxad lived five and thirty years, and begat Salah. And Arphaxad lived after he begat Salah four hundred and three years, and begat sons and daughters. And Salah lived thirty years, and begat Eber. And Salah lived after he begat Eber four hundred and three years, and begat sons and daughters.

From that time, the faith of God's people for longevity had started to dwindle through infiltration of fear in addition to the deteriorative conditions on the earth after the flood, which was not the same as it was before the flood. However, we are to occupy all spares by the profession of our faith of life until Jesus comes (Luke 19:13). We are to dethrone the prince of the powers of the air by meeting Jesus Christ in the air through the Word of God that is resident in our hearts and comes out of our mouths. Numbers 14:28 declares, "Say unto them, as truly as I live, saith the Lord, as ye have spoken in mine ears, so will I do to you."

And Ephesians 2:2 affirms, "Wherein in time past ye walked according to the course of this world, according to the prince of the power of the air, the spirit that now worketh in the children of disobedience."

It is time to meet the Lord in the air every day and not only to wait until the day of rapture. You cannot meet the Lord in the air and meet with the prince of the power of the air at the same time. This spirit cannot work in the children of obedience. It only works in the children of disobedience. First Thessalonians 4:17 states, "Then we which are alive and remain shall be caught up together with them in the clouds, to meet the Lord in the air: and so shall we ever be with the Lord."

Choosing Jesus is key to walking in God's wisdom. The wisdom of God which can only be accessible by believing and doing the Word of God that will cancel every appointment with death because it's impossible for any of us to obey God's Word without the Holy Spirit. We might desire to obey it, but we cannot do so in the energy of the flesh. Romans 7:18–20 describes the dilemma this way:

> For I know that in me (that is, in my flesh,) dwelleth no good thing: for to will is present with me; but how to perform that which is good I find not. For the good that I would I do not: but the evil which I would not, that I do. Now if I do that I would not, it is no more I that do it, but sin that dwelleth in me.

Adam and Eve would have lived forever if they had eaten of the tree of life. As believers, we can eat of that tree every day by spending time in the Word of God. Jesus revealed to Simeon by the Holy Spirit that he would not see death until he held Jesus in the flesh in his arms (Luke 2:26). He cancelled every generational appointment with death until he held Jesus in his arms. There is a generation that will repeat the same. They will not see death until they see Jesus step down from eternity to the earth and be caught up to meet him in the air. Luke 2:26 declares, "And it was revealed unto him by the Holy Ghost, that he should not see death, before he had seen the Lord's Christ."

Jesus affirms in Luke 9:27 that some will not see death until they see the kingdom of God which was enacted on the day of Pentecost. Jesus Christ by His Word cancels their appointment with death: "But I tell you of a truth, there be some standing here, which shall not taste of death, till they see the kingdom of God."

The Lord Jesus Christ said to Peter in John 21:21–24 that what if he desires that John, the Apostle whom the Lord loves did not see death? Jesus never said He would not see death, but what if He did not want him to see death? And that word alone everyone began to proclaim in conjunction with the love of God in the heart of John and made him the only apostle who historians say died naturally and peacefully.[126]

John 21:21–24 declares:

> Peter seeing him saith to Jesus, Lord, and what shall this man do? Jesus saith unto him, If I will that he tarry till I come, what is that to thee? follow thou me. Then went this saying abroad among the brethren, that that disciple should not die: yet Jesus said not unto him, He shall not die; but, If I will that he tarry till I come, what is that to thee? This is the disciple which testifieth of these things and wrote these things: and we know that his testimony is true.

The Word of God in Psalms 91:16 will manifest in our lives for as long as we dwell in the secret place of the Most High, observing God's covenant, and we will abide under the shadow of the Almighty. The Word declares, "With long life will I satisfy him, and shew him my salvation."

The low level of purity both in motive and actions in the church today is a result of a lack of a continuous increasing revelation of the resurrection of Christ and how it benefits us now and in eternity. Apostle John declares in 1 John 3:2–3:

> Beloved, now are we the sons of God, and it doth not yet appear what we shall be: but we

---

[126] "Ephesus! History, Information, and Pictures of Ephesus Ancient City, St John in Ephesus," Accessed June 1, 2020, https://www.ephesus.us/ephesus/st_john_in_ephesus.htm.

know that, when he shall appear, we shall be like
him; for we shall see him as he is. And every man
that hath this hope in him purifieth himself, even
as he is pure.

Furthermore, we must determine to increase in our personal
revelation of the resurrection so as to bear witness of the reality and
power thereof both in miracles and godly conduct and so live above
the fear and sting of death (1 Cor. 15:55; Heb. 2:14,15),

The resurrection of Christ signifies to us the ultimate triumph
of good over evil, righteousness over sin, light over darkness, wisdom
over ignorance, healing over sickness, and prosperity over poverty.
The resurrection of Christ gives us the hope that we will ultimately
be victorious in our Christian lives, no matter the present difficulties
or problems we may be currently facing.

By revelation of and faith in the "now" resurrection of Jesus
Christ, we can overcome every attack of Satan, the adversary, and
cancel every appointment with death (John 16:33).

We do not have to wait until the final resurrection when we
receive an eternal glorified body to experience the resurrection power
of the Lord Jesus Christ. We can receive a measure of it in this life in
our present physical bodies. Paul declares in 2 Corinthians 4:10–11:

Always bearing about in the body the dying
of the Lord Jesus, that the life also of Jesus might
be made manifest in our body. For we which live
are always delivered unto death for Jesus's sake,
that the life also of Jesus might be made manifest
in our mortal flesh.

This power of His resurrection is firstly manifested in our physical bodies to dominate the sin nature, making it possible to live a
pure and holy life in which our physical bodies have been exercised
or trained to love righteousness and hate sin (Ps. 45:7; Heb. 1:9,
5:14). This resurrection power is manifested in the life of Peter and
Paul, even when people were healed, delivered, and even raised from

the dead after making physical contact with their bodies or clothes (Mark 5:27–30; Matt. 14:36; Acts 19:11–12, 20:10–11).

Sometime ago, the world was in chaos because of Napoleon Bonaparte who almost conquered the world. Everything fell before him. At Waterloo in Belgium, he suffered defeat at the hands of the Duke of Wellington, bringing an end to the Napoleonic era of European history. The British feared that soon their homeland would be invaded by the troops of France. In one last effort to stop the tremendous rush of Napoleon's army, they sent their greatest general. General Wellington invaded the heartland of Europe. The people waited as the forces were joined at Waterloo. Eagerly, they followed the watchman on the tower of Winchester Cathedral as he looked out over the English Channel in the fog, waiting for some sign of a ship to bring them news of the outcome.

The hope of England rested on that report. Finally, as the fog lifted just a little bit, the watchman saw a ship blinking the signal of what had happened. The letters were taken down, Wellington defeated. The fog sank, and with it all the hope of England. The people quivered at the thought that soon they would hear the tramp of French troops upon their land. However, an hour or so later, the fog lifted, and again, the message was sent forth: "Wellington defeated enemy!"

A wild shout of glee went out all over England; that feared invasion never came. The British army, which included Belgian, Dutch, and German troops, was commanded by Arthur Wellesley, Duke of Wellington, who had gained prominence fighting against the French during the Peninsular War.

In a critical blunder, Napoleon waited until midday to give the command to attack in order to let the waterlogged ground dry after the previous night's rainstorm. The delay gave Blucher's remaining troops—who by some accounts numbered more than thirty thousand—time to march to Waterloo and join the battle later that day.

Although Napoleon's troops mounted a strong attack against the British, the arrival of the Prussians turned the tide against the French. The French emperor's outnumbered army retreated in chaos. By some estimates, the French suffered more than thirty-three thousand casualties (including dead, wounded, or taken prisoner), while

British and Prussian casualties numbered more than twenty-two thousand.

Ultimately, the Battle of Waterloo marked the end of Napoleon's storied military career. He reportedly rode away from the battle in tears.[127]

There is a great hero whose name is Jesus. On a hill outside the city wall of Jerusalem, He went forth to take on the combined forces of death, hell, and Satan. And on the third day, as the sun began to break over that lonely sepulcher, a new light came with a dazzling radiance. The huge stone that blocked the door began to move back as if by some unseen hand. Those Roman troops were startled by the appearance of the messengers resplendent in white. Then, out of the darkness of that tomb, out of the very pit of hell itself, there stepped forth one who was dead and could now say, "I am He that was dead and, behold, I am alive forevermore and have the keys of death and of hell!" Word went out through all of Jerusalem.

Jesus has the keys. He proved that He has the keys of both death and hell, for He unlocked both and arose victorious. Death could not hold its prey. Hell could not hold its prey. God made all of us His resurrection and the life, giving us power to cancel every appointment with death. Oh, death, where is your sting? Oh grave, where is your victory? Oh, gates of hell, you shall not prevail, for the Redeemer of Israel and the Savior of the world holds in His triumphant hand the keys. Revelations 1:8 declares, "I am he that liveth, and was dead; and, behold, I am alive for evermore, amen; and have the keys of hell and of death."

At one time, He was dead, but now the grave is empty, and He is alive. He is the living God forever and ever. And this ever living one has the keys, and He lives in us. John 14:19 states, "Yet a little while, and the world seeth me no more; but ye see me: because I live, ye shall live also."

We commonly think of keys being used to lock or unlock doors, but there is another sense in which the word *key* is used. Many times,

---

[127] "Napoleonic Wars, European History" *Encyclopedia Britannica*, 2020, Accessed April 28, 2020, https://www.britannica.com/event/Napoleonic-Wars.

when we say we have the key to a thing, we mean that we have the solution to a problem. Jesus was saying to John and to us all that He has the solution to death and hell and the grave. He has all the problems connected with it unraveled and solved. He had worked out the problem for Himself and overcame in it. Christ has the key and shall ultimately bring every man into the fullness of His life. Christ has the power to redeem, and He has the keys of death and hell.

Not only do the firstborn among many brethren possess the keys of death and hell, but He shares them with His overcomers who are partakers of His eternal life. Jesus said to Peter, "You are Peter, and upon this rock I will build My Church and the gates of hell shall not prevail against it" (Matt. 16:18).

The gates of hell have not prevailed against our Lord Jesus Christ, and they shall not prevail against His Church. What are the "gates" of hell? Gates are used either to bar entrance or prevent exit. Jacob stood at the gate of heaven and was not aware of it (Gen. 28:17).

Jesus Christ, the captain of the well-fought fight, the greatest general of all times, has come and has had a greater victory than any of these. He has come not only into the opposition and hostility of this world, but He has gone into the very portals of hell. There He has taken on the most violent and the vilest of the underworld, and now He leads into the metropolis of the kingdom of God a great triumphal victory.

Anastasis: Standing Against COVID-19 Generational Impact

The impact of the novel coronavirus pandemic on every leader necessitates that we take fast and informed action to precisely gain an understanding of how each generation is experiencing and seeking to rebound from this perplexing phase in history.

The Word of God declares in Proverbs 30:11–14:

> There is a generation that curseth their
> father, and doth not bless their mother. There is

a generation that are pure in their own eyes, and yet is not washed from their filthiness. There is a generation, O how lofty are their eyes! and their eyelids are lifted up. There is a generation, whose teeth are as swords, and their jaw teeth as knives, to devour the poor from off the earth, and the needy from among men.

It is not possible for any pandemic to deter the will of God for any generation or the millennial generation in particular. David served his own generation by the will of God, and there is a generation of exploit that death or any pandemic cannot affect. David also declared in Psalms 22:30, "A seed shall serve him; it shall be accounted to the Lord for a generation."

God's chosen generation are here, and against the present data analysis and interpretation, no pandemic by whatever name it is called is greater than the Holy Spirit that lives on the inside of them or God's Word through which they live. They can never be silenced by COVID-19, and their future shall be great in Christ Jesus. They are the overcomer generation. Peter declares in 1 Peter 2:9, "But ye are a chosen generation, a royal priesthood, an holy nation, a peculiar people; that ye should shew forth the praises of him who hath called you out of darkness into his marvellous light."

Pyoria, et al., cited Edmund and Turner and Eyernab and Turner who connoted that the concept of generation has two basic meanings. Firstly, it means a familial generation or a social generation; that is, a cohort of people born in the same date range. However, a cohort does not constitute a generation by virtue of its age alone, other than in a statistical sense. And secondly, in the sociological use of the concept, a generation is thought to consist of a stratum who are born within a limited time range and who share not only the same date of birth but also similar sociocultural experiences.

They also cited Karl Mannheim who identified the three stages of generation formation. Mannheim specified that the first premise for the formation of a generation is membership of the same age group, but that alone is not enough, for there must also exist some social and cultural factor that most people in the age group share in common. Mannheim detailed that youth is a particularly strategic time for the development of generational consciousness, and he also realized that the key experience is shared by a certain cohort and at once unites and divides generations. According to him, the third stage of generation formation involves drawing together people from a certain age cohort to pursue a common goal or way of life here that the generation is mobilized.[128]

According to Pew Research, the Traditionalists or Silent Generation are born between 1928 and 1945. The Baby Boomers are born between 1946 and 1964. The Generation X are born between 1965 and 1980. The Millennials are born between 1981 and 1996, while Generation Z—or iGen or Centennials—are born between 1997 and present.[129]

Slicing the generational topography from Baby Boomers who witnessed the assassination of President Kennedy in the United States or the event of September 11, 2001, to the millennials, we can observe that both Gen X and Gen Z are now seriously agitated by the coronavirus pandemic. From the pathological study of different generational phases, it was inferred that millennials perceived COVID-19 as suffering another traumatic event which was a reminder to post 9/11 memories. Gen X now plans to delay retirement much longer, and many are facing the new challenge of taking care of their children and parents in addition to working from home.

The impact of COVID-19 on Gen Z—who at this moment in their lives have their assessments and track being shaped—is that this will be the first global event of their lives of which they have no reference point, unlike the other generations, and thus have no single clue on how to respond in the way older generations do. Whether it is the Millennials or Gen Z, it's all about knowing the God of Abraham, Isaac, and Jacob who is ever faithful to a thousand generations (Deut. 7:9).

---

[128] Pyoria, et al, "The Millennial Generation: A New Breed of Labor? *Sage Journals*, 2017, Accessed June 3, 2020, https://journals.sagepub.com/doi/full/10.1177/2158244017697158#articleCitationDownloadContainer.

[129] "Generations and Age," Pew Research Center, Accessed June 1, 2020, https://www.pewresearch.org/topics/generations-and-age/.

Judges 2:10 alerts, "And also all that generation were gathered unto their fathers: and there arose another generation after them, which knew not the Lord, nor yet the works which he had done for Israel."

Case in point, the COVID-19 has not only altered Gen Z's mode of schooling but also their mobility and personal finances. They are also being quarantined at home with food shortages at grocery stores and are unable to get their driver's licenses at the appropriate age. The result is that this newest generation, Gen Z, will come of age in a world where virtual classes and restaurant delivery are not just normal but often the only option and where businesses and brands completely overhaul how they interconnect, participate, and market to shoppers and potential workforces.

Hillary Hoffower indicated that how you handle the coronavirus pandemic depends upon your age because coronavirus risk increases with age. People over sixty years are at a greater risk of becoming seriously ill than younger people who do not have underlying health conditions, and those who do have preexisting conditions are also at higher risk. According to Hoffower, people who are in their eighties or nineties, known as the silent and greatest generation, are even at the highest risk.

These risk groups combined with life stage and identity have left the biggest generations facing the pandemic on their own terms. The younger generations, like Generation Z, think the coronavirus is not as serious as it is, which is reflected in their crowding beaches during March 2020 for spring break. Meanwhile, Millennials are worried about their parents, many of whom fall into the aforementioned high-risk group.

Hoffower specified that Generation X had stated that they are the only generation well-equipped to handle the pandemic because they have survived several world crises and need to serve as a role model to both their children and high-risk parents, whereas Baby Boomers, who fall into these high-risk groups, are having trouble staying indoors because they just do not feel their age. She added that Generation Z received several backlashes for ignoring coronavirus warnings and social distancing rules as many college students were crowding beaches from Florida to Texas to liven up their spring break, and spring breakers were also spotted partying on booze cruises in The Bahamas.

Hoffower cited a spring breaker who opinionated that the coronavirus is not a big deal, and the threat of being dead from coronavirus cannot stop him from living life "because you only have one." YOLO: You Only Live Once. A group of seventy spring breakers that chartered a plane from Texas to Cabo in mid-March had forty-four of them tested positive for the coronavirus, and although millennials are not partying, that does not stop their anxiety as they work from home and watch Hulu while yelling at their parents not to go outside, forcing many of them to realize the fact that their parents are aging and could be considered at-risk individuals.[130]

Zamira Rahim explicated that Generation Z are now graduating into a labor market devastated by the global pandemic. Workers of this cohort are more likely than older generations to work in industries shut down by social distancing restrictions according to Amanda Barroso and Rakesh Kochhar from Pew Research Center.[131] She elucidated that Generation Z's future prospects look gloomy, and as the Resolution Foundation's analysis had suggested, layoffs that are linked to the coronavirus pandemic could affect the young people's pay and job prospects in the long-term as in the United Kingdom. The economy could shrink by 14 percent in the year 2020 while unemployment is expected to hit 9 percent.

Rahim described the impact of unemployment in a recession as being particularly severe on those who have just left school where only

---

[130] Hillary Hoffower, "From Gen Z Spring Breakers to Toilet Paper-Hoarding Boomers, the Coronavirus Pandemic is a Case study in Generational Differences. Here's How Each Generation Is Dealing with It," *Business Insider*, 2020, Accessed May 17, 2020, https://www.businessinsider.com/coronavirus-generational-effects-millennials-gen-z-baby-boomers-2020-4.

[131] Amanda Barroso and Rakesh Kochhar, "Young Workers Likely to be Hard Hit as COVID-19 Strikes a Blow to Restaurants and Other Service Sector Jobs," Pew Research Center, *Fact Tank News in the Numbers*, 2020, Accessed May 18, 2020, https://www.pewresearch.org/fact-tank/2020/03/27/young-workers-likely-to-be-hard-hit-as-covid-19-strikes-a-blow-to-restaurants-and-other-service-sector-jobs/.

fewer jobs and internships are available to younger people searching for work, especially in sectors such as hospitality, travel, and retail, which provide large numbers of entry level roles.[132]

Andrew Van Dam acknowledged that after accounting for the present crisis, the average Millennial has experienced slower economic growth since entering the workforce than any other generation in US history, and Millennials will certainly bear the pandemic economic scars for the rest of their lives in the form of lower earnings, lower wealth, and delayed milestones, such as homeownership.

Additionally, he noted that losses are particularly acute on the jobs front, and in particular, one brutal month of the coronavirus set the labor market back to the turn of the millennium. He explained that the last time there were about 131 million jobs was January 2000, and for Millennials who came of age then, it is as if all the plodding expansions and jobless recoveries of their namesake epoch evaporated in weeks. He continued that the milestones will get even more dire in the next jobs report, but for now, the economic regression back to Y2K is a fitting symbol for a generation that more than any other has been shaped by recession.

Van Dam explicated that the losses were not merely symbolic but that the recession steamrolled younger workers. Just as Millennials were entering their prime working years, the oldest millennials are nearing forty while the youngest are in their mid-twenties.

Proportionally, the even younger generation, known as Zoomers, suffered worse than all of them. A third of their jobs vaporized in two months in 2020. But Gen Z is only just entering the labor force, while the oldest Zoomers are in their early twenties. According to Van Dam, at the beginning of 2019, Millennials became the largest generation in the US full-time workforce, surpassing Gen X. But the coronavirus crisis walloped Millennials so disproportionately that

---

[132] Zamira Rachim, "Why Gen Z Will Be Hit the Hardest by the Financial Fallout from Coronavirus," *CNN Business* (2020), https://www.cnn.com/2020/05/13/business/coronavirus-generation-z-jobs-intl-gbr/index.html (accessed May 17, 2020).

they're probably giving the top generational spot back to Gen X in the next month or two.

Millennials, suffering through high unemployment during the recession, ended up less likely to work for high-paying employers and less likely to complete as much education as workers in places where the recession did not hit as hard. He also noted that Millennials had to settle for worse jobs early in their careers, depressing their lifetime earnings potential. Millennials had much less of a financial cushion than previous generations did at their age, Kent said, even though they had been doing many things right. Millennials are getting married later and having children later and at an age when Boomers and Gen X are building equity, and they have no housing net worth, and they are the most educated, most diverse generation in history, at least until Zoomers pass them and those distinctions come with burdens.[133]

Emily Wilson observed that COVID-19 has changed the workplace for good, which is a complete disruption of the typical workplace that came at a time when the oldest members of Generation Z are entering the workforce. She explained that companies around the globe already know that office setups and expectations have changed radically, and COVID-19 has presented an opportunity for employers to get prepared for what the next generation of employees may want in a job or career. Presently, Gen Z accounts for a staggering one-third of the world's population, and this cohort wants significantly different things from employers, compared to previous generations. She added that salary comes up as the most important factor in deciding which job to pick for Gen Z but to a much lesser extent than all other generations.

He cited Deloitte who discovered that nearly two-thirds (65 percent) of Gen Z lists their employment as a key part of their identity, and in order to align with this eco and politically conscious gen-

---

[133] Andrew Van Dam, "Millennials Are the Unluckiest Generation in US History," *The Washington Post, Democracy Dies in Darkness*, 2020, Accessed June 1, 2020, https://www.msn.com/en-us/news/markets/the-unluckiest-generation-in-us-history/ar-BB14EOM7.

eration, companies would benefit from becoming more value-driven and provide more than just a paycheck to enable Gen Z to connect with their work. And because Gen Z want a company they can believe in, companies need to work toward the greater good because members of Gen Z prioritize companies that positively impact society. These could be causes such as climate change, sustainability, accessibility to health care, and ending poverty.

However, caring about challenges the world is facing is just one piece of the puzzle. Companies must also prove they're acting to impact change in order to attract the most diverse generation the world has ever seen.

Wilson stressed that while many organizations have shied away from offering flexible working arrangements, the flexibility that Gen Z craves from the workplace is being tested organically due to COVID-19, so also after the global pandemic is over, some flexible practices may still remain. Presently, many organizations that once feared their at-home workers would be walking their dog and doing laundry are learning that remote employees are exhibiting strong job performance. Gen Z has certainly taken note of these changing business dynamics.

Zoom has taken the place of cross-country meetings, and retailers have adapted to curbside pickup when local authorities require them to keep doors closed to customers. Business as usual has been turned on its head, and this will impact the dynamics Gen Z will expect as they enter the workforce. Furthermore, he emphasized that a rise in flexibility may change the way companies approach their workforce where part-time positions might gain popularity to make space for employees to have more community involvement and creative side projects. And once employees return to offices, varied schedules that foster social distancing could appeal to Gen Z and especially to those living in cities who are now profited by less time spent commuting or commuting at off-peak hours, and they can now devote more time to the things that they enjoy outside of work.

Additionally, he observed that some companies are giving mental health days, crisis days, or hazard pay to account for more difficult working conditions. This focus on employee well-being will need to stick around post-pandemic as the effects of this strange time might be long-lasting. Wilson elucidated that the swift transition to remote work will enable Gen Z to avoid crowded city centers and live in more remote areas that allow them to be closer to nature and other things they're passionate about. She stated that mandatory work from home policies have proven that employees can still be productive anywhere with a strong Internet connection, and thus, Gen Z might break with the tradition of moving to a cramped apartment in the city when they're first starting out in their careers.

Wilson concluded that there is a level of uncertainty that remains for all workers as we navigate a very uncertain time, although some future Gen Z workforce may be less selective in their job searches given the high rate of unemployment. However, as companies rethink what they stand for and gear up to welcome a new generation into their ranks, it's clear that there is plenty more work to do as we are already in a great time of learning both on the employee and employer side. And when we enter a post-COVID-19 world, work is going to look quite different, and predictably, Gen Z will be among the first to reap the benefits.[134]

It will then be an understatement to conclude that coronavirus pandemic does not have any generational implications. Different generations comprehend and interpret COVID-19 in different perspectives, especially as it relates to global economy fallout and future prospects.

According to Billy McMahan, Generation Z has been referred to as "iGen." The term alludes to the fact that they are the first generation that has grown up in the age of the smartphone. He buttressed that they are deeply rooted within the heart, and the mind of a Gen Z-er is a desire to change the world and the idea that each person has something unique to offer the world is commonplace. They have something inside them that says the world as we know it is less than

---

[134] Emily Wilson, "How COVID-19 Will Change Gen Z's Approach to the Workplace," *Forbes: SAP BrandVoice Innovation*, 2020, Accessed June 15, 2020, https://www.forbes.com/sites/sap/2020/06/11/how-covid-19-changes-gen-z-approach-to-the-workplace/#4c66966742ea.

what it could be. He added that Generation Z is quick to jump in on social issues, and it is easy to move them into action if it means that it would really make a difference.

McMahan observed that Generation Z-ers are hooked to their screens, and this characteristic is not only about the smartphone, but it also includes computers for school, TVs when they get home, and the time they spend gaming. He documented that 57 percent of teens are reported to be using a screen of some kind for four hours a day.[135] Twenty-six percent of that 57 percent admit to spending more than eight hours per day on their screen, and these numbers are staggering.

In addition to the amount of time they are spending using some form of technology, it is incredible and is important to understand the trends of how Generation Z is connecting with the Church. What is it that is bringing them in? What is it that is making them stick? What are the things they are hungry for? God has handcrafted each one of us. Each one of us is created to be in community and relationship with Him. What is that this generation is longing for that will draw them toward Him?

Besides the supported idea that Generation Z is made up of strong multitaskers, and they have the ability to do more than one thing at a time, it is fairly uncommon to see a young person only doing one thing at a time. But for previous generations, multitasking has been an inhibitor, but Generation Z can do it well, which can be seen through the ability to listen and be truly investing in a conversation while also working on homework or through scrolling social media platforms. As a result of growing up in the age of the smartphone, Generation Z has been trained to handle multiple things at the same time. Their proficiency in multitasking is a cause for excitement in working with them.

---

[135] Vicki Rideout and Michael B. Robb, "The Common Sense Cense: Media Use by Tweens and Teens," Accessed June 9, 2020, https://www.commonsensemedia.org/sites/default/files/uploads/research/2019-census-8-to-18-full-report-updated.pdf.

McMahan disclosed that Generation Z is open to guidance or coaching. They are open to having someone walk with them through learning experiences, and surprisingly, they are open to input on how to do different things. Generation Z has been considered to be the first truly post-Christ American generation, and having a post-Christian worldview means they think they know what Christians have to offer and have refused it. He narrated that a larger percentage of this generation would identify themselves as atheist than any generation, and many teens use negative experiences they had or heard about as reasons for not following the beliefs of the Church. But unfortunately, much of Generation Z is gaining their understanding of what Christianity is from politicians and celebrity figures.

Additionally, McMahan specified that every generation has issues that seem to plague their generation, and just like previous generations, the emerging generation has its own unique challenges which have to do with the context in which Gen Z-ers are being reared, and in order to effectively minister and serve these young people, it is helpful to understand the issues they are facing, just as it is in an established trust between two people. And after trust is established, then they are open to guidance.

This presents a huge opportunity for growth of intergenerational discipleship with members of Generation Z. On the contrary, previous generations have been very closed off to the idea of being coached.

He added that the need among members of Generation Z is great, and while Christians have been commissioned as followers of Jesus to make Him known, they should also know that they are in the midst of a battle and that the enemy will do all he can to keep a generation from coming to our Lord, and truly, Generation Z is living under a worldview that tells them that they need to be perfect, that they need to work and strive, and their personal value drops if they fall short.

In his explanation, he specified that through the history of world missions, we have seen missionaries give up everything and actively pursue the people that God led them to. We have seen the examples of William Carey going to India, Hudson Taylor to China, and Jim

Elliot to Ecuador. We have seen the example of A. B. Simpson, who would stand and preach at the docks in New York City as people arrived in the New World. We even saw Paul's desire to get to Rome.

Time and time again, Christian leaders have placed themselves in places and positions to reach people with the Good News of Jesus. McMahan asked, what does that look like here and now as we try to reach Generation Z here in America? He answered that we must discover what it is that could capture the heart and mind of Generation Z. How could these barriers be removed so that Gen Z-ers would reframe their current understanding of Jesus and the Church?

McMahan acknowledges the potential of Generation Z as they are the largest generation and most diverse, strongest in multitasking, and most adaptable generation ever whose capture to truly change the world is greater than any previous generation, but their problem is that they are hurting, and the enemy is waging war against them through isolation, anxiety, and depression. They do need Jesus followers who can help guide the way by sharing their lives. They need people who are willing to risk and share their journey with God, including both the good moments and the worst moments. Generation Z needs seasoned Jesus followers to help them recognize and unlock their true potential. He concluded that we should build our church systems in a way that will welcome them home to a Father that is sprinting shamelessly toward them.[136]

Anastasis: COVID-19 and Neo-Leadership Concepts

The COVID-19 pandemic has tried every faculty of humanity ranging from our personal lives, families, jobs, communities, companies, nations, and the entire world. While the world has suffered many crises in times past, the COVID-19 pandemic is unique. It is not like the days of the Great Recession where those who lost

---

[136] Billy McMahan, Morris et al., ed., "Igniting Hope Among Gen Z," *Great Commission Research Journal. Church Music's Influence on Church Growth* (Madison, MS: Great Commission Research Network, 2020), 105–122.

their jobs can still hang out for discussion at a coffee shop and be refreshed, but social distancing and quarantines have swallowed all those possibilities. There arises new guiding principles, theories, concepts, and models for leaders to equalize ethical demands with the need for practical effectiveness and economic sanity after this crisis.

There are new steps to be taken going forward through a global post-COVID-19 directive to help guide the policies needed to rebuild economies, world trade, and our societies. There must be capable intellectuals who can formulate guidelines for how public and private leaders can best approach stability and growth for the social and future economy of the world.

The twenty-first century leaders must now be flexible on policies, and demonstrating acts of consideration and empathy are the most needed during this unprecedented pandemic season. They will determine the most appropriate objectives and strategies and guide the populace toward delivering successful objectives and satisfy the expectations of all the stakeholders and the needs of populations. It is during this time that the world needs leaders that focus on sustainability of natural resources and care for people.

Courageous COVID-19 leaders cannot deny that there is a problem that must be fixed; neither could they just admit that there is a problem and then politicize it, but they must provide solutions from investing heavily into vaccines, preventing the spread of the virus through social distancing, regular handwashing, and wearing of masks; also by promoting the use of tracking and tracing technologies, while still believing that the miraculous hand of the Almighty God will save, heal, and deliver. They must opt for pragmatic and audacious change that reconciles with those who are hardest hit by the pandemic so as to acknowledge our human dependency on one another and how deeply we need each other. This crisis is just the beginning of sorrows, and God's elect leaders must be adequately prepared.

The Word of God declares in Mark 13:8, 20, 27:

> For nation shall rise against nation, and
> kingdom against kingdom: and there shall be

earthquakes in divers' places, and there shall be famines and troubles: these are the beginnings of sorrows.

And except that the Lord had shortened those days, no flesh should be saved: but for the elect's sake, whom he hath chosen, he hath shortened the days.

And then shall he send his angels and shall gather together his elect from the four winds, from the uttermost part of the earth to the uttermost part of heaven.

Clay Scroggins explained that self-leadership demands that you know more about yourself than anyone else, and one needs a PhD in one's self, and in order to become well-versed in the ins and outs of one's self, there is the greatest need to observe and understand the distractions and noises in one's life by learning the scientific method. Scroggins added that leadership involves an internal versus external dynamic, and good leaders learn to manage external factors well by responding effectively to even the most abrupt external changes. He enumerated that external factors will always fight to become the dominant proxy for determining success, and a growing leader is as healthy as one's emotional self-awareness who will resist the proxies on his or her life and keep focus on what matters most.[137]

David Bowman stated that one needs AQ to achieve success in life. He explained that most people believe it will take a combination of Intelligence Quotient (IQ) and Emotional Intelligence (EQ). He cited Paul Stoltz who explained that the biggest factor in determining your success is your Adversity Quotient (AQ).

Stoltz added that only few people have heard of AQ, but it is the individuals with high AQ that are most likely to achieve their

---

[137] Clay Scroggings, *How to Lead in a World of Distraction. Maximizing Your Influence by Turning Down the Noise* (Grand Rapids: Zondervan Reflective, 2020), 50–80.

visions.[138] Adversity Quotient (AQ) is the measure of your ability to go through a rough patch in life and come out without losing your mind. AQ determines who will give up in the face of troubles, who will abandon their family, or who will consider suicide.

Daniel Montgomery elucidated that our bodies are wired for balance, and they will do anything they can to make up for depletions in other parts of us (spiritually, emotionally, and mentally). He added that being mindful of our bodies directly relates to our experience of the world because God has designed us to interpret the world through sensations, urges, movements, emotions, images, memories, and thoughts, and once we become mindful of how these physical aspects are processed in our bodies, we can begin to balance our bodies interpretations of the information.

Montgomery clarified that the human nervous system is built around the balance of two opposing actions which are the sympathetic nervous system that is associated with the fight-or-flight response that is as a result of the release of cortisol (stress chemicals) throughout the bloodstream; and the second is the parasympathetic nervous system that is associated with relaxation, digestion, and regeneration. He noted that these two parts are meant to work in a rhythmic alternation that supports healthy rhythms of alertness and restfulness that benefits physical and mental health.[139]

Nicolas Fischbach advocated that fire, flood, earthquake, or lack of energy supply are four historical horsemen of standard business continuity planning, and these four generally affect an individual site, office, or business function and are typically isolated, short-term, or acute incidents which the company can quickly start to recover from in order to get "back to normal." This is why business continuity plans are also often known as "disaster recovery plans."

---

[138] David Bowman, "This Is What You Really Need for Personal Success," Nexus Business Solutions, 2020, Accessed June 1, 2020, https://nexusbusiness.com/adversity-quotient-personal-success/.

[139] Daniel Montgomery, *How to Be Present in an Absent World: A Leader's Guide to Showing Up, Paying Attention, and Becoming Fully Human* (Grand Rapids, Zondervan Reflective, 2020), 168–169.

He explained that when normal metamorphosis from normal to baseline in the world that has gotten more connected while the extended enterprise has become more expansive and most plans did not account for a longer-term disruption that is widespread across the enterprise or globe such as with COVID-19 pandemic, then organizations are presented with challenges that have never been faced before. Opportunities arise to come through the event so as to evolve stronger than before.

Fischbach elucidated that as shelter-in-place orders expand across the globe, companies that are able to do so are sending large numbers of employees to work from home on an extended basis. While working from home or working remotely has become increasingly prevalent over the last few years with the growing gig economy, today's massive remote work model is unparalleled. In addition to the device-busy home Internet setup, the possible use of a shared family computer, and targeted phishing, it is possible to end up with pathways for bad actors to find their way in. Now more than ever, the risk of a breach is very tangible when security is neglected at the human level. He advised that IT security and information protection must be on organizational executive team radar and that different groups will need different tools or access in order to work effectively from home. The customer support teams may need an extra monitor, finance teams will need a local copy of confidential data, and the developers that have been reliant on Linux desktops will now need to quickly find a suitable at-home replacement as network jitter is making remote connections ineffective.

He also stated that for the CEO, it is a unique platform that can be used to set the strategy, the business direction, and the culture of the company. What the CEO cares about, the rest of the company cares about. Once the company is past the first-wave war room stage, it will be up to the CEO to ensure that the business of safeguarding company assets gets a seat at the table. This is not just about risk management; it's about recognizing that these functions are contributing to the business's success. He noted that this is a good time to update and expand the business continuity plan to include what was learned during this time and address the company's new ways of working.

Fischbach buttressed that in the midst of trying to navigate through uncharted business territory during this pandemic, the goal for every company should be to come out on the other side stronger and more secure than before.[140]

Leaders in every stratum of life must understand meticulous strategies and tools that work best for a work-from-home scenario as well as to drive sales and marketing goals across generations.

COVID-19 has affected organizations, communities, and individuals across the world. It is the most significant global change mockup of the century. It has many mysteries in history and has resulted into the collapse of many organizations. However, some organizations will be spared due to their positioning as essential businesses, but all will be transformed for a very long time by this experience. The choices made by senior organizational leaders will shape the future of their establishments.

Ira Chaleff advocated that self-management encompasses the nuts and bolts of effective leadership or followership, which though it's mundane and pedestrian, yet it is a critical skill, and the courageous follower must be prepared to do this hard work involved in being personally well organized. Chaleff encouraged that the management of our life and health is even more fundamental than management of our work if we are to be reliable team members and a source of support for our leaders. We must do our jobs and not become our jobs. He added that managing our life and health is not a marginal issue, but in the long run, it can make the difference between brilliantly contributing to the common purpose and blowing up, fizzling out in the attempt. But leaders occupy their positions

---

[140] Nicholas Fischbach, "Moving Business Continuity to Safeguard the New Normal: Reinventing Cybersecurity," Global CTO, Forcepoint WSJ, 2020, Accessed June 2, 2020, https://partners.wsj.com/forcepoint/reinventing-cybersecurity/moving-beyond-business-continuity-to-safeguard-the-new-normal/?utm_medium=content_discovery&utm_source=taboola&utm_content=&utm_term=%7Bmsn-msn-home%7D&tblci=GiBP9uR5Lo8racJi58rMyD-63mAa6XcHGppMxUU5mPCfbCCCrok8.

because of some constellations of strength that are of great value to the organization.

He stated that an incident in which old successful leadership behavior clashes with a changed environment can provide a courageous follower the opportunity to discuss these changes with the leader, and the fallout from the incident may provide a ripe opportunity for helping the leader reexamine behavior. He also explained that great leaders face challenges, and they often encounter relentless opposition while seeking a path that will achieve their organization's purpose. The biographies of Winston Churchill, Martin Luther King Jr., and Ghandi are filled with years of patience-wearing struggle and setbacks; likewise, many lesser famous leaders also labor for years or decades before they see their dreams fulfilled.[141]

The post-COVID-19 world will require extreme toughness from organizations, societies, and nations. Leadership agility becomes more crucial than ever. Scottie Andrew reported that coronavirus will surge again when the summer ends in the year 2020. According to infectious disease experts, they are almost certain about that, but they do not know how severe the resurgence will be.

Andrew cited Mike Ryan who had offered one bleak hypothesis for what the next few months of coronavirus could look like. Ryan stated that while still living through the first wave of the pandemic, and cases are still rising, infections could jump up suddenly and significantly "at any time." He noted that a second peak would not unfold as neatly or gradually as a wave. A new peak would mean a sudden spike in cases, which could overburden health care systems again and possibly cause a greater number of deaths. He clarified that the second peak could be worse than the first.

In a second peak scenario, coronavirus cases would spike sharply and quickly until they reach a new high, likely after a period when the rate of infection remains fairly stable. In a second wave, infections may unfold more gradually and impact different regions of the world at different times. Andrew narrated that in both a second peak

---

[141] Ira Chaleff, *The Courageous Follower: Standing Up to and For Our Leaders* (Oakland: Berret-Koehler Publishers, Inc, 2009), 46–89

scenario and one in which we "flatten the curve," the same number of people could be infected, and only timing counts.

A second peak would mean that many more people are infected with coronavirus at the same time and during flu season, which would overburden health care systems.[142]

When confronted with a crisis such as COVID-19, leaders must not act in an unacquainted way. Crises such as this demand that leaders take an emergency reaction plan and acclimatize with it as new evidence and factors gradually evolve. Following coronavirus pandemic, many leaders are confronted with troublesome changes that have never been experienced.

Routines and the familiars are obstructed, prompting leaders to begin to discover new equilibrium in daily activities such as at work, social lives, mental, and even physical health.

For many, a superfluity of distressing feelings has surfaced: anxiety, worry, fear, frustration, sadness, anger, panic, helplessness, uncertainty, skepticism, confusion, stress, and even losses. The ripple effect of all these will impact the behavior of the leader and the organization regarding how they perceive the world, how they perceive themselves, and how they relate to others.

Truly, the coronavirus pandemic has distorted every aspect of the leader and the organizational structure. From approach to work, to collaborations with friends and family, and the constant news of the coronavirus and its spread, it has had great impact in the infinitesimal daily transactions of the leader, and the COVID-19 pandemic has brought an overnight change and disruption to organizations, companies, industries, and even the world at large. At this moment, each leader must learn to insulate their organization with tough adaptability against the heat from the metamorphosis. The COVID-19 pandemic has introduced to our world new challenges, new circumstances, and new uncertainties. Jobs are mutating, atten-

---

[142] Scottie Andrews, "What a Second Peak of Coronavirus Could Look Like," *CNN*, 2020, Accessed May 28, 2020, https://www.msn.com/en-us/health/health-news/what-a-second-peak-of-coronavirus-could-look-like/ar-BB14Gg-mi?ocid=mailsignout.

uating, and vanishing, just as coworkers, teammates, and technology are shifting.

To survive the gigantic dearth that this pandemic has brought, the leader must be irrepressible, both personally and professionally. The leader must see himself or herself arriving at the triumphant side of life. Effective leaders understand that success requires more than just coping with change and that the goal is not just to hang in but to accept that change is happening and so arm one's self with provable strategies to solve the unforeseen circumstances. They will always shift their comportment to acclimatizing with new situations and trials.

Leaders who display adjustable leadership seek new and pioneering ways to solve problems, master new skills, and view disorder as a challenge rather than a threat and possess enough skills needed to prevail through uncertain times. Strategic planning must be adapted for our organization to handle the changes and aligning within the group and inspiring fresh commitment from our people.

We must adequately confront obstacles against leading effectively in an uncertain world and readily take care of our mental and physical health so that we can reach our full potential in our God-given assignment whether as an entrepreneur, an attorney, a medical doctor, or a clergy. The Bible declares in Philippians 4:8, "Finally, brethren, whatsoever things are true, whatsoeverthings are honest, whatsoever things are just, whatsoeverthings are pure, whatsoever things are lovely, whatsoeverthings are of good report; if there be any virtue, and if there be any praise, think on these things." We must not forget that during this hard time and more than before, bodily exercise still profits little, but godliness is profitable unto all things (1 Tim. 4:8).

Leaders must not be distracted with mundane things that they forget what is really important. Obviously, COVID-19 and all that it entails has introduced other complications and pressures to an already full plate, but we must not lose track of who we are in Christ Jesus and never allow one's self to degenerate into a Christ-less entity. Jesus stated in Matthew 6:31–33:

> Therefore take no thought, saying, what shall we eat? or, what shall we drink? or,

Wherewithal shall we be clothed? For after all these things do the Gentiles seek:) for your heavenly Father knoweth that ye have need of all these things. But seek ye first the kingdom of God, and his righteousness; and all these things shall be added unto you.

Furthermore, as the world enters the unacquainted terrain in navigating the COVID-19 pandemic, a band of the global workforce has risen to setting up shop to work from home. With new emphasis on telecommuting comes a new need for virtual leadership. Teams need a strategy for thinking differently, communicating digitally, and making sure people feel included and connected in order to effectively manage their people and projects remotely, and as a leader, your organization will be looking up to you for direction, enthusiasm, and creativeness. These are times when the leader must implement strategic decisions that may change the course of the organization in addition to providing intentional guidance.

Therefore, organizations that are most efficient at creating new leadership capabilities across different functions are intentional, calculated, and focused on effectively linking that development to business results. Employees throughout the organization expect each other to engage, change, innovate, and move forward. Traditional leadership development will lag behind to support this kind of agility at the new workplace. The leader must bear in mind that as the coronavirus pandemic continues to cause uncertainty for businesses and organizations, employees are coming to grips with an unfamiliar work life. For many, the typical workday is punctuated with new challenges that include time-outs for homeschooling children, navigating the complexities of sharing a workspace with a spouse or partner, and ensuring the household's basic needs are met.

The reality of life post-COVID-19 has not fully sunk in yet, and its consequences for our businesses, organizations, economy, and society will play out over the rest of 2020 and beyond. It is imperative for leaders to educate and familiarize themselves with the new normal and navigate through it to achieving effectiveness. This connotes going beyond receiving information just from the media so as not to be engulfed into the melodrama that characterizes the social media in particular and thus transfers the same inadequate information to our employees.

Paul declares in 2 Timothy 2:15, 4:13:

> Study to shew thyself approved unto God, a workman that needeth not to be ashamed, rightly dividing the word of truth.
>
> The cloke that I left at Troas with Carpus, when thou comest, bring with thee, and the books, but especially the parchments.

We must understand the trajectory of the new challenges and how to overcome the same by studying relevant books. God's Word declares that every other thing and circumstances may change, but our God still remains the same yesterday, today, and forever, and only His truth will prevail (Mal. 3:8; Heb 13:8).

Daniel reinforces the need for us to give an undivided attention to all that is in the book. Daniel 9:2–4 declares:

> In the first year of his reign I, Daniel understood by books the number of the years, whereof the word of the Lord came to Jeremiah the prophet, that he would accomplish seventy years in the desolations of Jerusalem. And I set my face unto the Lord God, to seek by prayer and supplications, with fasting, and sackcloth, and ashes. And I prayed unto the Lord my God, and made my confession, and said, O Lord, the great and dreadful God, keeping the covenant and mercy to them that love him, and to them that keep his commandments.

Jonathan Falwell explained that apologetics involve the art of persuasion and the defense of the Christian faith. He buttressed that the concept is derived from the Greek word *apologia,* meaning "to give answer." Falwell explicated that while it is necessary for the Holy Spirit to illuminate our minds to God's truth, He does so by appealing to both the sacred text and to human reasoning; thus, faith and reason are allies in the quest for truth. He noted that in classical Christian orthodoxy, faith precedes reason, but it does not eliminate it. Christianity is not a mindless religion of mystical experiences that are devoid of reasonable conclusions but the most-reasoned faculty-based religion on the planet.

Falwell added that it is one thing to believe in and defend the inspiration of Scripture, but it is another matter altogether to read it, understand t, and internalize its truths, knowing that the inspired text can affect our daily lives as we study it and pally it. Falwell stated that real Christianity must be rooted in biblical truth and lived in the reality of life's challenges. The Bible speaks with the same authority it does in telling us how to get through life as it does in telling us how to get to heaven. Furthermore, Falwell observed that understanding God has always been a challenge to the human mind, and despite our human limitations, the Bible clearly tells us that we fallible beings can know the infallible God.[143]

It is extremely vital to speak God's blessings from the Book of Life all the days of your life. Every morning, when you wake up, you must start praising God and begin to walk in the footsteps of David from Psalm 103. These new generational leaders must arm themselves to the new realities of cancelling appointments with death of any kind. Proverbs 3:1–2 declares, "My son, forget not my law; but let thine heart keep my commandments. For length of days, and long life, and peace, shall they add to thee."

Moses documented in Deuteronomy 11:18–21:

> Therefore shall ye lay up these my words
> in your heart and in your soul, and bind them
> for a sign upon your hand, that they may be as

---

[143] Jonathan Falwell, *InnovateChurch: Innovative Leadership for the Next Generation Church* (Nashville: B&H Publishing Group, 2008) 205–208.

> frontlets between your eyes. And ye shall teach them your children, speaking of them when thou sittest in thine house, and when thou walkest by the way, when thou liest down, and when thou risest up. And thou shalt write them upon the door posts of thine house, and upon thy gates. That your days may be multiplied, and the days of your children, in the land which the Lord sware unto your fathers to give them, as the days of heaven upon the earth.

Resurrection (anastasis) is not reincarnation. We have one life here on earth, and when that life is over, we will face one of two kinds of judgement (2 Cor. 5:10). Those who have not received Jesus as Lord and Savior will stand before the Great White Throne of God for judgment appointed by God. Hebrews 9:27 clearly states, "It is appointed into men once to die, but after this the judgement."

That is why it is important that in this life, you do that which is right, and you begin by making Jesus Christ your Lord and Savior and avoid the stress of guilt. Love everyone. Avoid hatred or harboring ill will against any. Micah 6:8 declares, "He hath shewed thee, O man, what is good; and what doth the Lord require of thee, but to do justly, and to love mercy, and to walk humbly with thy God?"

Zechariah 8:16–17 states:

> These are the things that ye shall do; Speak ye every man the truth to his neighbour; execute the judgment of truth and peace in your gates. And let none of you imagine evil in your hearts against his neighbour; and love no false oath: for all these are things that I hate, saith the Lord.

You must be lively, pleasant, peaceful and joyful. The road map to accessing the peace of God is by prayer and supplication with thanksgiving (Phil. 4:6–7) while access to God's joy is by being a carrier of God's presence through a joyful praise (Ps. 16:11, 22:3; Neh. 8:10).

David declares in Psalms 34:12–14, "What man is he that desireth life, and loveth many days, that he may see good. Keep thy tongue from evil, and thy lips from speaking guile. Depart from evil, and do good; seek peace, and pursue it." Whatever makes those who are not believers to live beyond one hundred must give believers better hope who have the quickening eternal life-giving power of the Holy Spirit residing in them.

Anastasis: The Fruit of the Spirit Antioxidant

Researchers concluded that in the right quantities, antioxidants from a range of colorful vegetables and fruits combat everything from cancer to wrinkles. They are valiant defenders that protect us from the toxic world around us by working inside our bodies. They are substances that can prevent or slow damage to cells caused by free radicals, unstable molecules that the body produces as a reaction to environmental and other pressures. Antioxidants are said to help neutralize free radicals in our bodies, and this is thought to boost overall health.

While antioxidants are great, the protective power of the fruit of the spirit is greater. The fruit of the spirit is love, joy, peace, patience, kindness, goodness, faithfulness, gentleness, and self-control. These God-nature characteristics are spiritual forces at work, much like antioxidants, so that when they are released into our lives, our youth will be renewed like the eagle's. The fruit of the spirit protects us from the effects of the evil effect of this fallen world. It defends us from the attacks of the devil, and it helps keeps us from death. Unlike natural antioxidants, we cannot obtain the fruit of the spirit from the outside, but for every believer, spiritual antioxidants effervesce within us from the wellspring of our reborn spirits. They flow like a river from the inner man.

According to *Harvard Health Publishing*, some vitamins and minerals, including vitamins C and E and the minerals copper, zinc, and selenium serve as antioxidants in addition to other vital roles. The publication defines *antioxidant* as a general term for any compound that can counteract unstable molecules called free radicals that damage DNA, cell membranes, and other parts of cells. Because free radicals lack a full complement of electrons, they steal electrons from other molecules and damage those molecules in the process. Antioxidants neutralize free radicals by giving up some of their own electrons. In making this sacrifice, they act as a natural "off" switch for the free radicals which help break a chain reaction that can affect other molecules in the cell and other cells in the body.

The publication noted that it is important to recognize that the term *antioxidant* reflects a chemical property rather than a specific nutritional property. While free radicals are damaging by their very nature, they are an inescapable part of life. The body generates free radicals in response to environmental insults, such as tobacco smoke, ultraviolet rays, and air pollution, but they are also a natural byproduct of normal processes in cells. When the immune system musters to fight intruders, for example, the oxygen it uses spins off an army of free radicals that destroy viruses, bacteria, and damaged body cells in an oxidative burst. Some normal production of free radicals also occurs during exercise. This appears to be necessary in order to induce some of the beneficial effects of regular physical activity, such as sensitizing your muscle cells to insulin.

Furthermore, the publication informs that because free radicals are so pervasive, the body needs an adequate supply of antioxidants to disarm them. The body's cells naturally produce some powerful antioxidants, such as alpha lipoic acid and glutathione. The foods one eats also supplies other antioxidants, such as vitamins C and E. Plants are full of compounds known as phytochemicals or "plant chemicals," many of which seem to have antioxidant properties as well. For example, after vitamin C has "quenched" a free radical by donating electrons to it, a phytochemical called hesperitin (found in oranges and other citrus fruits) restores the vitamin C to its active antioxidant form. Carotenoids (such as lycopene in tomatoes and lutein in kale) and flavonoids (such as flavanols in cocoa, anthocyanins in blueberries, quercetin in apples and onions, and catechins in green tea) are also antioxidants.[144]

The Bible connotes that a merry heart will do much good to our bodies, just like medicine (Prov. 17:22), and medical science agrees that it is wholesome for your well-being to be merry, relaxed, cheerful, and sanguine. It is really bad for your health to be angry, sorrowful, anxious, envious, and pessimistic.

Just as natural antioxidants and other valuable nutrients are most potent when they come from fresh foods, they have been recently connected to the plant on which they grow. The divine life within us is most potent when we are connected to Jesus Christ, our spiritual Vine. Our fruit is more robust when our fellowship with Jesus is fresh and we are staying in contact with Him by obeying His Word. We have the fruit of the spirit within us because of our union with Jesus. It is a supernatural byproduct of His divine life within us. Our fruit is more robust when our fellowship with Jesus is fresh and we are staying in contact with Him.

Medical science has connected depression to diseases such as heart disease, osteoporosis, and cancer. Joy, on the other hand, has a tremendously positive effect on your health. Stress is the number one hazard to human health today, which is why every child of God must stop stressing out and live in the peace that comes from being joined with Jesus.

The National Institutes of Health (NIH) publication explains that for years, scientists have known about the relationship between depression and heart disease, and at least a quarter of cardiac patients suffer with depression, and adults with depression often develop heart disease. NIH publication commented on the puzzle: Is depression a causal risk factor for heart disease? Is it a warning sign because depressed people engage in behaviors that increase the risks for heart disease? Is depression just a secondary event prompted by the trauma of major medical problems, such as heart surgery?

---

[144] "Understanding Antioxidants," *Harvard Health Publishing*, Harvard Medical School, Trusted Advice for a Healthier Life, Accessed June 2, 2020, https://www.health.harvard.edu/staying-healthy/understanding-antioxidants.

The publication cited the World Health Organization who documented that 350 million people suffer from depression worldwide, and 17.3 million die of heart disease each year, making it the number one global cause of death. The publication also cited Jesse Stewart who specified that thirty years of epidemiological data reveal that depression does predict the development of heart disease. In the publication, it was connoted that researchers agree that while the pathways are not completely understood, there are many likely explanations to the biology of depression, such as autonomic nervous system dysfunction, elevated cortisol levels, and elevated markers of inflammation.[145]

Any believer that the enemy wants to give an exit notice out of this world through depression, sickness, pain, and other unforeseen challenges of life must never abandon the good fight of faith and never surrender to death. Such must submit themselves to God, His Word, and resist the devil, including the spirit of death and hell, and he will flee (James 4:7). You have a covenant right of living peacefully in health on this planet Earth, serving the Lord until you are satisfied in regard to the perfect timing of the Lord who makes all things beautiful in His own time or at best until we are changed in the twinkle of an eye and caught up to meet the Lord in the air (1 Cor. 15:51–52; 1 Thess. 4:17) in good health, vitality, peace, joy, and abundant life.

David declares in Psalms 104, 4, 116:8–9, 118:17:

> Who redeemeth thy life from destruction; who crowneth thee with lovingkindness and tender mercies.
>
> For thou hast delivered my soul from death, mine eyes from tears, and my feet from falling. I will walk before the Lord in the land of the living.
>
> I shall not die, but live, and declare the works of the Lord.

---

[145] "Heart Disease and Depression: A Two-Way Relationship," National Institutes of Health—National Heart, Lung, and Blood Institute, 2017, Accessed June 2, 2020, https://www.nhlbi.nih.gov/news/2017/heart-disease-and-depression-two-way-relationship.

The Scriptures declare that the death of the righteous in one of victory and triumph. They confirm again and again that for the believer, it is not a painful end but a glorious promotion.

Psalms 116:15 declares, "Precious in the sight of the Lord is the death of his saints." The Hebrew word translated "precious" in the verse refers to an item of great worth or value such as a precious gem. It speaks of something that has honor, glory, and splendor. The word can also refer to something rare or difficult to find. Hebrew commentary chooses the definition as the most appropriate and explains it as death by divine kiss. No wonder Balaam cried out, "Let me die the death of the righteous" (Num. 23:10).

Genesis 35:8, 35:29, 49:33 state:

> Then Abraham gave up the ghost, and died in a good old age, an old man, and full of years; and was gathered to his people.
>
> And Isaac gave up the ghost, and died, and was gathered unto his people, being old and full of days: and his sons Esau and Jacob buried him.
>
> And when Jacob had made an end of commanding his sons, he gathered up his feet into the bed, and yielded up the ghost, and was gathered unto his people.

Deuteronomy 32:48–50, 34:4–7 also declare:

> And the Lord spake unto Moses that selfsame day, saying, get thee up into this mountain Abarim, unto mount Nebo, which is in the land of Moab, that is over against Jericho; and behold the land of Canaan, which I give unto the children of Israel for a possession. And die in the mount whither thou goest up, and be gathered unto thy people; as Aaron thy brother died in mount Hor, and was gathered unto his people.

> And the Lord said unto him, This is the land which I sware unto Abraham, unto Isaac, and unto Jacob, saying, I will give it unto thy seed: I have caused thee to see it with thine eyes, but thou shalt not go over thither. So Moses the servant of the Lord died there in the land of Moab, according to the word of the Lord. And he buried him in a valley in the land of Moab, over against Bethpeor: but no man knoweth of his sepulchre unto this day. And Moses was a hundred and twenty years old when he died: his eye was not dim, nor his natural force abated.

Just as Jesus Christ gave up the ghost, so we can receive His Holy Ghost through the law of giving and receiving (John 19:30). These men gave up their spirits and were gathered unto their people. They depicted how to leave this world never by demonic eviction but in a divine style. They finished out their lives, decided they were satisfied, and shrugged off their physical bodies the way you throw off an old coat. They truly cancel appointment with death.

Paul the aged (Philem. 1:9) has death under his perfect control as he declares in Philippians 1:21–24:

> For to me to live is Christ, and to die is gain. But if I live in the flesh, this is the fruit of my labour: yet what I shall choose I wot not. For I am in a strait betwixt two, having a desire to depart, and to be with Christ; which is far better. Nevertheless, to abide in the flesh is more needful for you.

Paul stated in 2 Timothy 1:10, "But is now made manifest by the appearing of our Saviour Jesus Christ, who hath abolished death, and hath brought life and immortality to light through the gospel." Like the Patriarchs who lived thousands of years before them, Peter (2 Pet. 1:13–14) and Paul (2 Tim. 4:7) knew when their missions on earth had been consummated. They sensed when it was time to go, and when the time came, they took off in victory. They stayed around until they were satisfied, and when they sensed the season had come for them to depart, they left this earth in peace and victory, and believers must check out of the earth in good old age before Jesus returns while those who live in Christ will be changed in a moment, in the twinkling of an eye and be caught up to meet the Lord in the air.

Anastasis: The Spirit that Raised Jesus Christ from the Dead

While the soul and spirit are so closely related that it is sometimes difficult to distinguish accurately between them, there seems to be only one logical conclusion, namely that "soul" and "spirit" are not the same. The Bible does make a distinction. Man is a tri-une being because he is created in the image of God. "God said, let us make man in Our image" (Gen. 1:26). We know that God is a Trinity. "The grace of the Lord Jesus Christ, and the love of God, and the communion of the Holy Ghost, be with you all. Amen" (2 Cor. 13:14). Our Lord Himself said in what we call "The Great Commission or Missio Dei," "Go ye therefore, and teach all nations, baptizing them in the name of the Father, and of the Son, and of the Holy Ghost" (Matthew 28:19).

We were created in the image of God, so man is likewise a trinity. He has a spiritual nature that is separate and distinct from the body in which it dwells. First Thessalonians 5:23 states, "I pray God your whole spirit and soul and body be preserved blameless unto the coming of our Lord Jesus Christ." And Hebrews 4:12 buttressed, "For the word of God is quick, and powerful, and sharper than any two-edged sword, piercing even to the dividing asunder of soul and spirit, and of the joints and marrow (body), and is a discerner of the thoughts and intents of the heart."

We use the "body" to touch the physical world through the five senses of sight, smell, hearing, taste, and touch. The soul is the seat of the mind, will, and emotions.

In the mind, there is the womb of memory (subconscious past), the womb of contemplation which processes the "now" (present), and imagination which deals with the future. What goes into the subconscious mind determines how one interprets life, which is the reason why we must renew our minds with the Word of God (Rom. 12:2).

The womb of memory contains, among many other things, past sins or transgression which must be cleansed by faith in the blood of Jesus Christ. David prayed to God to blot out his transgression (Ps. 51:1). He also affirms this blessedness in Psalms 32:1–2, "Blessed is he whose transgression is forgiven, whose sin is covered. Blessed is the man unto whom the Lord imputeth not iniquity, and in whose spirit, there is no guile."

The womb of contemplation is about the life we live now which must be by the living Word of God. Paul described in Galatians 2:20, "I am crucified with Christ: nevertheless I live; yet not I, but Christ liveth in me: and the life which I now live in the flesh I live by the faith of the Son of God, who loved me, and gave himself for me."

It is the life we are living now in the world by faith. Now faith is (Heb. 11:1) for the just shall live by faith (Hab. 2:4; Rom. 1:17; Gal. 3:11; Heb. 10:38). The womb of imagination is about the future, which must be impregnated with the declaration of the more sure word of prophecy (2 Pet. 1:19). We are to write the vision (Hab. 2:2) and meditate on the Word to embrace our glorious future as dictated by God's Word (Joshua 1:8; Prov. 23:7; Phil. 4:8).

The gates of the soul are imagination, conscience, memory, reason, and affections. The "Spirit" receives impressions of outward and material things through the soul. In his unfallen state the spirit of man was illuminated from heaven by the Holy Spirit, but when all the human race fell inside Adam, sin closed the window of the spirit, pulled down the curtain, and the boardroom of the spirit became a death chamber and remains so in every unregenerate heart until the life and light-giving power of the Holy Spirit through hearing and responding to God's Word floods that chamber with the life and light.

Therefore, the spirit of man, being the sphere of God-consciousness, is the inner or private office of man where the work of regeneration takes place. The Bible declares in Proverbs 20:27, "The spirit of man is the candle of the Lord, searching all the inward parts of the belly." The natural man or common sense does not have the capacity to comprehend the things of the Spirit of God, "for they are foolishness unto him; neither can he know them, because they are spiritually discerned" (1 Corinthians 2:14).

The human spirit requires the transformation that can only come by faith in God's Word through the regeneration power of Jesus Christ before there can be an understanding of the things of God. Man's spiritual nature must be renewed before there is a true conception of godly living. The only thing that stands as a watch at the door of man's spirit is his "own will," and when the will is surrendered to God, the Holy Spirit takes up His abode in the spirit of man. And when that transaction takes place, the Spirit will bear witness with your spirit that you are now a child of God (Romans 8:16).

However, to will to do God's Word might not be any difficulty, but to actually perform is the nitty-gritty. Paul described this in in Romans 7:18, "For I know that in me (that is, in my flesh,) dwelleth no good thing: for to will is present with me; but how to perform that which is good I find not." If many will yield their will to the Spirit of God, then He will renew their human spirits. This is where you start to begin to even understand God's Word. The deep things of God never will be understood by the world outside of Jesus Christ. Jesus informs us in Matthew 7:6, "Give not that which is holy unto the dogs, neither cast ye your pearls before swine."

The spirit of the unregenerate man has no more capacity to appreciate the things of God than a dog has to appreciate holy things or a hog a genuine pearl necklace. The Bible teaches that "the dog is turned to his own vomit again; and the sow that was washed to her wallowing in the mire" (2 Peter 2:22). This they did because the dog was a dog and the sow was a sow. No amount of religion or church activity can change the spirit of the unregenerate man. You cannot change the skin of an Ethiopian nor the color of the skin of a leopard (Jer. 13:23).

Anastasis: Moving from Mortality (Humanity) to Immortality (Divinity)

According to *Merriam-Webster Dictionary*, the word *immortal* means exemption from death. Paul declares in 1 Corinthians 15:19, "If in this life only we have hope in Christ, we are of all men most miserable." He also pronounced in 2 Corinthians 5:1, "We know that if our earthly house of this tabernacle were dissolved, we have a building of God, a house not made with hands, eternal in the heavens."

Salmond explained that the belief in a future life was so associated in ancient times with the Nile Valley that the Egyptians had the repute of being the first people who taught the immortality of the soul. He added that the ancient people of Egypt two thousand years before Christ firmly believed that the gods of Egypt had become a countless multitude as every hour had its special divinity. He elucidated that the papyrus rolls recovered from Egyptian tombs, the inscriptions on statues and walls, and the writing on sepulchral cases and wrappings reveal most of Egyptian doctrine of immortality.

He noted that for Egyptians, the title given to coffin in one of the oldest inscriptions is the "chest of the living" because they believed from first to last with an intense belief in the continuance of life. Salmond expounded that the persistence of life, the exchange between death and life, the thought that life must live, and that personal life here means a personal survival hereafter is a constant element of the Egyptian faith. He emphasized the Egyptian art of embalming grew out of their belief in immortality. Their conception of a future life originated the idea and construction of the pyramids, one of the wonders of the world. These huge monuments were erected because it was believed that the soul returned to the body and required an eternal abode. So the mighty pyramids and Egyptian mummies tell us of the ancient belief in a deathless soul.[146]

The immortal souls of saints and the ferocious alike have voiced a hope in life beyond the grave. Through six millenniums of human history, man has looked upon immortality as a reality. Universally believed, it is the most indestructible of all instincts and the most penetrating of all intuitions. Every man's soul is immortal and can never be annihilated. Even though the soul that sins dies to the divine but is alive to sin and hell (Ezek. 18:4). Jesus said in Matthew 10:28, "Fear not them which kill the body, but are not able to kill the soul; but rather fear him which is able to destroy both soul and body in hell."

Daniel Montgomery stated that from quixotic quests for the "fountain of youth" to pseudoscientific practices like bathing in blood or having sex with virgins, humans have had a long odd history of trying to put off death. He added that in recent decades, some have turned to a host of fanciful options from cryogenic freezing to parabiosis, which is a theoretical treatment that transfers plasma from young donors to older recipients while some leaders continue to spend billions attempting to eliminate death, and others have learned to embrace their inevitable date with the reaper as a catalyst for better living in the present.

Montgomery buttressed that Christians are right to perceive death as an enemy. However, Christ's victory on the cross tell us about how to overcome that foe. He noted that Stoicism is ultimately a form of fatalism that denies biblical teaching about God and the true nature of created reality, including life and death. He added that from skyscrapers to social networks, everything we do is an attempt to transcend our finite existence and find some scrap meaning that will last beyond the grave and that terror management theory for Christians will be problematic if it is understood sociologically as an attempt to reduce the organs of our faith to a mere revolt against mortality because the more death-conscious Christians are, the closer

---

[146] Ibid., 120–134.

they will cleave to values, systems, and behaviors that give them a sense of transcendence.[147]

Death is the last enemy that will be destroyed. There is death of the body (Heb. 9:27), there is spiritual death which the Bible refers to as "dead in trespasses and sins" (Eph. 2:1), and "alienated from the life of God" (Eph. 4:18). There is also eternal death or exile from God which 2 Thessalonians 1:9 described as punishment with everlasting destruction from the presence of the Lord (2 Thess. 1:8–9). Revelation 21:8 declares, "But the fearful, and unbelieving, and the abominable, and murderers, and whoremongers, and sorcerers, and idolaters, and all liars, shall have their part in the lake which burneth with fire and brimstone: which is the second death."

The body of our first parent, as God created him, was an immortal body created to endless existence, and their disobedience to God brought the degenerative effect of death into the body (Gen. 2:17; Rom. 5:12; Heb. 9:27). Overall, the human race, having received its natural life from Adam, hangs the sentence of death. Mortality is the curse upon our race as the result of sin. The body of man does not possess immortality by nature, but he is a mortal being that is subject to death. However, the purpose of the coming of our Lord Jesus Christ was to offer redemption to the fallen race, and the only way that man could escape the sentence of death was by "the appearing of our Lord Jesus…who only hath immortality" (1 Tim. 6:14, 16)?

The soul of man, though retaining endless existence, became morally degenerate. After the fall, his body became corruptible, and his spirit lost all relationship with God. But the immortal God became mortal and "obedient unto death" (Phil. 2:8) that He might redeem the soul of man, restore his spirit to right relationship with God, and make his body heir to incorruptibility. This is the triumph of the cross of Christ and "that through death, He might destroy him that had the power of death (that is, the devil) and deliver them who, through fear of death, were all their lifetime subject to bondage." (Heb. 2:14–15). First Corinthians 15:22 announces, "For as in Adam all die, even so in Christ shall all be made alive."

---

[147] Ibid., 74–76.

The moment the sinner accepts Jesus Christ as Lord and Savior, he receives eternal life which is the gift of God. John 3:36 and 20:31 declare:

> He that believeth on me hath everlasting life: and he that believeth not the Son shall not see life; but the wrath of God abideth on him.
>
> But these are written, that ye might believe that Jesus is the Christ, the Son of God; and that believing ye might have life through His Name.

Immediately upon the Holy Spirit's taking residence in man's spirit, the soul receives eternal life. But the body, even though it has become heir to immortality and incorruptibility, must die.

The only possibility the Christian has over his body is escaping death and the grave. At the return of Christ, we will be caught up to meet Him in the air. God, through redemption, has offered man a way out of disease, pain, and disability which is the consummation of the redemption. Paul described this in Romans 8:23, "We ourselves groan within ourselves, waiting for the adoption, to wit, the redemption of our body." Redemption is ever continuous. The redemption of the spirit is past; redemption of the soul is presently at work as we receive the engrafted Word of God; while the redemption of the body is still in the future.

All three component parts of man must be united. It can only be possible as man is restored once again to the image and likeness of God which was demonstrated when Jesus Christ, the immortal one, became mortal by His death. But death gave up in His resurrection from death and the grave to immortality, and the same is guaranteed for every redeemed child of God. As every child of first Adam dies, so will every child of the second or last Adam (Jesus Christ) be raised and never to die again. Romans 8:11 declares, "But if the Spirit of him that raised up Jesus from the dead dwell in you, he that raised up Christ from the dead shall also quicken your mortal bodies by his Spirit that dwelleth in you."

Death cannot triumph over those who are redeemed by the blood of Jesus Christ. Paul states in 1 Corinthians 15:53–54:

> For this corruptible must put on incorruption, and this mortal must put on immortality. So, when this corruptible shall have put on incorruption, and this mortal shall put on immortality, then shall be brought to pass the saying that is written, death is swallowed up in victory.

There could be no fear of death for God's children.

The biblical conception of immortality originates with man being in right relation to God, and such relationship he cannot attain by human effort. Man must acknowledge the immortal Christ as his only hope for life after death. Without the Cross of Christ, there could have been no redemption for the fallen race, and without that redemption, there can be no hope for the life that is immortal. The Lord has promised to change our vile bodies that we may be fashioned like unto His glorious body, according to the working whereby He is able even to subdue all things unto Himself (Phil. 3:20, 21). Regarding resurrection, Job 19:25–26 declares, "For I know that my Redeemer liveth, and that He shall stand at the latter day upon the earth: And though after my skin worms destroy this body, yet in my flesh shall I see God."

David was confident of a future life that he confessed in Psalm 16:9, 17:15, "My flesh also shall rest in hope…I shall be satisfied, when I awake, with Thy likeness." The human body will literarily resurrect from death and the grave, and those who have passed on out of this world are presently sleeping away from the world. Jesus said to His disciples in John 11:11–13, "Our friend Lazarus sleepeth; but I go that I may awake him out of sleep. Then said His disciples, Lord, if he sleeps, he shall do well. Howbeit Jesus spake of his death."

The martyrdom of Stephen was likened to sleeping (Acts 7:60). For as his body went to its death, earth was retroceding, but heaven's gate was approaching. He knew that he was entering into another sphere of the living. He prayed, "Lord Jesus, receive my spirit" (Acts 7:59). He did not seek to postpone death or to fight it off from his murderers. He thus remembered the words of Jesus in Luke 12:24, "Be not afraid of them that kill the body, and after that have no more that they can do."

This assurance of immortality and eternal life enable him to bear suffering, face all opposition, and die for the sake of the gospel. Paul commented of the five hundred brethren who had seen Christ alive after His resurrection that "some are fallen asleep" (1 Cor. 15:6). His comforting message to the believers at Thessalonica was, "I would not have you to be ignorant, brethren, concerning them which are asleep" (1 Thess. 4:13). The Apostle Peter, speaking of Old Testament saints, said, "The fathers fell asleep" (2 Pet. 3:4).

Moses and David were informed that they would sleep like their fathers (Deut. 31:16; 2 Sam. 12). While the body, which is the earthly tabernacle, sleeps, the spirit of the believer will depart from the body to be with Christ. Paul corroborates in Philippians 1:23, "For I am in a strait betwixt two, having a desire to depart, and to be with Christ; which is far better." The believer exchanges the vile body for the glorified body at the coming of Jesus Christ. Philippians 3:21 declares, "Who shall change our vile body, that it may be fashioned like unto his glorious body, according to the working whereby he is able even to subdue all things unto himself."

John explains further in 1 John 3:1–2:

> Behold, what manner of love the Father hath bestowed upon us, that we should be called the sons of God: therefore, the world knoweth us not, because it knew him not. Beloved, now are we the sons of God, and it doth not yet appear what we shall be: but we know that, when he shall appear, we shall be like him; for we shall see him as he is. And every man that hath this hope in him purifieth himself, even as he is pure.

Christ shall "change our vile body" (Phil. 3:21) means He will transfigure our vile body which is the same as the process of metamorphosis, a remarkable change in the form and structure of a living body. Jesus was transfigured before Peter, James, and John (Matt. 17:2). Christ's post-resurrection transfigured or metamorphosed body does not have any physical barrier. He came into the room to meet His disciples behind shut doors (John 20:19).

Biologically speaking, the change of a caterpillar into a butterfly is spoken of as "metamorphosis." The ugly, repulsive caterpillar is confined to a tomb which it spins for itself. While in the cocoon, there is an apparently dead and formless substance. But after the warm sun of spring has beaten its golden rays upon that cocoon, there comes forth a beautiful butterfly. Though the butterfly is different in appearance from the caterpillar, we recognize the beautiful winged insect as being the same as the caterpillar. It is the same living creature, yet different.

So also is the resurrection of the body. Now we have a body of humiliation or vile body as a result of the sin of Adam which degenerates the former glorious body of Adam to a sinful body. Paul declares in Romans 7:18, "For I know that in me (that is, in my flesh,) dwelleth no good thing: for to will is present with me; but how to perform that which is good I find not."

In our present bodies of humiliation, we are unfit for the glories of heaven and God's presence because flesh cannot inherit the kingdom, but we look for the Lord to turn our bodies of humiliation like unto His own glorious body at His Second Coming. This will be the same recognizable Christ but wonderfully and gloriously changed. First Corinthians 15:38 says, "But God giveth it a body as it hath pleased Him, and to every seed his own body."

Anastasis: Receiving Believers' Crown of Reward

The Judgment Seat of Christ will be a crowning day for those Christians who will receive rewards for their works (2 Cor. 5:10). Revelation 3:11, 22:12 declare:

> Behold, I come quickly: hold that fast which
> thou hast, that no man take thy crown.

> And, behold, I come quickly; and My
> reward is with Me, to give every man according
> as his work shall be.

The rewards and crowns that we receive upon meeting the Lord will be ours for all eternity as precious gifts of loving gratitude shared by the One who made it possible to earn them, Jesus Christ. These crowns are incorruptible crowns (1 Cor. 9:25–27), which is the victor's crown conferred on believers with self-discipline which is the ability to say "No" when necessary. The incorruptible crown for the Christian is the victor's crown for those who keep under the body and bring it into subjection. If an athlete must subject himself to many months of rigid discipline and training to obtain a corruptible crown, how much more should we bring our bodies into subjection for a crown that is incorruptible. Life is full of good things that take our focus off Christ, but it is imperative for us to choose appropriately.

The crown of rejoicing (1 Thess. 2:19–20) will be awarded to those who bring sinners to Christ by reaching out to others beyond reach so heaven could be their portion. It is the crown of souls winning. Every time an individual is converted, there is joy in heaven, and our hope at the Judgment Seat of Christ resides in how many souls are in heaven because of our prayers, gifts, preaching, and personal work. The crown of righteousness (2 Tim. 4:8) is for those who long for the appearing of their savior, Jesus Christ, when He comes in the heavenly cloud.

The righteous God will give it to the righteous. The crown of life (James 1:12; Rev. 2:10) is for the believer who is victorious over persecution, temptation, and sometimes martyrdom. The God of reward has prepared a martyr's crown for those who paid the precious price of their life and died proclaiming the Gospel of Christ. The crown of glory (1 Pet. 5:2–5) is for the fivefold ministers' under-shepherds, including deacons, ministry team leaders, Sunday school teachers, and everyone that servants lead. We must give ourselves without ostentation to the care of the sheep of His pasture for the crown of unfading glory from the Chief Shepherd.

There will be joy and rejoicing for those who receive the crowns as there will be sorrow, tears, and disappointments for those who will not receive them. John declares in 1 John 2:28, "And now, little children, abide in Him; that, when He shall appear, we may have confidence, and not be ashamed before Him at His coming."

Paul detailed in 1 Corinthians 3:12–15:

> Now if any man builds upon this foundation gold, silver, precious stones, wood, hay, stubble. Every man's work shall be made manifest: for the day shall declare it, because it shall be revealed by fire; and the fire shall try every man's work of what sort it is. If any man's work abides which he hath built thereupon, he shall receive a reward. If any man's work shall be burned, he shall suffer loss: but he himself shall be saved; yet so as by fire.

Colossians 3:23, 24 declares, "And whatsoever ye do, do it heartily, as to the Lord, and not unto men; knowing that of the Lord ye shall receive the reward of the inheritance: for ye serve the Lord Jesus Christ;" while Hebrews 6:10 buttressed, "For God is not unrighteous to forget your work and labour of love."

First Thessalonians 5:2 declares, "For yourselves know perfectly that the day of the Lord so cometh as a thief in the night." That is why we are to be sober and to be vigilant (1 Pet. 5:8), fully alert in our walk with God. We are not to serve God with apathy or half-hearted efforts but rather serve Him passionately. Jesus will return at any moment, like a thief in the night (2 Pet. 3:10). We are to be motivated in our service and in living holy unto God as we look forward to this day.

There is a perfect and immutable home for us where everything will echo the glory and the holiness of God (Rev. 21:1–2, 22:19), where our fellowship with God and one another will surpass anything we have known on earth. Jesus said in Matthew 8:8, "Blessed are the pure in heart; for they shall see God." We will also be in fellowship with the "innumerable company of angels, the general assembly and church of the firstborn, and to the spirits of just men made perfect" (Heb. 12:22–24). Paul speaks of "the whole family in heaven and earth" (Eph. 3:15).

Heaven is our eternal home. There shall be no more sea (Rev. 21:1), and God's will, will be done here on earth as it is in heaven (Matt. 6:10, 18:19). The earth and its fullness are the Lord's, who is the head of the body, the husband of the Church, and by virtue of our union with our husband, the head and husband of the Church, it also belongs to us (Ps. 24:1). All who go there are one family with God as their Father, but according to Paul's letter in 1 Corinthians 13:9–10, 12:

> For we know in part, and we prophesy in part. But when that which is perfect is come, then that which is in part shall be done away.
>
> For now we see through a glass, darkly; but then face to face: now I know in part; but then shall I know even as also I am known.

In regard to tasting of the powers of the world to come, Elvis Mbonye explained that man is an epitomized creation of the eternal Creator that has similar qualities, attributes, and potencies of God. He added that there is a coming age where man will live in full awareness of these attributes. However, man can have a foretaste of all these if he closes out to this present world of limitations, awakens to God, moves upward from glory to glory, and walks in the illumination within the spirit. He highlighted that the world does not know how to access the "powers of the age to come," although it has attempted to do so by increasing interest in spiritualism, psyche phenomena, and the occult in desperation for mystical powers that transcend reason.

Mbonye explicated that the stage is set for the delivery of true spirituality to the world, which is not the sense-ruled stereotype that is stripped of the supernatural. He alluded that civilization has failed to meet the full needs of man because of the failure of the type of Christianity we have offered that has resulted in a mass of humanity not knowing the real God and do not know how to find Him. He added that we are making a rediscovery of the secret of God-consciousness, which is our God-conscious level of existence in which we find transcendent powers and wisdom rising to the cognizant level that is revealing to humanity the solution to contemporary problems.[148]

There is also a *"now"* heaven for the redeemed, a present reality of enjoying the blessings of heaven, a foretaste of the glory of heaven. Hebrew 6:5 states that, "And have tasted the good word of God, and the powers of the world to come." Paul declares in Ephesians 2:6 regarding our *"now"* heavenly position in Christ Jesus, "And hath raised us up together, and made us sit together in heavenly places in Christ Jesus." For in Him we live, move, and have our being, and our lives are now hidden in Christ Jesus (Acts 17:18; Col. 3:3).

Enoch walked with God for he was not, and God took him (Gen. 5:22, 24; Heb. 11:5). Elisha was translated to heaven in a whirlwind (2 Kings 2:1, 11). Philip did not necessarily have to die or wait for the Lord's Second Coming before the Spirit of the Lord caught him up, and was in Azotus without physically walking to Azotus, travel by land, sea, nor air (Acts 8:40). We shall be also be caught up to meet the Lord in the air, just as they all tasted of the powers of the world to come. First Thessalonians 4:17 declares, "Then we which are alive and remain shall be caught up together with them in the clouds, to meet the Lord in the air: and so shall we ever be with the Lord."

Anastasis: The Swallowing up of Death by Jesus Christ

Hosea 6:1–3 states:

> Come, and let us return unto the Lord: for he hath torn, and he will heal us; he hath smitten, and he will bind us up. After two days will he revive us: in the third day he will raise us up, and

---

[148] Elvis A. Mbonye, *Tasting of the Powers of the Age to Come* (UK: Xlibris Corporation, 2012), 37.

we shall live in his sight. Then shall we know, if
we follow on to know the Lord: his going forth is
prepared as the morning; and he shall come unto
us as the rain, as the latter and former rain unto
the earth.

The Bible catalogued ten people that were raised back to life
from the dead, excluding Jesus Christ who truly resurrected without
any human agent. The New Testament reveals that there were others
who came back to life in addition to the ten individuals who are specifically named in the scriptures. The Gospel of Luke confirmed this
in Luke 7:22, declaring:

Then Jesus answering said unto them, Go
your way, and tell John what things ye have seen
and heard; how that the blind see, the lame walk,
the lepers are cleansed, the deaf hear, the dead are
raised, to the poor the gospel is preached.

Through Jesus Christ's sacrificial death, burial, and resurrection, He conquered sin forever, making it possible for all believers
to possess eternal life. The Lord has promised all believers that we
will be raised from the dead at the Second Coming of Jesus Christ,
but unbelievers will be raised unto damnation. John 5:28–29 clearly
enumerated:

Marvel not at this: for the hour is coming,
in the which all that are in the graves shall hear
his voice. And shall come forth; they that have
done good, unto the resurrection of life; and
they that have done evil, unto the resurrection of
damnation.

When the hand of the Lord rested upon Ezekiel, he was carried
by the spirit of the Lord into the valley that was full of bones that
were very dry and disjointed. Prophet Ezekiel was commanded by

the Lord to prophesy specifically unto the dry bones because they shall live. He was not supposed to speak to God but to the dry bones. The prophecy brought forth a noise, then a shaking followed by bone coming to bone. Sinews and flesh appeared on them and were all covered with skin, but there was no breath in them. The prophet was commanded again to prophesy unto the four winds of heaven to breath upon the slain, and he did, and they lived and appeared as an exceeding great army (Ezek. 37:1–14).

In this same resurrection vein, these ten individuals were raised back to life after being dead but to die again. However, Jesus's resurrection was entirely different in that He was the only one who actually resurrected and is never to die again. His name is called "The Resurrection and the Life." Jesus was not raised by any prophet or any human being but by the Holy Spirit of God. Romans 8:11 implies, "But if the Spirit of him that raised up Jesus from the dead dwell in you, he that raised up Christ from the dead shall also quicken your mortal bodies by his Spirit that dwelleth in you."

The widow of Zarephath's son was raised by Elijah. While the Lord sent the prophet to the home of the widow which was a pagan city, unexpectedly, the woman's son grew sick and died. She had thought that Elijah had come to bring God's wrath on her for her sin. However, Elijah carried the boy into the loft and laid him on the bed and stretched himself out on the body of the boy three times. He cried out to God for the boy's life to return. God heard Elijah's prayers, and the child's life came back, and Elijah carried him downstairs. The woman declared, "Now by this I know that thou art a man of God, and that the word of the Lord in thy mouth is truth" (1 Kings 17:17–24).

The Shunammite woman's son was raised by Elisha. He was Elijah's spiritual protégé who had received the double anointing that was on Elijah. The Shunamite woman and her husband built an upper room for Elisha in tehri house in Shunem, and he prayed for the woman who had been barren to have a son. Several years later, the boy complained of a pain in the head and then died (1 Kings 17:17–24). The woman raced to Mount Carmel to meet Elisha who sent his servant ahead with his staff, but the boy did not respond.

Finally, Elisha went to the room that the couple bult for him where they lay the boy, and he stretched himself on the dead boy who they laid on the bed they had provided Elisha as He cried out to the Lord with his mouth to the mouth of the dead boy, eyes to eyes, hands to hands. The boy's body grew warm, then he sneezed seven times and opened his eyes. When Elisha presented the boy back to his mother, she fell and bowed to the ground (2 Kings 4:18–37).

The Israelite man who was about to be buried was hurriedly thrown into the tomb where Elisha had been buried. This happened as the Moabite raiders attacked Israel, thereby interrupting a funeral. But as soon as the body of the Israelite man touched Elisha's bones, the dead man came to life and stood up on his feet. This miracle was a foreshadowing of how Christ's death and resurrection turned the grave into the passageway to new life (2 Kings 13:20–21).

The widow of Nain's son was raised to life at the funeral procession at the town gate of the village of Nain. Jesus and his disciples met the procession where mourners were sorrowfully crying because the boy was the only son of this widow. When Jesus saw her, he had compassion on her and touched the platform that held the body and then spoke to the body of the young man to get up. The son sat up and began talking, and all the people were astounded. Praising God, they hollered:

> And there came a fear on all: and they glorified God, saying, that a great prophet is risen up among us; and, That God hath visited his people. And this rumour of him went forth throughout all Judaea, and throughout all the region round about. (Luke 7:11–17)

Jairus's twelve-year-old daughter had been sick. Jairus was a leader in the synagogue and had begged Jesus, who was in Capernaum, to come to him to heal the daughter, but while Jesus was on the way, a messenger said not to bother Jesus anymore because the girl had died. But Jesus said to Jairus, "Don't be afraid; only believe, and your daughter will be healed." On arrival at the house, Jesus told the mourners that the girl was not dead but only sleeping. Immediately, they laughed him to scorn, and Jesus put them all out of the room and took the girl by her hand, saying, "Maid, arise."

Immediately her spirit returned, and she was raised up to life again. Jesus ordered her parents to give her food to eat but not to tell anyone what had happened (Luke 8:49–56).

Lazarus of Bethany was one of the family of three that were very close to Jesus. The names of his sisters were Martha and Mary. They had informed Jesus Christ that Lazarus was sick, and interestingly, Jesus stayed back two more days where he was. Jesus told his disciples that Lazarus was sleeping but later told them he had died. When he and his disciples finally arrived at Bethany, Lazarus had been in the tomb for four days. Martha met them outside the village where Jesus told her, "Your brother will rise again. I am the resurrection and the life." They approached the tomb where Jesus wept, and afterward, he instructed that they should remove the stone of the tomb where they laid him away. After giving thanks to God, He commanded Lazarus to come forth, and he came out instantly and walked out wrapped in burial cloths. He commanded that they should lose him and let him go (John 11:1–44).

After Jesus Christ died on the cross, there was an earthquake that opened up many graves and tombs in Jerusalem. This happened after Jesus resurrected (anastasis) from the dead. The saints in Jerusalem who had died earlier were raised back to life and appeared to many in the city. Matthew is imprecise in his Gospel about how many rose and what happened to them afterward. Bible scholars believe they rose from the dead but waited for the resurrection of Jesus Christ to be able to go to the holy Jerusalem, then to the Jerusalem that will come down from heaven. The first proposition is that if they were saints, they must have possessed the Holy Spirit.

David acknowledged the presence of the Holy Spirit in his life (Ps. 51:11) and pleaded with God not to take it away, meaning these saints would have already witnessed being "caught up" unto glory, and maybe the elders who John saw in the book of Revelation were some of these saints.

The second proposition is that it maybe they went back to their homes where many acquaintances saw them, and this would be a startling experience for their relatives and friends, and maybe they eventually died again, and their families buried them again along with all the other saints who died. They also await in their graves the resurrection to a new spirit life of glory (Matt. 27:50–54).

Tabitha or Dorcas was a woman that everyone loved in the city of Joppa. She was always doing good, helping the poor, and making garments for others. But one day, Tabitha, whose Greek name was Dorcas (Greek), became sick and died. Women washed her body and then placed her corpse in the room on the upstairs. Afterward, they sent for Apostle Peter who was in the nearby town, Lydda. Clearing everyone from the room, Peter fell to his knees and prayed and said to her, "Tabitha, get up." She sat up, and Peter gave her to her friends, alive. News spread like wildfire. Many people believed in Jesus because of it (Acts 9:36–42).

Paul was raised from the dead after being stoned in the city of Lystra. After Paul and Barnabas arrived in Iconium, they were able to preach the Gospel to a great multitude both of the Jews and also Greeks who believed the Lord, but they had a problem with the unbelieving Jews who stirred up riots and assaults among the Gentiles against these two apostles and created a division among the people. Therefore, Paul and Barnabas fled to Lystra and Derbe, cities of Lycaonia, and healed an impotent man after receiving faith to be healed from hearing God's Word.

In the speech of Lycaonia, the people lifted up their voices after seeing this miracle and said, "The gods are come down to us in the likeness of men." However, certain Jews from Antioch and Iconium came over and persuaded the people to stone Paul, and after drawing him out of the city, assuming that he had been dead, with the disciples standing all around him, he rose up and came into the city and the next day departed with Barnabas to Derbe (Acts 14:1–20).

It was assumed that at this time when Paul died, he was caught up to the third heaven which he referred to as paradise (2 Cor. 12:1–4). The second letter of Paul to the Corinthians stated, "Are they ministers of Christ? (I speak as a fool) I am more; in labours more abundant, in stripes above measure, in prisons more frequent, in deaths oft."

In this experience, Apostle Paul enters immediately into heaven and was at home with the Lord. We Christians are citizens of heaven. Philippians 3:20 declares, "For our conversation is in heaven; from whence also we look for the Saviour, the Lord Jesus Christ;" while Hebrews 3:1 affirms that we have become "partakers of the heavenly calling."

Eutychus was in a packed third-story room in Troas. The hour was late. Many oil lamps made the quarters warm, and the Apostle Paul was preaching for a very long time. While sitting on a windowsill, Eutychus dozed off and fell out of the window and was pronounced dead. Paul the preacher rushed outside and threw himself on the lifeless body just like Elijah and Elisha had done in the Old Testament. Paul went back upstairs, broke bread, and ate and preached for a long while, even till daybreak, and departed while Eutychus came back to life, and the people were comforted and took him home alive (Acts 20:7–12).

In all of these ten different encounters, Jesus Christ stood out in that He had no human instrumentality to raise him up to life as in the case of the son of the widow of Zarephath, the Shunammite woman's son, the widow of Nain's son, Eutychus, or Tabitha or Dorcas. There was no bone of Elisha that raised Jesus, and Jesus Himself had raised Jairus's twelve-year-old daughter, Lazarus of Bethany, and there were no disciples that surrounded Jesus as in the case of Paul. There was no human being that died and then produced tremors that would cause the dead body of Jesus to resurrect as in the case of many whose graves and tombs were opened in Jerusalem.

Several men conspired to murder Jesus Christ. After a mock trial, he was scourged and taken to Golgotha Hill outside Jerusalem where Roman soldiers nailed him to a cross. But it was all part of God's plan of salvation for humanity. After Jesus died, his lifeless body was placed in the tomb of Joseph of Arimathea where a seal was attached. Soldiers guarded the place, but on the third day, without any man to roll away the stone as in the case of Lazarus, the angel of the Lord came down in an earthquake to roll away the stone from the door and sat upon it. Mary Magdalene and others thus had access into the tomb that they found empty (Matt. 28:2).

The angel said Jesus had resurrected from the dead. He appeared first to Mary Magdalene, then to His apostles, and then to many others around the city (Matt. 28:1–20; Mark 16:1–20; Luke 24:1–49; John 20:1–21:25).

Matthew 28:5–10 declares:

> And the angel answered and said unto the women, Fear not ye: for I know that ye seek Jesus, which was crucified. He is not here: for he is risen, as he said. Come, see the place where the Lord lay. And go quickly and tell his disciples that he is risen from the dead; and, behold, he goeth before you into Galilee; there shall ye see him: lo, I have told you. And they departed quickly from the sepulcher with fear and great joy; and did run to bring his disciples word. And as they went to tell his disciples, behold, Jesus met them, saying, All hail. And they came and held him by the feet and worshipped him. Then said Jesus unto them, Be not afraid: go tell my brethren that they go into Galilee, and there shall they see me.

Revelation 20:4–5 states:

> And I saw thrones, and they sat upon them, and judgment was given unto them: and I saw the souls of them that were beheaded for the witness of Jesus, and for the word of God, and which had not worshipped the beast, neither his image, neither had received his mark upon their foreheads, or in their hands; and they lived and reigned with Christ a thousand years…this is the first resurrection.

The key word here is *first*—the *first* resurrection. The Greek word used here is *protos* and literally means "first" or "foremost;" that is, foremost in reference to time, place, order, or importance. It also implies that there are other orders to follow, but this is first and distinctive in its resolve. While others can follow in due time, they can never have that special honor and purpose of being the first to be born.

There is going to be a physical resurrection, and our bodies will get back up from their dissolution and the grave, just by observing the pattern of Jesus Christ and how He resurrected from the dead. Jesus Christ is our original blueprint of the first resurrection. He is the prime example, the forerunner, the pattern of our redemption and destiny. That is why all of God's saints will experience this same resurrection into glory as exemplified in those Old Testament saints' dead bodies in the grave that were raised back to life.

Matthew 27:52–53 accounts that "the graves were opened, and many bodies of the saints which slept arose, and came out of the graves after His resurrection, and went into the holy city, and appeared unto many." This historical and undeniable event occurred because of the resurrection of Jesus Christ. Dead bodies literally arose and walked out of their tombs at the resurrection of Jesus Christ, and they were seen by many according to that scripture to confirm that there would be a first resurrection experience.

Practically, resurrection always happened after death, and the first person that death was introduced to was Adam in the garden. Genesis 2:17 stated, "But of the tree of the knowledge of good and evil, thou shalt not eat of it, for in the day that thou eatest thereof thou shalt surely die."

The Lord had said in Ezekiel 18:4, 20, "Behold, all souls are mine; as the soul of the father, so also the soul of the son is mine: the soul that sinneth, it shall die… The soul that sinneth, it shall die."

Adam and Eve's souls literally died immediately. They disobeyed God by eating from the forbidden tree. His soul died to God who is Spirit. His soul died to God who is the way, the truth, and the life. His soul died to God who is our righteousness. His soul died to God who is our healer. His soul died to God is the Most High, and Adam became the "most low" or the lowest. His soul died to God who is Holy and just in all of His ways. Ephesians 2:1 attested, "And you hath he quickened, who were dead in trespasses and sins." Likewise, Colossians 2:13, "And you, being dead in your sins and the uncircumcision of your flesh, hath he quickened together with him, having forgiven you all trespasses."

Jesus Christ said, "Let the dead bury the dead" (Matt. 8:22), meaning anyone that is not saved is living but dead, and these dead (who are living) are dead souls. Apostle John said, "He that have the Son have life, and he that does not have the Son of God does not have life" (1 John 5:12).

Jesus Christ makes it clear in John 3:36, "He that believeth on the Son hath everlasting life: and he that believeth not the Son shall not see life; but the wrath of God abideth on him."

Revelation 3:1 stated, "Thou hast a name that thou livest and art dead." Likewise, 1 Timothy 5:6, James 5:20, and 1 John 3:14, respectively, "She that liveth in pleasure, is dead while she liveth… shall save a soul from death…He that loveth not his brother abideth in death."

There are still many that though they have experienced the salvation of their spirit, they are yet to experience the regeneration of their soul; thus, their soul is still dead. After our spirit has been saved, the soul must be fully redeemed, transformed, and raised up to live in His sight, for that is the first resurrection. The body, on the other hand, cannot be changed until "the thousand years are finished," and this literarily means until the day of the Lord in our lives is consummated and has totally done its work in us.

The Lord will surely perfect everything that concerns us. Jesus declares in Luke 13:32, "And he said unto them, go ye, and tell that fox, Behold, I cast out devils, and I do cures today and tomorrow, and the third day I shall be perfected." We are thoroughly being made alive as a new people, conformed to His image through obedience to God's Word, because we have risen in newness of life and are seeking those things which are above where Christ sits at the right hand of God, therefore experiencing the first resurrection.

Paul's desire was to know Jesus Christ and the power of His resurrection and the fellowship of His suffering being made conformable unto His death. First Corinthians 1:24 declares that, "Christ is the power of God." That Christ, who is the power of God, even the power of His resurrection has made new men and women of tens of millions. He has turned them right around and set their faces toward God. This is impossible with men and all of his doctrines and denominational walls, but it is now made possible by the resurrection power of God.

The four key victories of the battles of Alexander the Great, which include the battle of the Granicus (May 334 BC), the battle of Issus (November 5, 333 BC), the battle of Gaugamela (October 1, 331 BC), the Battle of the Persian gate (January 330 BC),[149] and the eight battles of Julius Caesar and the tribal leaders of Gaul (modern-day France), which include the battle of Bibracte, battle of Vosges, battle of the Sabis River, battle of Morbihan Gulf, the Gallic Wars, battle at Gergovia, battle at Lutetia Parisiorum, and the battle at Alesia where most of these battles were won by the Romans under Julius Caesar,[150] including Napoleon Bonaparte's sixty battles where he lost only seven.[151] the Napoleonic Wars spanning through a period of twelve years comprising several major conflicts with Napoleon Bonaparte militaristically emboldened the French Empire and various coalitions of European allies, a period marked by relentless war and the emergence of large-scale gun use that led to some of history's bloodiest military confrontations.

---

[149] Tristan Hughes, "The 4 Key Victories of Alexander the Great's Persian Campaign," HistoryHit, 2018, Accessed June 11, 2020, https://www.historyhit.com/key-victories-of-alexander-the-greats-persian-campaign/.

[150] N. S. Gill, "Winners and Losers of Julius Caesar's Gallic War Battles. The Battle Near Dijon and the Battle of Bibracte Make this List," ThoughtCo, 2019, Accessed June 11, 2020, https://www.thoughtco.com/caesars-gallic-war-the-battles-117531.

[151] HistoryExtra, "Napoleon Bonaparte's Greatest Triumphs and Disasters," *BBC History Magazine, BBC History Revealed*, and *BBC World Histories Magazine*, 2017, Accessed June 11, 2020, https://www.historyextra.com/period/georgian/napoleon-greatest-battle-triumph-disaster-victory-defeat/.

Battles such as the Pyramids (July 21, 1798), the battle of Marengo (June 14, 1800), the battle of Trafalgar (October 21, 1805), the battle of Austerlitz (December 2, 1805), the battle of Jena-Auerstädt (October 14, 1806), the battle of Rolica (August 17, 1808), the battle of Borodino (September 7, 1812), the battle of Leipzig (October 16–19, 1813), the battle of Ligny (June 16, 1815), and the battle of Waterloo (June 18, 1815), Napoleon's final battle,-[152]can never be compared to battle of Jesus Christ over death and hell manifested through His resurrection power.

The military power of these men could reduce men to feigned submission, but it could not access the inner nature and change the secret heart and will and soul. This is what Jesus Christ has done for us over and over again. Have you ever tried to reform any soul held in the grasp of some aberration, obsession, or sin? Intention after intention, you urge the damage he is doing to himself, his self-respect, public opinion, the love of friends and family, his place in this world or the next, all in futility. For a moment, the hopeless sinful feet make a subtle battle to lift themselves out of the mire and then sink back deeper. A sense of hopelessness and despondency comes over you, and you feel as if no good thing can ever come out of you.

But through an encounter with Jesus Christ of Nazareth, you receive a new heart, a new will, and a new mind and you become a new creation as you become transformed gradually to the image and likeness of Jesus Christ.

To shatter a man's defiance, to reverse his will, to turn the tides of his heart of which the Lord said it's evil and desperately wicked, to reprogram and reedit his mind; to sterilize his emotions and desires; to make him love what formerly he hated as in loving righteousness and hating iniquity; to set his soul triumphantly grander to sin, feebleness, sorrow and death; to translate him into the kingdom of the

---

[152] Harry Atkins, "10 Key Battles in the Napoleonic Wars," HistoryHit, 2019, Accessed June 11, 2020, https://www.historyhit.com/key-battles-in-the-napoleonic-wars/.

Son and position his seating in the heavenly places; to make him an intrepid son of the Most High with a calling to glory and virtue—whosoever can work these transformations in the life of that man is sturdy beyond all that the mighty of the earth can ever fabricate. This is what our Lord Jesus Christ has done for us, and He is still doing it up till today, and He shall reign until all enemies are under His feet (Heb. 1:13, 10:13).

We are to follow Jesus's footsteps of resurrection as His brethren. This is because as the father has sent Jesus, so has He sent us (John 17:18, 20:21), and since we abide in Him, we are to walk even as He walked (1 John 2:6). Hebrews 2:11 declares, "For both he that sanctifieth and they who are sanctified are all of one: for which cause he is not ashamed to call them brethren."

David declares in Psalms 23, "He restoreth my soul," and this is what God is doing in the first resurrection. He is presently restoring our souls. This is the power of His resurrection that Paul was referring to in Philippians 3:10 in the Amplified version:

> And this, so that I may know Him (experientially, becoming more thoroughly acquainted with Him, understanding the remarkable wonders of His Person more completely) and (in that same way experience) the power of His resurrection (which overflows and is active in believers), and (that I may share) the fellowship of His sufferings, by being continually conformed (inwardly into His likeness even) to His death (dying as He did).

This first resurrection is made available to all of us in this present time. This first resurrection breaks every appointment with death and destroys the fangs of COVID-19 and other future pandemics. Jesus Christ was resurrected, never to die again. He is alive forever more, and because He lives, we shall live also. Jesus said in the Gospel of John 10:17–18, 14:19:

> Therefore doth my Father love me, because I lay down my life, that I might take it again. No man taketh it from me, but I lay it down of myself. I have power to lay it down, and I have power to take it again. This commandment have I received of my Father.
>
> Yet a little while, and the world seeth me no more; but ye see me: because I live, ye shall live also.

CHAPTER 9

COVID-19 Testimonies

Experts have warned that there is no such thing as 100 percent precision, effectiveness, and reliability of missile defense systems due to human errors or other factors. God's divine missile defense system is the only one that is 100 percent sure and can never miss the target because He is our faithful creator. He is a man of war that can never lose a battle or miss His target. The defensive mighty power of God's divine missile defense system is matchless, and it is domiciled in His Word.

Edward and Kelly Mrkvicka cited C. H. Spurgeon who described God's power as God Himself who is self-existent, self-sustained, which the mightiest men cannot add so much as a shadow of increased power to the omnipotent one. He added that God sits on no buttressed throne and leans on no assisting arm. His court is not maintained by the courtier nor does it borrow its splendor from His creatures. Spurgeon described God's power as God Himself, the great central source and originator of all power.[153]

Testimonies of Eternal Life

At this junction, the questions you want to ask yourself are, can Christ the power of God make you live? Has He made you survive

---

[153] Edward F. Mrkvicka, Jr. and Kelly H. Mrkvicka, *The Plot to Kill God* (Denver: Outskirts Press, Inc, 2015), 26.

the COVID-19 pandemic? And is He able to keep you during the next coronavirus wave or other pandemics? Are you ready to live? Do you want to fulfill your days? Can He help you to cancel every appointment you have with death? Revelation 1:18 declares, "I am he that liveth, and was dead; and, behold, I am alive for evermore, Amen; and have the keys of hell and of death."

Paul asked in 1 Corinthians 15:55, "O death, where is thy sting? O grave, where is thy victory?"

Death is an enemy and the last enemy (1 Cor. 15:26) that must be destroyed by the end-time or last days army of God. The Church is the invisible body of Christ, and Jesus is the head of that body. Paul admonishes the Colossian church for not holding fast to the head. The head nourishes and supports the whole body through the joints and ligaments, and it grows the way God wants it to grow (Col. 2: 19). The last part of the body of Christ is the feet. How beautiful are the feet of them that preach the gospel of peace and bring the glad tidings of good tidings (Rom. 10: 15)? There is a feet church that is practically involved in soul-winning who will place all enemies, including death the last enemy under their feet victoriously before the second return of our Lord Jesus Christ. Ephesians 1:22 declares, "And hath put all things under his feet, and gave him to be the head over all things to the church."

All enemies, including death, the last enemy, must be placed under the feet of the Church or generation, the last days army of God. The Bible advocated in 1 Corinthians 15:25, 27 and Hebrews 2:8:

> For he must reign, till he hath put all ene-
> mies under his feet.
> For he hath put all things under his feet.
> But when he saith all things are put under him, it
> is manifest that he is excepted, which did put all
> things under him.
> Thou hast put all things in subjection under
> his feet. For in that he put all in subjection under
> him, he left nothing that is not put under him.
> But now we see not yet all things put under him.

Satan formerly had the power of death. But Jesus "through death, destroyed him that had the power of death, and that is the devil." And now Satan, the devil, the adversary, the accuser of the brethren, and that old serpent is under your feet. That means the power of death is among the powers of the devil you have been covenanted to trample under your feet. Jesus said in Luke 10:19, "Behold, I give unto you power to tread on serpents and scorpions, and over all the power of the enemy: and nothing shall by any means hurt you."

Command and speak to every power of hell in your life that they no longer have power over you, because Satan, their master, is under your feet. Say, "Death, you have no more power to hurt me. God has empowered me to trample you under my feet. He has empowered me by His Word and by His Holy Spirit to trample you under my feet. You cannot have me and my household. COVID-19, you cannot hurt me anymore or kill me because I am of God, and I have overcome you. The greater one is in me, so you must bow to the words of Jesus coming forth out of my mouth. You must bow to my will and authority, in Jesus Christ's name."

A very long life is not a special privilege. It is a common covenant right. It is not a gift but a choice. What joy it would be for you to reach the age of 120 and see your children's children even to the fourth generation. It is wisdom to partake of all that the Lord has packaged for you.

Proverbs 3:13–18 states:

> Happy is the man that findeth wisdom, and the man that getteth understanding. For the merchandise of it is better than the merchandise of silver, and the gain thereof than fine gold. She is more precious than rubies: and all the things thou canst desire are not to be compared unto her. Length of days is in her right hand; and in her left-hand riches and honour. Her ways are ways of pleasantness, and all her paths are peace. She is a tree of life to them that lay hold upon her: and happy is everyone that retaineth her.

Death was swallowed up in victory about two thousand years ago. All you need to walk in that victory now is enlightenment. Death is not your friend; it is an enemy.

Our security is in the secrets of God. Every kingdom secret guarantees earthly security. Every light from heaven shatters darkness on the earth. You are not created to die like men, nor were you born to fall like one of the princes. You are different from others. You are "a peculiar people." You are not meant to die like a beast or have a burial like that of an ass.

Psalms 82:6–7 declares, "I have said, Ye are gods; and all of you are children of the Most High. But ye shall die like men and fall like one of the princes."

Psalms 49:12, 20 state, "Nevertheless man being in honour abideth not: he is like the beasts that perish… Man that is in honour, and understandeth not, is like the beasts that perish."

Jeremiah 22:19 added, "He shall be buried with the burial of an ass, drawn and cast forth beyond the gates of Jerusalem."

As earlier stated, Jesus Christ now has the keys of death and the grave; they are no longer with Satan. He is no more in charge. Legally, he lost the battle two thousand years ago. Jesus demonstrated the defeat in an open show. He went down, the graves opened, and then the dead saints came out and walked on the streets of Jerusalem. Colossians 2:15 puts it this way, "And having spoiled principalities and powers, he made a show of them openly, triumphing over them in it."

Satan has lost the power to kill. He lost it two thousand years ago. You no longer need to live at his mercy if you are a child of God. Jesus has the keys and will not use it against you.

God is a covenant-keeping God who kept His covenant of long life with the patriarchs of old. We are of the bloodline of Abraham through Christ Jesus. Galatians 3:29 states, "And if ye be Christ's, then are ye Abraham's seed, and heirs according to the promise."

If the Lord could give these patriarchs long life as well as perfect health, then you too can live long and in perfect health. The Lord has designed a very long life for you that coronavirus or any other pandemic, disease, or sickness cannot terminate as long as you fulfill your part of the covenant. The lines have fallen, and the enemy has no power to terminate it, so long as you do what you're expected to do. Surely, the lines are fallen unto us in pleasant places, and yes, we all have a goodly heritage (Ps. 16:6). If you are a child of the Almighty God, you do have a goodly heritage.

The Testimony of Abraham

Jeremiah 6:16 stated that, "Thus saith the Lord, stand ye in the ways, and see, and ask for the old paths, where is the good way, and walk therein, and ye shall find rest for your souls."

The Lord had promised Abraham that he would go to his fathers in peace and be buried in a good old age (Gen. 15:15). Did God fulfill His promise? Let us consider the age of Abraham from the scriptures. Genesis 25:7–8 declares, "And these are the days of the years of Abraham's life which he lived, a hundred threescore and fifteen years. Then Abraham gave up the ghost, and died in a good old age, an old man, and full of years; and was gathered to his people."

Why are you contemplating death at the age of seventy while Abraham was 175 years old at his death? Your appointment with death is hereby cancelled as you belief the truth in Jesus Christ's name.

The Testimony of Isaac

Genesis 35:28 states, "And the days of Isaac were a hundred and four score years. And Isaac gave up the ghost, and died, and was gathered unto his people, being old and full of days: and his sons Esau and Jacob buried him."

Isaac was 180 years old when he was gathered unto his people. The Bible did not specifically say that they died but that they were gathered unto their people.

The Bible declares in Galatians 4:28, "Now we, brethren, as Isaac was, are the children of promise." So we are partakers of Isaac's blessings, promises, and heritage. We are the present-day Isaacs.

The Testimony of Jacob

Genesis 47:28 declares regarding Jacob, "And Jacob lived in the land of Egypt seventeen years: so the whole age of Jacob was an hundred forty and seven years." At the age of 130, he still rode on a chariot to Egypt from the land of Canaan (Gen. 47:9). The God of Abraham, Isaac, and Jacob is still alive. Therefore, you have no reason to allow Satan that is under your feet to terminate your life abruptly from this earth. These are the days when those who will not be caught up with Jesus but exit this earth to heaven, the abode of Jesus, will say like Simeon (his name means the one who has ears to hear) who the Lord said will never taste death until he had seen the Lord Christ, "Now thou thy servant depart in peace" (Luke 2:25–30).

The Testimony of Joseph

Genesis 50:26 accounted, "So Joseph died, being an hundred and ten years old: and they embalmed him, and he was put in a coffin in Egypt."

The Testimony of Moses

Deuteronomy 34:7 declares, "And Moses was an hundred and twenty years old when he died: his eye was not dim, nor his natural force abated." But to prove that God is the God of the living and not the dead, Moses showed up in the mountain of transfiguration alongside with Elijah with our transfigured Lord, Jesus Christ (Mark 9:1–4).

Jesus made it clear in Matthew 22:31–33:

> But as touching the resurrection of the dead, have ye not read that which was spoken unto you by God, saying, I am the God of Abraham, and the God of Isaac, and the God of Jacob? God is not the God of the dead, but of the living. And when the multitude heard this, they were astonished at his doctrine.

The Testimony of Joshua

The book of Joshua 24:29 declares, "And it came to pass after these things, that Joshua the son of Nun, the servant of the Lord, died, being an hundred and ten years old."

We serve a covenant-keeping God. Jeremiah 33:20–21 likens the covenant keeping power of God in this way:

> If ye can break my covenant of the day, and my covenant of the night, and that there should not be day and night in their season. Then may also my covenant be broken with David my servant, that he should not have a son to reign upon his throne; and with the Levites the priests, my ministers.

Joshua departed at 110 years, and we are the last days Joshua generation. All our covenant fathers lived very long on earth because they were kept by God.

First Peter 1:5 declares, "[W]ho are kept by the power of God through faith unto salvation ready to be revealed in the last time."

The Testimonies during COVID-19 Pandemic

God is the only one that receives all the glory and honor regarding few of the miracles and testimonies that are catalogued in this book. Space will not permit us to detail the rest. There is no iota of glory that is credited to man but only to our wonder-working God, Jesus Christ. He is the same yesterday, today and forever (Heb. 13:8). I join my voice to declare Psalms 115:1 here that, "Not unto us, O Lord, not unto us, but unto thy name give glory, for thy mercy, and for thy truth's sake."

Anytime anyone receives the Word that God sent through His sent servant/son and acts on it, they are healed and delivered from their destructions, and we call these miracles (Ps. 107:20). Additionally, only God can confirm the sent Word. Mark 16:20 declares, "And they went forth, and preached everywhere, the Lord working with them, and confirming the word with signs following. Amen."

When God's servant declares God's Word, it will turn to testimony to those who receive it. The anointing of God must rest on the anointed. To preserve the human instrument that God used for the miracle, we must acknowledge God for every minute miracle. The Lord will never share His glory with no individual, group, or race. The one leper that returned to glorify God for His healing was made whole, and we know Jesus asked for the remaining nine.

Every testimony written in this book and the ones that are not written are accredited to God and God alone. We must be intentional about giving God all the thanksgiving, praise, and worship.

Luke 17:17–19 explains, "And Jesus answering said, were there not ten cleansed? but where are the nine. There are not found that returned to give glory to God, save this stranger. And he said unto him, Arise, go thy way: thy faith hath made thee whole."

These testimonies are pointers for you to believe that the same God who did the same for these individuals will also do it for you. The Scriptu3res declare in Revelation 12:11, "And they overcame him by the blood of the Lamb, and by the word of their testimony;

and they loved not their lives unto the death." David declares about God's testimonies in his lives in Psalms 119:24, 31, 46, 95, 111:

> Thy testimonies also are my delight and my counselors.
> I have stuck unto thy testimonies: O Lord, put me not to shame.
> I will speak of thy testimonies also before kings, and will not be ashamed.
> The wicked have waited for me to destroy me: but I will consider thy testimonies.
> Thy testimonies have I taken as an heritage forever: for they are the rejoicing of my heart.

The Testimony of Undefeated Lion during COVID-19

You are redeemed and anointed to go well in life. You are not permitted to go slow or grow weak or be defeated by COVID-19 or any other pandemic. The Bible says in Proverbs 30:29–30, "There be three things which go well, yea, four are comely in going. A lion which is strongest among beasts, and turneth not away for any."

Jesus Christ of Nazareth is not only the lamb that was slain for our sins, He is also a courageous lion. His spiritual weapon of mass destruction never misses the target. He also has lion-like children, for as He is, so are we in the world (1 John 4:17). As the Father has sent us, so has Jesus Christ sent us (John 17:18, 20:21). First John 3:1–2 declares:

> Behold, what manner of love the Father hath bestowed upon us, that we should be called the sons of God: therefore, the world knoweth us not, because it knew him not. Beloved, now are we the sons of God, and it doth not yet appear what we shall be: but we know that, when he shall appear, we shall be like him; for we shall see him as he is.

There is an undefeatable lion nature in you that is bold (Prov. 28:1). That lion-like nature makes you walk in confidence, dares anything, and is never afraid. It makes you to be unstoppable and a risk-taker. The lion believes any animal is food for him and considers that any opportunity is worth giving a trial and never lets it slip from its hands. Jesus Christ, the lion of the tribe of Judah, lives in you. He is Lord over the church of God. He is the head of the church of God, and we are His body.

The elephant might be the biggest in the jungle, the giraffe might be the tallest, the fox might be the wisest and the cheetah the fastest; no one can assume the position of the lion as the king of the jungle, even without any of these abilities. You might not be the fastest, the wisest, the smartest, or the most brilliant—all you need is courage of a lion. God commanded Joshua to be courageous.

Joshua 1:6, 7, 9 advocates:

> Be strong and of a good courage: for unto this people shalt thou divide for an inheritance the land, which I sware unto their fathers.
>
> Only be thou strong and very courageous.
>
> Have not I commanded thee? Be strong and of a good courage; be not afraid, neither be thou dismayed: for the Lord thy God is with thee whithersoever thou goest.

You need the "will" to try, step out, and step forward and believe the Lord. Imagine, male lions sleep an average of twenty hours per day. The females, on the other hand, do all of the really hard work of killing the prey, which the males then appropriate for themselves. The main danger males face is fighting off other males that want to take over their pride and territory. The females get about sixteen to nineteen hours of shuteye. The lionesses spend more time hunting and taking care of cubs, which is why they get slightly less sleep. And following a large meal, lions may even sleep up to twenty-four hours.

You do not necessarily have to be huge to be a champion, a winner, a redeemer, a remnant of God, or an overcomer over COVID-19, sicknesses, and diseases. Imagine the elephant that works for twenty hours and only eats grass. Wild elephants sleep at night for an average of two hours, making them the lightest-known snoozers of any mammal. Those in captivity spend much of their time asleep lying down, but they also sometimes sleep standing. Your life's strategy matters most in your approach to circumstances and situations for you to be a champion or winner always, especially over pandemics. You must begin to manifest your lion-like nature against coronavirus and all other sickness and disease. The wisdom of rest makes the lion rejuvenate.

Exodus 31:16–17 declares:

> Wherefore the children of Israel shall keep the sabbath, to observe the sabbath throughout their generations, for a perpetual covenant. It is a sign between me and the children of Israel for ever: for in six days the Lord made heaven and earth, and on the seventh day he rested, and was refreshed.

According to Health Essentials, Dr. Walia explained that depriving yourself of shut-eye has a negative impact on your health, such as lack of alertness, excessive daytime sleepiness, impaired memory, relationship stress, low-quality of life where you become less likely to participate in normal daily activities or to exercise, and greater likelihood of car accident.[154]

Additionally, from the reports funded by the National Institutes of Health documented in *The National Academies* publication, it was estimated that fifty to seventy million Americans chronically suffer from a disorder of sleep and wakefulness, hindering daily functioning, and adversely affecting health and longevity, which means there are around ninety distinct sleep disorders, and most are marked by one of

---

[154] Health Essentials, "Here's What Happens When You Don't Get Enough Sleep (And How Much You Really Need a Night)," Cleveland Clinic, 2020, Accessed June 11, 2020, https://health.clevelandclinic.org/happens-body-dont-get-enough-sleep/.

these symptoms: excessive daytime sleepiness, difficulty initiating or maintaining sleep, and abnormal events occurring during sleep.

The publication recorded that the cumulative long-term effects of sleep loss and sleep disorders have been associated with a wide range of deleterious health consequences, including an increased risk of hypertension, diabetes, obesity, depression, heart attack, and stroke. Decades of research proved that the case can be confidently made that sleep loss and sleep disorders have profound and widespread effects on human health disorders.[155]

Cancelling appointments with death by God's covenant of eternal life demand that you take time off to refresh yourself. Working without resting is destructive. God said observing the Sabbath or taking a rest is a sign or covenant with Him forever. Additionally, not giving cognizance to good health care, thereby living in poor health care is self-destructive.

Consider the story of Epaphroditus in Philippians 2:25–30, "For the work of Christ he was nigh unto death, not regarding his life." Epaphroditus would have actually died if God had not had mercy on him, just because he did not regard his life. This is to say every covenant child of God must have a health care mentality. Know what to eat and in what measure and when to eat so you don't give room to the enemy to rob you of your life. Divine life requires divine sense. Divine health is impossible without divine sense.

To be refreshed, you must rest. Cutting off rest will cut you off, and the individual will be retired or expired. Whenever you overdrive yourself, you end up in the grave. If you refuse to rest, you will be laid to rest by others. Jacob said in Genesis 33:13, "My lord knoweth that the children are tender, and the flocks and herds with young are with me: and if men should overdrive them one day, all the flock will die."

---

[155] Reports Funded by National Institute of Health, "Sleep Disorders and Sleep Deprivation: An Unmet Public Health Problem," *The National Academies*, 2006, Accessed June 11, 2020, https://www.ncbi.nlm.nih.gov/books/NBK19961/.

GRA Global Metamorphoo Prayer Line Testimonies

GRA Global Metamorphoo Prayer Line is a mandate given by the Lord from Obadiah 1:17, "But upon mount Zion shall be deliverance, and there shall be holiness; and the house of Jacob shall possess their possessions."

In the midst of a pandemic where there have been over thirty-three million cases and over a million deaths due to the coronavirus, God has been exceedingly faithful to God's Remnant Assembly worldwide. God used this time to bring many of His children back to Him during our Metamorphoo Prayer Line. Additionally, during the time of the lockdown, not only were there testimonies of healing, promotion, debt cancellation, preservation of death, success in businesses, careers, families, etc., but most importantly, there were testimonies of mass salvation. God moved in our midst like never before with over 350 people from all over the world, including the United States, the Caribbean, Africa, Europe, and Asia where people were miraculously healed from COVID-19 by the mercy and grace of God!

Through prophetic instructions, such as the partaking of Holy Communion, the anointing, and the power of the prophetic mantle and by launching our faith to another dimension, many lives were sustained, and we give God the highest praise! Though many people showed drastic symptoms of COVID-19, God, in His mercy, miraculously healed them all. There were no records of death in our midst throughout this time, and we know that this is only due to God's marvelous power! God surely is the lifter up of our heads, and we know that these are His mighty acts. During the time that many were unemployed, many members of God's Remnant Assembly were miraculously promoted and received jobs with wonderful benefits. God gave us abundant joy during this time, and all the praise and glory belongs to Him.

*****

I praise God for total restoration and healing of my family. In Nigeria alone, there have been 55,632 cases and 1,070 deaths due to COVID-19. My father is a medical doctor in Nigeria, and because he is a health care professional, he was likely to expose himself to the virus because he is constantly treating patients. My dad was diagnosed with COVID-19, and the virus spread to my mom, niece, brother, and two other individuals who were all living together. I thank God for His faithfulness because my family were not a part of any negative statistics of death. After following prophetic instructions and by believing the prayers of my Father in the Lord in regards to my family, the six individuals who were once diagnosed with COVID-19 are now *completely healed!* My dad is eating, thinking, and communicating normally. *God is wonderful!* The devil has been dealt another lethal blow and failed. *Hallelujah!*

—Bro. S.

Since I started my job, I always obeyed every instruction from God's Word from the GRA Metamorphoo Daily Prayer Line that came forth. One night, we prayed over grape juice that we receive as the blood of Jesus Christ by faith (Matt. 26:28; 1 Cor. 11:25). I brought the emblem and poured it on the ground of the facility where I worked and prayed that because I am here, there will be no cases of COVID-19. Weeks after, they decided to test everyone (including the 177 elderly residents and employees) for COVID-19. The result came back that no one in the whole building tested positive, including all the elderly and employees. This is a miracle because many elderly people living at several assisted residential houses have tested positive across the country. Other branches of the same company where I work have had many individuals who tested positive. I give God all the praise for the continuous preservation from COVID-19. I know it was due to following the prophetic instructions during the prayer line that kept me, the employees, and the elderly protected from COVID-19. Exodus 12:13 declares, "And the blood shall be to you for a token upon the houses where ye are: and when I see the blood, I will pass over you, and the plague shall not be upon you to destroy you, when I smite the land of Egypt."

—Sis. D.

I received great news this morning from the doctor's office. My test results for COVID-19 came back negative. I am so grateful and happy to reunite with my family whom I have been quarantined away from for the past twenty-four days. Thank you all of God's Remnant Assembly for praying for and with me. I will never be the same again. I thank God that my mother-in-law and I were not a part of the 340,000+ number of people who died. I truly believe God brought me to the GRA Metamorphoo Daily Prayer Line for many reasons. On May 13, our Father in the Lord made a prophetic decree, and I was healed the next day, May 14. I regained my strength, energy, breath, my lungs cleared up, and immediately, all the mucus due to the virus left my body. I am grateful to Jesus Christ. My husband and I are worshipping together. Additionally, my husband and both of my children did not get the virus. I'm humbled and grateful for God's mercy. I give God all the glory and all the praise. We're overwhelmed! Thank you, Lord. Psalm 117:23 declares, "This is the Lord's doing; it is marvellous in our eyes."

—Sis. K.

My husband's name is Yefrin from the Dominican Republic. We called GRA Metamorphoo Daily Prayer Line from the Dominican Republic and have been watching God's Remnant Assembly's Sunday services on YouTube and were incredibly blessed by the Word of God. A couple of weeks ago, I was feeling fatigued, weak, and tired. It was very bad. Two weeks later, my husband and I went to the hospital to be tested for COVID-19. Glory be to God, my husband tested negative, even though he had been exposed to it through his mom who tested positive for it. Although my husband tested negative, I tested positive for COVID-19, but I thank God that through the prayers and prophetic decrees released during the prayer line, that we believe was "Yea" and "Amen" for us, we were healed. Indeed, God answers by fire. Later, when I went for a checkup, the doctors said my immune system had been fighting the virus. I am so grateful to God. The Bible attested in 1 Corinthians 1:20, "For all the promises of God in him are yea, and in him Amen, unto the glory of God by us."

—Sis. Y.

Glory be to God. My wife and I began to feel very strong in the Lord. For a whole week, we could not do anything. We were coughing, sneezing, and had a high body temperature. We had thought this was malaria and took malaria medications but kept on connecting to the God's Remnant Assembly's Metamorphoo Prayer Line, and we obeyed every prophetic instruction that came forth. Afterward, our Father in the Lord decreed God's Word of healing over our lives, and we were immediately healed. We are grateful to God for His divine healing. First Peter 2:24 states, "Who his own self bares our sins in his own body on the tree, that we, being dead to sins, should live unto righteousness: by whose stripes ye were healed."

—Bro. D. and Sis. A.

On one Monday morning, I began to feel discomfort in my throat as if my tonsils were inflamed. It hurt to the point that I could not swallow anything nor was I able to speak or sing. Immediately, I went to the doctor who diagnosed me with COVID-19. He asked me to take the test, although I told him there should not be any assumption. He also diagnosed me with strep throat. I did the COVID-19 test, and after the test, I began to sing praises and worship songs with some of my sisters in the Lord. Jesus inhabited our praises, and I received my healing instantly. Also, one of my sisters who had been sick received her healing, and I received a call from the doctor that my results for strep throat and COVID-19 were negative. Blessed be the name of the Lord for this birthday gift and for the word of faith on the GRA Metamorphoo daily prayer line.

—Sis. C.

I had a roommate in the fall of 2019 who shared with me that she had never seen her menstrual cycle as a freshman in college. She should have had seen her period. Many months later, during GRA's fifty days of fasting in the year 2020, during prayer in my dorm, the Holy Spirit instructed me to pray for her and anoint her bed with the anointed oil and pray over by my Father in the Lord. Although I felt reluctant to do so because I did not want her to feel bad, thank God, I did pray with her privately in the bathroom, and then I told her to sing and thank God. We sang praises to God, and I told her the prayers wouldn't work, except she believed. To the glory of God, after returning from winter break approximately one month after, she said, "Oh, Lisa, I forgot to tell you that I finally got my menstrual cycle a few days ago." My jaw dropped. I asked her how long she'd been having the problem, and she said she had been going to the gynecologist for about four years, and they had been giving her medication for that long. I was greatly amazed at the power of the Almighty God. To Him alone be the glory. Additionally, I had not been able to sleep, suffering insomnia for a long time, but my case was called on the Metamorphoo GRA Prayer Line, and from that day, I experienced a miracle after believing God's Word spoken to me. I have been sleeping well henceforth. All glory to God.

—Sis. L.

I am giving all the glory to God for His divine healing and restoration in my life. I happened to work in a high-risk COVID-19 environment. We took all precautionary measures to avoid being infected, but a colleague in my office tested positive on the thirtieth of May. My office was then shut down, and everyone was told to isolate themselves and go for the COVID-19 test. Three of us tested positive, and they told me the news. I burst into laughter because I know COVID-19 cannot be my portion. God said so in His Word that we daily receive through Metamorphoo Prayer Line all the way from Nigeria, and the power of God's Word coming from our Father in the Lord had vanquished all foes. I told the lady that broke the news to me that I would do the test again, although she had started to console me to take heart. I said to myself, "COVID-19 cannot dwell in my body where the Holy Ghost inhabits and not with a surer word of prophecy filled with consuming fire coming from our Father in the Lord." I refused to inform anyone about this situation so as not to corrupt my faith with their fear, although I quarantined myself. To the praise and the glory of God, I was able to do another test a few days after, and the result came out negative. This can only be God and God alone. Blessed be His Holy name forever and ever.

—Bro. A.

As of September 7, 2020, there have been over 190,000 deaths in the United States due to COVID-19. I am currently an official at a penitentiary in Maryland who was previously exposed to the coronavirus. During this time, I was told to self-isolate from my family and those at my workplace! Unfortunately, my family also ended up being exposed to the virus, but I give God glory because He is forever faithful. During the time many were battling with drastic symptoms from the virus, God miraculously healed my family. I followed every prophetic instruction from my Father in the Lord during the Metamorphoo prayer line, and my Father in the Lord also personally prayed for me. I give God all of the glory and praise because God sustained my health and that of my family. We are all healed from COVID-19 and are extremely thankful! Additionally, during the pandemic, many have been unemployed. In fact, the unemployment rate in the United States is one of the highest of at all time, but in the midst of this difficulty, God is continuously prospering my business like never before. This is indeed the doing of the Lord, and it is marvelous in our eyes! Hallelujah.

—Bro. N.

I just want to give God all the glory and praise for all the marvelous things He has done! The doctors informed us that there was a cancerous tissue found in my mom's left breast the last week of May 2020. Glory be to God, my mom had a successful procedure two weeks later in June when she also removed her gall bladder, removed due to gall stones causing her extreme pain. The following month in July, my mom received a call from the hospital saying that they found another cancerous tumor in her liver. The doctors informed us that this was a serious issue, but I trusted in God because with God, all things are possible, including the healing of my mom. We sent a prayer request to my parents in the Lord in regard to the situation. During our Metamorphoo line, we were given prophetic instructions by our Father in the Lord, and by faith and obedience, I anointed my mom with the anointing oil and gave her the water made wine and prayed over to drink. There have been many marvelous testimonies of miraculous healing, and I trusted that God would do the same for my mom. Glory be to God, when my mom went for another scan to see the development and current status of the cancerous tumor in her liver, the doctors found that there was nothing there! Our God is faithful, and the doctors could not find the tumor. It had disappeared. Glory be to God in the highest.

—Bro. B.

God's faithfulness is ever true. I have been calling the Metamorphoo Prayer Line all the way from Ohio! I sent a prayer request about my health conditions and asked to be prayed for speedy health recovery. I had been losing a drastic amount of blood from my body and was not receiving enough oxygen, causing me constant shortness of breath. At the hospital, I was given blood transfusions in order to compensate, and this was extremely painful for me. On a Sunday, I was unable to join the prayer line and was told that the church prayed for me. I am here to testify that God truly honored the prayers made over me by our parents in the Lord and everyone at God's Remnant Assembly! A couple days after, I was able to go home and was even released earlier than my actually set date because God healed me! I am grateful because my condition miraculously got better, and I had a chance to recover at home. I believe that through the church's prayers, God healed me. I am extremely thankful to each and every one who prayed for me during this time, and I am glad this has given me an opportunity to experience the Lord in a new light. I give God all of the glory and praise! He is truly wonderful. *Hallelujah!*

—Sis. H.

During GRA Metamorphoo Prayer Line, our Father in the Lord instructed us to read Isaiah 54, Psalm 121, Colossians 1 and 2 if we had problems sleeping. Prior to sleeping, I took a shower, read what we were instructed to read, and I listened to praise and worship music. Because of this, I slept pleasantly and peacefully like never before after a long time of having sleep problems. Praise ye, Lord. Psalms 127:2 declares, "[F]or so he giveth his beloved sleep."

—Bro. J.

After our Father in the Lord decreed restoration of health during the Jeremiah 33:3 prayer line, two weeks later, I noticed my heart, kidney, and erectile problems were gone. Even the occasional symptoms of COVID-19 are not there anymore. Praise God. Exodus 15:26 declares, "And said, If thou wilt diligently hearken to the voice of the Lord thy God, and wilt do that which is right in his sight, and wilt give ear to his commandments, and keep all his statutes, I will put none of these diseases upon thee, which I have brought upon the Egyptians: for I am the Lord that healeth thee."

—Bro. J.

A few months ago, my skin had a tremendous breakout. My hands were extremely dry to the point where my skin was splitting open. The cuts became worse, and pus-filled pimples grew at the site. My entire face, forehead, and ears also broke out in a rash. My lips were also extremely dry to the point that liquid was coming out the cracks. This was a very scary experience, but I thank Jehovah Rapha, the Lord, my Healer! I had made an appointment to see a doctor who prescribed me an ointment and cream for my face and hands. We have been taught by our Father in the Lord at God's Remnant Assembly that it is only God that can make medications work. I prayed that God would allow the cream to work for me and also anointed my hands with anointing oil and put it in the areas where I was affected. Glory be to God, the rashes on my face and other parts of my body are completely gone, and the eczema on my hands is controlled. My God is wonderful. Hallelujah!

—Sis C.

I want to especially thank God for His faithfulness in the life of my family. A few weeks ago, I sent in a prayer request to the God's Remnant Assembly's line asking for a prayer in regards to my parents. At that moment, my mom was ready to divorce my dad. I have been asking and trusting God to send peace to my household because for a while, my parents were not in good terms nor speaking. To the glory of God, I came home from work one day to see my parents talking, eating from the same plate and spending quality time with each other. I'm extremely grateful because for the first time in weeks, there has not been any shouting, yelling, malice and anger in our house. God is truly marvelous and I bless His holy name! Hallelujah!

—Sis C.

About two weeks ago during GRA Metamorphoo Daily Prayer Line, our Father in the Lord had us place the blood of Jesus over ourselves. My brother was not near me so I placed the blood of Jesus by faith over a picture of him. The next day, he took an IT certification test that he had failed previously when he studied for 2 months and passed it. Later that day he got a temporary job offer making $54 an hour, which is more than what he was previously earning. I give God all the glory and praise. Psalms 75:6 declares, "For promotion cometh neither from the east, nor from the west, nor from the south."

—Sis. A.

During GRA Metamorphoo Daily Prayer Line, our Father in the Lord decreed that my star would continue to shine and that it's time for me to arise and shine by the Holy Spirit. The next day, I went to the car dealership by faith and was able to buy a 2020 Ford Mustang without having a job yet. This is truly a testimony to me, and I give God all of the glory. Isaiah 60:1 declares, "Arise, shine; for thy light is come, and the glory of the Lord is risen upon thee."

—Bro. A.

The Lord allowed me to start back my classes against all contradictions. Additionally, the Lord reduce the amount I had to pay for my classes. Furthermore, I was favored at my job this week and I received an additional $582 to my paycheck. Praise the Lord. Psalms 5:12 declares "For You, O Lord, will bless the righteous; With favor You will surround him as with a shield."

—Sis. K.

My grandmother called and said she was not feeling well, and her blood pressure was high. The doctor called her and recommended that she should go and pick up a medication. We went to get her from her house, and we brought her to our house and glory be to God because of the blood covenant of Jesus Christ upon the ground of our house none of the infection cannot enter our house where the blood of Jesus was speaking protection. The next day my grandmother was bouncing with energy, no more single symptom. Additionally, we checked her blood pressure and it was back to normal. Hebrews 12:24, "And to Jesus the mediator of the new covenant, and to the blood of sprinkling, that speaketh better things than that of Abel."

—Bro. P.

For two weeks I had a very severe headache, I had never had a headache like that in my entire life, it was followed by fever, cough, sore throat and a running nose. I bought flu medicine and pain medicine, but the medicine was not working, as I was feeling more fatigued. For 2 days, I could not smell or taste. After partaking of the "water made wine mystery" by faith (John 2:9, 4:46) and the "bread of life" prayed over during the Jeremiah 33:3 prayer line (Matt. 26:26), amazingly the next day I realized that I didn't have any of those symptoms anymore! Both myself and another sister had the same symptoms and we were instantly healed after that. Glory to God. Hebrews 13:8 stated, "Jesus Christ the same yesterday, and today, and forever."

—Sis. O.

I was diagnosed with COVID-19, and since receiving the news, I began experiencing a few symptoms. I recently started calling GRA Metamorphoo Daily prayer line consistently and I thank God for total healing! After last night's anointing service, I put some of the anointing oil in water and took a bath. Afterwards, I added some of the anointing oil into my lotion and used it. I placed the mantle that was prayed over under my pillow and went to bed believing in my heart that I would wake up healed and delivered. I woke up healed and delivered! No more pain or shortness of breath, my energy is returning, and likewise my appetite. I am now able to do things I could not do before, such as standing up for long periods of time, walking faster and talking in full sentences without losing my breath. The greatest testimony of all, was that my husband and my

Children have not experienced any symptoms at all. Thank God for this miraculous healing. Psalms 138:8 declares, "The Lord will perfect that which concerneth me: thy mercy, O Lord, endureth forever: forsake not the works of thine own hands."

—Sis. K.

My mother is a nurse and came home with coronavirus-like symptoms. She had a fever and was very weak. She bought flu medicine and wanted to self-medicate, claiming she had allergies. When she realized we all call in to pray on GRA Metamorphoo prayer line, she would always eavesdrop into the prayer line and silently be saying Amen to all the prophetic decrees. By virtue of her connecting into the prayers she was miraculously and instantly healed to the glory of God. James 5:15 declares, "And the prayer of faith shall save the sick, and the Lord shall raise him up; and if he has committed sins, they shall be forgiven him."

—Sis. E.

I have been experiencing a few symptoms of the corona virus. My body was aching and while on the prayer line the pain became worse and I began to cough up bloody mucus. I felt so weak, I could barely pray or even say Amen. When we started to pray again, I gathered my strength and began to pray in the Holy Spirit with all of my power and might. I also took anoint myself and the mucus came up clearer and clearer until it was completely gone. My body ached less and less. I went to bed still feeling some aches, but not as bad as before. I prayed to God and believed that I was already healed. I placed the mantle under my pillow and went to sleep. The following morning, I woke up completely pain free, freshly energized and the migraine I had before was completely gone. I give God all the glory for his goodness and mercy. Psalms 118:1 declares, "O give thanks unto the Lord; for he is good: because his mercy endureth forever."

—Sis. K.

I want to thank God for His healing power in my mom's life. A few weeks ago, the doctors said my mom had the coronavirus in addition to pneumonia. When she told us, I quickly remembered the prophetic decree by my Father in the Lord that no one here will lose their life nor will any of our families lose their life. That day, I poured the anointing oil on her pillow, and put a prophetic mantle under her mattress. Both were prayed over during GRA Metamorphoo Daily prayer line. My Father in the Lord instructed me to put a Bible under her pillow and opened it to Psalms 91 to help my faith (2 Cor. 1:24) and he released a prophetic word over my family. The very next day, her story changed. She immediately began to feel better, and now she is totally healed from the coronavirus. Hallelujah and I give God all the praise. Numbers 31:49 stated, "And they said unto Moses, thy servants have taken the sum of the men of war which are under our charge, and there lacketh not one man of us."

—Bro B.

My dad was coughing these past few days and last night he had a fever that was over a hundred degrees. By faith, I anointed him with oil and by the following morning, I told him to partake of the Holy Communion. To my shocking surprise his temperature went back to normal to the praise and glory of God. Additionally, I had a balance of $830 from my school. My Father in the Lord decreed that our debts would be canceled in Jesus name and instructed that we write a letter to ask for our debt to be erased. I had earlier written to my school multiple times which they refused but this time around they instantly reduced the bill to $378. Ephesians 5:20 declares, "Giving thanks always for all things unto God and the Father in the name of our Lord Jesus Christ."

—Sis. A.

I suddenly developed a sore throat which went very bad for three days. However, after GRA Metamorphoo Daily prayer line, I believed the water I am holding had been turned to God's wine that will bring change into this situation. Thankfully to God, when I woke up and the pain had vanished. Praise the Lord. The Bible says in Psalms 30:5, "For his anger endureth but a moment; in his favour is life: weeping may endure for a night but joy cometh in the morning."

—Sis. A.

I want to thank God for totally healing me. During the week of March 17, I started having an itchy throat which I didn't take seriously. After I arrived at work, I noticed that the situation was getting worse. I also realized; I am having COVID-19 symptoms. I left work and went straight to the hospital. At the hospital, they informed me that I had acid reflux issues and gave me some help. In the evening, the symptoms felt worse and later that evening I started having terrible body aches, chills, itchy throat, and could not eat. The next morning, I went back to the hospital and they informed me that I had an upper respiratory infection and that I should go home. For about three days, the situations got worse and worse. When I noticed nothing was working, the Holy Spirit reminded me that I had done my own part and it is now time for Him to do His work. He reminded me of the decrees made by our Father in the Lord and the testimony shared of the woman in Africa who placed her tithe portfolio in front of her door when armed thieves raided her area and they dare not cross the line because she was a faithful tither. The Lord also reminded me of the prophetic word of my Father in the Lord especially when the Holy Spirit spoke through his and said that no true sons and daughters of God's Remnant Assembly will be knocked down by coronavirus according to Numbers 31:49. I proclaimed that since I am a faithful tither and I believe the Word of the Lord spoken by our My Father in the Lord from Numbers 31:49, the devourer is not permitted to devour me. That very night, I was comforted by that Word and left everything into the hands of GOD. When I woke up the next morning, my strength was automatically renewed. The aches, itchy throat and most of the symptoms were gone but the rest left during the day and by Sunday March 22, I was totally healed. God is truly faithful. The Word of God declares in Philippians 1:6, "Being confident of this very thing, that he which hath begun a good work in you will perform it until the day of Jesus Christ."

—Sis. O.

During GRA Metamorphoo Daily prayer line, our Father in the Lord gave a prophetic word that someone's career was being restored and instructed us to write letters to seek for debt cancellation during period of COVID-19. I wrote the letter, prayed over it and send it to the president and the financial department of my school asking for the financial hold on my status to be lifted so I can progress with my exams. The last time I communicated with the school officials, they said I must pay $15,000 before anything can be released but God turned the situation for me. I did not have the finances yet all of my school documents that I needed were released without me having to pay a dime. I give God glory. Second Corinthians 9:8 declares, "And God is able to make all grace abound toward you; that ye, always having all sufficiency in all things, may abound to every good work."

—Bro. S.

I called GRA Metamorphoo Daily prayer line all the way from Tanzania, and glory be to God, I was incredibly blessed. For a while, I could not sleep, and I was having demonic attacks and bad dreams. During the prayer line, we prayed over a mantle and our Father in the Lord made a decree. I went to sleep, and glory be to God, I am restored and renewed. Isaiah 54:14 declares, "In righteousness shalt thou be established: thou shalt be far from oppression; for thou shalt not fear: and from terror; for it shall not come near thee."

—Bro. R.

Just before cases of COVID-19 began to rise in Maryland, I was hospitalized for shortness of breath, wheezing, bad cough and flu like symptoms. At the hospital, they said it was an upper respiratory infection and a virus that they said they couldn't test because it would cost too much to run. I have never felt this kind of attack before. That week I ran to church for my Father in the Lord to pray over holy communion emblem for me which I began to eat. The hospital ran another test which was negative. Thanks be to God for the power that is in the blood of Jesus Christ. Ephesians 2:19 declares, "But now in Christ Jesus ye who sometimes were far off are made nigh by the blood of Christ."

—Sis. J.

I want to give God all the praise and glory for keeping me during the COVID-19 pandemic. On April 12th, I woke up and was not feeling well. By 3:00 p.m., I was in acute pain and complete distress, with severe shortness of breath, vomiting and diarrhea. My body became so weak that I could not hold my head up, speak full sentences or control any bodily movements. Over the phone, my father in the Lord made a decree over my life prior to going to the hospital. That evening, I called the prayer line while I was in the Emergency Room and while on the prayer line on the hospital bed, I received results from all the tests that I was "perfectly healthy" and couldn't find anything wrong. It's only by the grace of God through the Word of the Lord from my father in the Lord because I did not think I would make it. I give God all the glory and the praise for GRA Metamorphoo Daily prayer line. Isaiah 54:17 declares, "No weapon that is formed against thee shall prosper; and every tongue that shall rise against thee in judgment thou shalt condemn. This is the heritage of the servants of the Lord, and their righteousness is of me, saith the Lord."

—Sis. L.

Over a week ago, I received a call from someone whom I came in close contact with that someone in her household (a health care worker) tested positive for COVID-19. She also expressed that she was showing some of the symptoms. I tried my best to have faith in God and trust that He is on the throne even in the midst of this season we are in. 2 days later our thirteen-month-old started developing a fever. At first, it was low grade then increased. We had no hope at this point but to trust in the God we serve. The GRA Metamorphoo Daily prayer line was the tool God used for our faith to remain firm. Before the coronavirus pandemic, our daughters had their twelve-month regular checkup and we were told that they could possibly get a fever 7 days after the appointment, at the time the fever occurred it was eighteen days later. We called the nurse and we were told that the time has passed for any signs of fever to show. So, fear easily crept in through this message. Nonetheless, God is faithful. He destroyed the fever by the communion which we continuously partake of over the phone and we had solid faith in the more sure word of prophecy declared from our Father in the Lord from God's Word. We thank God for the Jeremiah 33:3 prayer line. Hebrews 13:20 declares, "Now the God of peace, that brought again from the dead our Lord Jesus, that great shepherd of the sheep, through the blood of the everlasting covenant."

—Sis. J.

A couple of days ago I was feeling feverish, my throat was feeling weird, and I was very tired. Later on, that night I got on the GRA Metamorphoo Daily prayer line, I recall the prayers centering around being a faithful tither so the Lord rebuke the devourer on our behalf. I told God that I am a faithful tither. The next day, all the symptoms were gone. Isaiah 41:21, "Produce your cause, saith the Lord; bring forth your strong reasons, saith the King of Jacob."

—Sis. M.

I am currently a teacher and it was just approved that teachers on cycle must be observed and passed with a high effective rating. This will greatly help toward getting our certification being paid for. If we are given an ineffective rating based on the observations throughout the school year, we would not be able to receive our official license to teach which comes with a major salary increase. Due to COVID-19 pandemic, administrators are not allowed to rate us ineffective. I give God all the glory because this is truly His favor. Being a teacher may not be the highest paying job, but during this time God has been very faithful to me. Ephesians 1:11 stated, "In whom also we have obtained an inheritance, being predestinated according to the purpose of him who worketh all things after the counsel of his own will."

—Sis. D.

During the week, I started experiencing some excruciating pain in my wrist. My hands were very weak, and it was hard for me to do many things. On Thursday evening during GRA Metamorphoo Daily prayer line, I cried out to God about the pain. When I woke up the next morning the pain was gone. I truly thank God for my perfect healing. Psalms 107:20 declares, "He sent his word, and healed them, and delivered them from their destructions."

—Sis. T.

I was recently diagnosed with coronavirus. I spoke with the doctors who gave the initial diagnosis. After connecting with GRA Metamorphoo Daily prayer line, they told me that I am "one of the blessed ones." Miraculously, I am officially cleared of any COVID-19. The doctor said my body has built antibodies against the virus. All symptoms are gone, and I no longer had fever and did not need to continue to self-quarantine. None of my family members were infected to the praise and glory of God. Thank you, Jesus for your Mercy and Grace. What has killed others was placed under my feet. Psalms 110:1 declares, "The Lord said unto my Lord, Sit thou at my right hand, until I make thine enemies thy footstool."

—Bro. A.

I want to give God glory for His divine favor in my life. The school I attended took me off enrollment because I could not pay for my classes. When I went to meet with financial aid officials, a lady there helped me to apply for multiple grants and on the spot, they gave me those grants. My account balance which was $24,077 was immediately dropped to $12,746 and I was reinstated back to classes. May our God be praised. First Peter 5:7 declares, "Casting all your care upon him; for he careth for you."

—Sis. J.

Throughout the week, I started to feel feverish and sharp pains in my throat. The enemy immediately rushed my head with thoughts of COVID-19 since I am taking care of my mom who had been sick with COVID-19. That night we prayed over the anointing oil and our Father in the Lord declared that when we wake up the following morning, the symptoms that we are currently feeling will be no more. To the glory of God, I have not felt feverish nor experience the sharp pain in my throat since. The fact that I have been able to remain strong in my faith, maintain true genuine peace, and not be discouraged with all that was going on is a testament to the Word of God coming from our Father in the Lord. I truly thank God. Psalms 55:22 stated, "Cast thy burden upon the Lord, and he shall sustain thee: he shall never suffer the righteous to be moved."

—Sis. C.

The very week that the quarantine began, I started working on that Sunday night. I am currently a concierge and work in buildings with older age group. At the beginning of the coronavirus pandemic, we were informed that seniors were more likely to be vulnerable to the virus. The first night I worked, I started to have a sore throat, I drank tea with ginger trying to get my throat feeling back to normal again, it evidently made it worse. The next night (Monday night), I made sure I dressed warmly and took Vicks for my nose, but my nose was still dripping as if I had cold or flu. On Tuesday night, I got massive headaches, with my nose still dripping, and my throat very sore. I asked God to heal me. The following morning, my nose was still stuffed, I could not breathe at all and was having a minor headache and cough. However, during the Jeremiah 33:3 prayer line, the Word of the God from my Father in the Lord pricked my heart as the focus was fighting oppression. I was fearful that I had COVID-19 but our Father in the Lord led us into powerful prayers that day and when I woke up, I did not have any symptoms of COVID-19, everything disappeared until this day. I give God all the glory. First Corinthians 6:20 declares, "For ye are bought with a price: therefore, glorify God in your body, and in your spirit, which are God's."

—Sis. C.

About three weeks ago, I went out for a run and when I came back, I saw about five to six birds that flew toward me at the front door of my house. Immediately I turned around and I screamed because it came to me unawares. That night I started having terrible fever, headache, loss of appetite and panic attacks to the point where I could not even go to sleep. That night, I woke up at 4:15

a.m. from a very terrible discomfort. During GRA Metamorphoo Daily prayer line, we had the prophetic mystery of the anointing oil and prophetic mantle to sleep. The Holy Spirit spoke through my Father in the Lord saying that as we sleep with the garment all the symptoms will disappear when we wake up in the morning. The next day all of my symptoms miraculously left me. Praise the Lord. Genesis 2:21–22 declares, "And the Lord God caused a deep sleep to fall upon Adam, and he slept: and he took one of his ribs and closed up the flesh instead thereof. And the rib, which the Lord God had taken from man, made he a woman, and brought her unto the man."

—Sis. C.

Throughout the week, I was having sharp pain in my right breast and I could feel something there which was hurting when I kept on touching it. During our GRA Metamorphoo Daily prayer line, our Father in the Lord decreed that any pain we had will be gone the next morning and to the glory of God, when I woke up, it was gone. Job 22:28 declares, "Thou shalt also decree a thing, and it shall be established unto thee: and the light shall shine upon thy ways."

—Sis. E.

I just want to thank God for divine healing. Before partaking of the water made wine (John 2:9, 4:46) prayed over during GRA Metamorphoo Daily prayer line, I had a major headache which was unbearable to the point where I could not move. I drank the water made into wine by faith and it was immediately gone. Hallelujah. Jeremiah 32:17, 27 declares, "Ah Lord God! behold, thou hast made the heaven and the earth by thy great power and stretched out arm, and there is nothing too hard for thee... Behold, I am the Lord, the God of all flesh: is there anything too hard for me?"

—Sis. F.

I want to give praise and glory to God. I had been calling GRA Metamorphoo Daily prayer line consistently from Kenya. But sometimes my daughter started developing fever and other COVID-19 symptoms. My husband and I thought it was just malaria fever or a relapsing fever. After about two days we took my daughter to the hospital and I had started having fever too and COVID-19 symptoms. Our Father in the Lord decreed over me, that whatsoever does not glorify God cannot be traceable to my body. The following day after the decree we were both made whole and to the glory of God when the result for COVID-19 came back we were both negative. We give God all the praise. Although we were challenged, Jesus Christ our overcomer brought us out of the challenges. Praise His Holy name. The Bible says in 1 John 5:4, "For whatsoever is born of God overcometh the world: and this is the victory that overcometh the world, even our faith."

—Sis. L.

I give God praise for His mercy upon my life. In the third week of March, I was in my office and I felt something was totally wrong. I felt sick all over my body, my temperature was very high and whenever I stood up, I felt like falling. It continually got worse by the hour. Knowing of the current COVID-19 pandemic, I started praying in tongues and pleading the blood of Jesus. By 6pm, I thought I had enough strength to drive home, which was less than thirteen miles away from my job. On my way back, I had to stop twice on the roadside because I was about to pass-out while driving. That night on the prayer line, my Father in the Lord told us to apply the blood of Jesus Christ to our doorposts, so I did, and I also drank the grape juice which is an emblem of the blood of Jesus Christ. The next morning, I applied the anointing oil all over my body and by the mercy and grace of God I have been instantly and permanently healed. Thank you, Lord Jesus. Mark 14:36 declares, "And he said, Abba, Father, all things are possible unto thee."

—Bro. F.

I am a registered nurse and I was working for an agency. We have been on the front line during the COVID-19 pandemic and I want to thank God that none of GRA Citadel of Miracle family had been a victim. Initially I was working for the position I applied for but the Lord tuned it around in a week. I have been very consistent on the GRA Metamorphoo Daily prayer line and I believe the Lord and the Word of God spoken by my Father in the Lord. I finally got a divine placement and the exact position that I applied for. I got God's unusual favor from left and right among this, is a payment of money close to two thousand dollars above my regular paycheck. I called the company to report this mistake and I was told it was really a mistake, but I should keep the money. God is forever faithful. Numbers 23:19 declares, "God is not a man, that he should lie; neither the son of man, that he should repent: hath he said, and shall he not do it? or hath he spoken, and shall he not make it good?"

—Sis. N.

Glory be to God, in the beginning of the week, I felt a sore throat coming on. I prayed before sleeping Monday night and woke up with no more sore throat but the same morning, I woke up feeling very weak but on Monday night during GRA Metamorphoo Daily prayer line, I receive and believe the prayer and the Word of the Lord is for me. Immediately after I finished drinking my bottle of water made wine prayed over during that Jeremiah 33:3 prayer line, I went to sleep in faith, and I keyed into God's Word that was declared. When woke up the foll0wing morning, all the body aches had surprisingly disappeared, and I have no more sore throat. First John 4:4 declares, "Ye are of God, little children, and have overcome them: because greater is he that is in you, than he that is in the world."

—Democratic Republic of the Congo

On November 16, 2019, our Father in the Lord, staff, and volunteers of Family Development & Samaritan Foundation visited Bakandia School in the Democratic Republic of the Congo to talk with students and distribute school supplies to over 1,200 students. As our Father in the Lord and the team were rounding up the distribution of the supplies, a young girl no older than ten years old, fainted in the midst of the crowd of students. One of FDSF male staff quickly picked her up and moved her away from the crowd to assess her state. The male staff quickly realized that the young girl had passed and informed our Father in the Lord of her situation. Our Father in the Lord requested that they bring the girl is presently in a state of comma alongside with his own bottle of water. He held the girl in his arm and called "Jesus." He then pours the water on the girl's face, saying, "this water is no longer water, but Jesus had made it wine of joy that brings resurrection." A moment later, the young girl jack back to life, opened her eyes and began to wipe the water from her face. The girl was handed over to her parents and teachers alive. All the glory belongs to Jesus Christ. Acts 20:9–12 declares, "And there sat in a window a certain young man named Eutychus, being fallen into a deep sleep: and as Paul was long preaching, he sunk down with sleep, and fell down from the third loft, and was taken up dead. And Paul went down, and fell on him, and embracing him said, Trouble not yourselves; for his life is in him. When he therefore was come up again, and had broken bread, and eaten, and talked a long while, even till break of day, so he departed. And they brought the young man alive and were not a little comforted."

—Sis. E.

After a brief crusade help by GRA Mission Squad at a village called "Honey Bush Village" in Nigeria, which was a very treacherous village where no gospel Church has ever existed. After everyone at the crusade surrendered their life to Jesus Christ, and as the missionary team were retuning into the mission van giving thanks to God, we heard a group of people crying out loud from the far distant thick forest. Our Father in the Lord was instructed by the Holy Spirit to trace were the crying was coming from. As we began to run, through the forest following a narrow path, we arrived at a very little village settlement where a woman of about sixty-five years old was laid on the floor dead, a big pot on firewood stove burning and some group of about twelve to fifteen elder women surrounded her and were weeping because she had died. Our Father in the Lord instructed all the women to stop weeping. Now these women do not understand English, but they responded to the instruction in English by being quiet. Then our Father in the Lord, announced to all them that, he knows some of them were witches and they were the brain behind the death of this woman. He said, that GRA Mission Squad just finished a crusade at a nearby village and we will not leave this village with a report that someone died in the nearby village. He told them that Jesus will raise the woman back to life as she was only sleeping. He asked that they bring the water that he was drinking and confessed that Jesus has turned this water to the wine of Joy. He poured the water on the woman on ground as we all began to give God thanks in the Spirit for raising the woman. Suddenly after about five minutes, the woman that had been laid cold on the ground being prepared for burial started sneezing and all the women started panicking but our father in the Lord instructed that the bring the woman on a chair to make her feel comfortable rather than laying on the bare ground. We started giving thanks to God and our Father in the Lord commanded that they give her food to eat. He also warned that those who refuse to give their life to Jesus Christ and will continue in wickedness such as witchcraft will experience the judgment of God from the God of vengeance. Later, the woman gave her life to Jesus Christ and changed her name to "Never die again." Praise ye the Lord. Acts 19:11–12 declares, "And God wrought special miracles by the hands of Paul. So that from his body were brought unto the sick handkerchiefs or aprons, and the diseases departed from them, and the evil spirits went out of them."

—Honey Forest Village

After our Father in the Lord had preached Jesus and on the power of the Holy Spirit, a man who had been deaf had his hearing popped open, those with excruciating pain in their body were delivered, a woman that sleeps and always wake up with severe back pain and numbness of the limbs received her instant healing. Migraine that feels as if the brain is burning and hurting were healing. Memory restored to those who suffers memory loss, heart palpitation ceased. Walking sticks were thrown away, the blind were healed. John 3:2 declares, "The same came to Jesus by night, and said unto him, Rabbi, we know that thou art a teacher come from God: for no man can do these miracles that thou doest, except God be with him."

—Ho Chi Minh, Vietnam

I thank God for divinely preserving my father's life. We had received a call that he had been rushed to the hospital due to heart failure. When we arrived at the hospital, he couldn't speak but was hooked up to a machine. I knew that we had been praying over his picture on the wall of fire (Zech. 2:5) and therefore no evil could befall him and I believe in the "More sure Word of Prophecy" that had been decreed by my Father in the Lord so I was rested that nothing would happen to him. I thank God for the life of my father because he is healed and well now. Praise be to the God who heals. The Scriptures declare in 2 Chronicles 32:8, "With him is an arm of flesh; but with us is the Lord our God to help us, and to fight our battles. And the people rested themselves upon the words of Hezekiah king of Judah."

—Sis. J

About three nights ago, I left the house to go to work. I currently work a night shift. I would always leave my son in the care of my aunt. That night I made sure my son was asleep before I left the house and I left him with my aunt, who was also asleep. I did not know that I forgot to lock the door when I left the house. At around 3:00 a.m. my son woke up and started looking for me. He left the room, went downstairs and went outside of the house. He stood in the middle of the road crying. My aunt was still in the house sleeping and she had absolutely no idea that he was outside. One of our neighbors' fiancée heard the crying of a baby and went to the window to see what was going on. She saw the child in the middle of the road and immediately went to her fiancé to call the police. When her fiancé; who is actually a friend to my husband saw my son in the middle of the road, he immediately recognized him and ran to get him from the middle of the road. While all this was happening, I had no idea because my job prohibits having our phone out on site. I give all the praise and glory to God that my son is here and alive. The Word of God declares in Lamentation 3:22–23, "It is of the Lord's mercies that we are not consumed, because his compassions fail not. They are new every morning: great is thy faithfulness."

—Sis. V.

When I was young, I used to be very sick every month, but since I have been a part of God's Remnant Assembly, Citadel of Miracle mandate, for the past seven years, I have not been sick at all. I thank God for perfect health. Psalms 125:1 says, "They that trust in the Lord shall be as mount Zion, which cannot be removed, but abideth forever."

—Sis. C.

Before being a part of God's Remnant Assembly, Citadel of Miracle mandate, I had been struggling with narcolepsy for several years but since I have joined this chariot GRA, I have been trusting God to give me strength in school and work. I used to be uncontrollably sleepy during school and work, and sometimes I would even fall asleep while driving. I told God that this must change. When I got this new job, I noticed that while I have been working, I have been awake, and alert and I have not felt sleepy. I have also been alerted while attending my classes, and my grades are better now in my master's program than they have ever been before. I thank the God of GRA for delivering me from this evil disease. Second Corinthians 1:20 declares, "Who delivered us from so great a death, and doth deliver: in whom we trust that he will yet deliver us."

—Sis. N.

My sister and her husband are into cassava (a type of potato in Africa) business, and where they left it to soak before processing it, someone went and put poison in it. When my sister started processing the cassava, the Holy Spirit told her not to process the cassava because it had been poisoned which was later tested and it was conformed that a poison had been added to it. Many in the village would have purchase the cassava and would have died. I thank the Lord God Almighty that I did not receive evil news from my hometown. Proverbs 1:17 declares, "Surely in vain the net is spread in the sight of any bird."

—Sis. D.

My brother who lives in Nigeria, was on his way to Port-Harcourt. He pulled over to the side of the road because his car had a problem. As he pulled over, a group of ten armed robbers attacked him and dragged him into the forest and tied his hands and feet. After taking his things they told him he must pay a certain amount of money in order to be released. I told my Father in the Lord immediately and he decreed he shall be released. I don't know how, but my brother was miraculously released without paying a single dime. Luke 10:19 declares, "Behold, I give unto you power to tread on serpents and scorpions, and over all the power of the enemy: and nothing shall by any means hurt you."

—Sis. M.

I thank God for protecting my granddaughter from being shot in Chicago last Sunday. She was approached by two gunmen but during the altercation we were at church praying against the plan and attack of the enemy against our self and family. I also thank God for not allowing my house to be burnt down through an incidence at that same time. The Word of God declares in Psalms 121:4, "Behold, he that keepeth Israel shall neither slumber nor sleep."

—Sis. B.

My brother drowned in the bathtub and died, I was paranoid, and it does not even cross my mind that I ought to call 911. I just remembered that I had the anointing oil that was prayed over and I hurriedly rushed to pour the oil on his head, and he jerk back to life. Interestingly he came back to life asking for what he needed to do in order to be saved and he gave his life to Jesus Christ immediately. Glory be to God in the Highest. Ephesians 3:20 declares, "Now unto him that is able to do exceedingly abundantly above all that we ask or think, according to the power that worketh in us."

—Sis. T.

A couple of weeks ago I went to my bank to make a transaction and realized there was a $6,000 increase as of the last time I checked it. I did not want to ask the teller any question, so I hurried out of the bank. I had an end of the year review with my superior, and I learned that my job had actually made an error which I was told I should not worry about. God reminded me that I had helped a brother of mine with $600 without expecting anything back and I received $6,000 miraculously. Praise ye the Lord! Luke 6:31 declares, "And as ye would that men should do to you, do ye also to them likewise."

—Bro. J.

I thank God for blessing my family with a new car. God instructed someone to bless us with the car of which we did not have to pay a single dime for. The individual just blessed us with thousands of dollars to purchase the new car. We were also blessed with $175,000 worth in baby gift cards. Only God could have done this! Hallelujah to the God who is faithful! Philippians 4:15–19 declares, "For even in Thessalonica ye sent once and again unto my necessity. Not because I desire a gift: but I desire fruit that may abound to your account. But I have all, and abound, I am full, having received of Epaphroditus the things which were sent from you, an odour of a sweet smell, a sacrifice acceptable, well pleasing to God. But my God shall supply all your need according to his riches in glory by Christ Jesus."

—Sis. E.

When I first came to God's Remnant Assembly, Citadel of Miracle, I had multiple growth in my head that I would have to constantly go to the hospital to drain out. One Sunday our Father in the Lord said he was going to pray for healing. On that particular Sunday I had bandages on my head. As our Father in the Lord began to pray, I began to feel something popping on my head. When I got home to change the bandages, my head was completely healed, and the growth was no longer there. Ever since the fasting period began, the medication I was supposed to take daily, I had not taken for four months as my physician discretion. Lastly, I was waiting to see our Mother in the Lord for a prayer for healing but while she was praying for another sister in the Lord, I overheard her decree healing over that individual and I received my own divine healing too without her having to lay hands on me. I thank God for supernatural healing. Mark 9:23 declares, "Jesus said unto him, If thou canst believe, all things are possible to him that believeth."

—Sis. B.

My sister was diagnosed with epilepsy and brain paralysis. I brought her picture and added it to God's Remnant Assembly wall of fire (A wall where photos of our loved ones are posted and prayed over weekly by the church, during our regular fasting and prayer day). Not long after, I got a call that she was completely healthy and sane. All glory to the Most High God. The Bible says in Mark 10:27, "And Jesus looking upon them saith, with men it is impossible, but not with God: for with God all things are possible."

—Sis. A.

One day as I was in a shower, I was hit by an unseen hand, and slumped to the floor. After few minutes, I felt physically ok, so I did not pay much attention to it. That night, my wife woke up and saw coming from my head which had soaked my pillow. She alerted the family when I could not seem to wake me up from sleep but at that same time, there was a fasting and prayer weekly meeting going on in God's Remnant Assembly during which the church prays over the wall of fire with my picture on that wall of fire. Before the night turned today, God gave me the breath of life, and I woke up completely healed and delivered. Hallelujah! Psalms 118:17 declares, "I shall not die, but live, and declare the works of the Lord."

—Bro. O.

I went for my routine doctor's appointment recently and I received a phone call afterwards that they found a growth in my breast. They wanted me to come back for a retest, but I said within myself that it is not necessary because my body is the temple of the Holy Spirit. Afterwards I called for an appointment for retest to prove the doctor wrong. Those doctors were amazed because after retesting they could not find the growth that they initially found in my breast. There is power in the blood of Jesus Christ. Romans 8:31 declares, "What shall we then say to these things? If God be for us, who can be against us?"

—Sis. G.

Before I got saved, I was sexually active with multiple women. One of the women contacted me and notified me that she was HIV positive. After I went and got tested at the clinic, the result came back positive for HIV. I began to feel very sick and worried for my future. God supernaturally brought me to God's Remnant Assembly. My father in the Lord openly prophesied that God would heal me during one of GRA services. He said, anyone with STD in their body should come to the front boldly and the healing from the Lord Jesus Christ will be given free of charge. I was one of those who went in faith and our Father in the Lord laid hands on me. I went to the clinic the same week and doctor's reports proved that I am now eternally free from HIV. John 8:36 declares, "If the Son therefore shall make you free, ye shall be free indeed."

—Bro. N.

I had a growth in my breast for about 6 months, but I trusted that the Lord would take care of it. During a particular service, God spoke through our Father in the Lord saying, "Anyone with a growth in their body should come to the front." Hands were laid on me and I completely forgot about the growth. On a Thursday morning during God's Remnant Assembly's Jeremiah 33:3 prayer line, a word came forth instructing someone to check their body because every growth had been destroyed. As I checked my body in faith, I realized that the growth had completely disappeared! Glory be to God. Matthew 15:13 declares, "But he answered and said, every plant, which my heavenly Father hath not planted, shall be rooted up."

—Sis. V.

Last month, I was having severe stomach pain. My doctor referred me for an ultrasound. Around that same time, our Father in the Lord made an altar call for people who were experiencing stomach pain to come out to be ministered to. I came out in faith and I felt that something came out of me. I went for an ultrasound to confirm it, and glory be to God, everything was perfect. Matthew 12:15 declares, "But when Jesus knew it, he withdrew himself from thence: and great multitudes followed him, and he healed them all."

—Sis. P.

There was a wart on my finger that had been there since last year and after our Father in the Lord laid hands on me it was completely gone. Also, I had a cyst in my body that completely disappeared at the same time. Glory be to God. First Thessalonians 5:18 says, "In everything give thanks: for this is the will of God in Christ Jesus concerning you."

—Sis. O.

On a Sunday during our breakthrough services, our Father in the Lord called out those that have been bleeding from different parts of the body, to lay hands on them. My son had been experiencing random nose bleeds for a while, and one time it was so severe that I had to take him to the hospital. I brought my son forward to be ministered to and since then he has not had any nose bleeds. Praise the Lord. The Bible says in Ephesians 5:20, "Giving thanks always for all things unto God and the Father in the name of our Lord Jesus Christ."

—Sis. V.

My mother was feeling dizzy last week, and she was complaining that she was feeling paralyzed. She called out of work, because every time she got up, she felt dizzy. That day as she was laying down, I was watching my Father in the Lord's message on YouTube. Through hearing the Word, she suddenly got up out of the bed, and said that she was feeling better because of the Word she heard from the YouTube message. May Our God be praised. Romans 10:17 declares, "So then faith cometh by hearing, and hearing by the word of God."

—Bro. N.

A few weeks ago, I had swollen lymph nodes. They were not painful; however, I knew within me that something was wrong. A couple of days ago, I visited a health expo where I was examined by a nurse practitioner who informed me that the symptoms, I was experiencing could either be for HIV, cancer, or that it may even be for both. That same night, I had night sweats and my lymph nodes grew larger than they were before. I knew that there was a chance I had contracted HIV because of my past life, so in fear I went to my Father in the Lord and told him of the situation. He instructed me to believe that the Lord has forgiven me all of my previous sins and I have confessed and repented of them all and ask me to begin to walk in the newness of life. He also told be partaking of the Holy communion severally. I went to visit the doctor for testing after a week of taking Holy Communion and all the results came out negative. Praise God for His divine healing. Romans 8:1 says, "There is therefore now no condemnation to them which are in Christ Jesus, who walk not after the flesh, but after the Spirit."

—Sis. M.

Earlier in the week, a bump appeared on my earlobe. I was unsure of the cause, so I immediately began to research what the cause could be. Knowing that I did not have health insurance, I began to fear the information I will find online. I quickly remembered that I had Holy communion materials and I began to take it. Surprisingly, by Wednesday the bump had completely disappeared. Praise to the Lord. Habakkuk 2:4 declares, "Behold, his soul which is lifted up is not upright in him: but the just shall live by his faith."

—Sis. T.

Recently, my niece called me from Nigeria asking me to join her in prayer for her husband. She explained to me that he had not had a bowel movement in three years, and his condition was becoming worse, as he had begun to swell. On Sunday, we observed the prophetic mystery of the anointing oil and the communion. As an act of faith, I smeared the anointing oil and the blood of Jesus Christ on the picture of my niece's family in Nigeria. After a few days, I spoke with my niece and she informed me that her husband has finally been having a pleasant bowel movement. His health has been restored back to normal. Hallelujah to the Lamb of God. Revelation 5:10 declares, "And hast made us unto our God kings and priests: and we shall reign on the earth."

—Sis. D.

I was experiencing strange discomfort and movement in my stomach and navel area. I would only feel this at night when I am going to sleep. It felt as if a baby was moving in my womb, but I am not pregnant. I was believing God for healing and during the service my Father in the Lord decreed that as we apply the anointing oil that every movement in someone's stomach would be destroyed. That night as I slept, I noticed a strange sensation went out of my body and has never returned. Praise the Lord. Psalms 22:46 declares, "Strangers shall fade away, and they shall be afraid out of their close places."

—Sis. J.

My grandmother was rushed to the hospital after she began to experience difficulty in breathing. At the emergency room, we were given reports that her vital organs were starting to shut down. When I got to church, I immediately told my Mother in the Lord and she prayed with me and anointed my hands with oil. I went to the hospital and laid hands on my grandmother, praying for her in faith. Glory be to God; she was instantly healed. Every expectation that she will die was cancelled to the glory of God. She has henceforth resumed her everyday normal life as if nothing ever happened! Praise the Lord. Psalms 79:11 declares, "Let the sighing of the prisoner come before thee; according to the greatness of thy power preserve thou those that are appointed to die."

—Sis. M.

My younger sister was complaining about a toothache that was extremely painful to the point that she was unable to sleep. I gave her some anointing oil and told her to apply it to her teeth. The toothache ceased immediately, and she was able to go to sleep. The Bible declares in 1 John 4:4, "Ye are of God, little children, and have overcome them: because greater is he that is in you, than he that is in the world."

—Sis. M.

During my first visit to God's Remnant Assembly, our Father in the Lord prayed over the anointing oil for everyone. Before attending that service, I had been experiencing a crucial back pain that went my doctor cannot diagnosed after several test and hospital visits. I applied the anointing oil and right after the pain vanished. All back-pain afflictions that I had been suffering, including bad dreams and nightmares ended ever since stepping my feet into God's Remnant Assembly, Citadel of Miracles. Jesus Christ did all for me. Exodus 14:14 declares, "The Lord shall fight for you, and ye shall hold your peace."

—Sis. X.

My niece was bleeding profusely after giving birth. Soon after that ordeal, her first son was diagnosed with cancer. In faith, I took all of their pictures and anointed them and prayed over them every Thursday during our prayers on the wall of fire. I bless the name of the Lord because my niece received complete healing. I also had another niece who was pregnant and at a point in time, her fetus stopped moving without any known cause. I thank God because the child was born safely and all thanks to God through the prayers, we pray here in God's Remnant Assembly. James 5:16 declares, "Confess your faults one to another, and pray one for another, that ye may be healed. The effectual fervent prayer of a righteous man availeth much."

—Dr. J.

I thank God for divine healing. My right arm and neck were hurting so bad that I could not write or move comfortably. That night, before going to bed, I rubbed my arm with anointing oil that had been prayed over during service, and when I woke up the pain was gone. I thank God for this perfect healing. Psalms 138:8 declares, "The Lord will perfect that which concerneth me: thy mercy, O Lord, endureth forever, forsake not the works of thine own hands."

—Sis. D.

I have had a sharp pain in my lower abdomen. But after I applied the anointing oil on my head and my lower abdomen, I received instant healing. I give God all the Glory and Praise. Isaiah 10:27 declares, "And it shall come to pass in that day, that his burden shall be taken away from off thy shoulder, and his yoke from off thy neck, and the yoke shall be destroyed because of the anointing."

—Sis. P.

God miraculously canceled a $44,000 debt that was placed under my name a couple of years ago. During the beginning of the week, our Father in the Lord prophesied that someone here would have a testimony by Thursday, and I received the Word in faith. That same week, an additional $10,000 was canceled. Praise the Lord. Matthew 12:28–30 declares, "Come unto me, all ye that labour and are heavy laden, and I will give you rest. Take my yoke upon you and learn of me; for I am meek and lowly in heart: and ye shall find rest unto your souls. For my yoke is easy, and my burden is light."

—Sis. M.

About two years ago my student status was terminated from Howard University after I had accrued a $40,000 debt on my account. I was told that I could not enroll into any class anymore until the debt was fully paid. I visited the financial aid office all the time, only to be put to shame. My Father in the Lord decreed over life during my thanks-giving celebration that in the next ninety days, all of my debt would be cancelled. I followed every prophetic instruction as revealed from the Word of God and held on only to God's Word. The Holy Spirit told me to visit the financial aid office and inquire about my debt. The lady who checked my account responded, "What debt?" Your account is completely cleared off." To the glory of God, I am now enrolled back in school. Hallelujah to the God of GRA, Citadel of Miracles. Exodus 15:1, 21 declares, "Then sang Moses and the chil-dren of Israel this song unto the Lord, and spake, saying, I will sing unto the Lord, for he hath triumphed gloriously: the horse and his rider hath he thrown into the sea... And Miriam answered them, sing ye to the Lord, for he hath triumphed gloriously; the horse and his rider hath he thrown into the sea."

—Sis. C.

In 2008, I borrowed $100,000 from the bank. In the past eleven years, I have only been able to pay about $6,000. I checked my credit report recently and saw that the loan was no longer on my record. I called the credit company and told them that the loan was missing, but they said there was no longer any bank loan on my record. I waited for three months and decided to check again, and to the praise and glory of God, it has been completely removed. Jehovah Jireh, my Great Provider has given me debt cancellation. Psalm 121 declares, "I will lift up mine eyes unto the hills, from whence cometh my help. My help cometh from the Lord, which made heaven and earth. He will not suffer thy foot to be moved: he that keepeth thee will not slumber. Behold, he that keepeth Israel shall neither slumber nor sleep. The Lord is thy keeper: The Lord is thy shade upon thy right hand. The sun shall not smite thee by day, nor the moon by night. The Lord shall preserve thee from all evil: he shall preserve thy soul. The Lord shall preserve thy going out and thy coming in from this time forth, and even for evermore."

—Sis. E.

I had a bill of $7,924 on my student account at Howard University. I brought the statement to my father in the Lord who decree the favor of the Lord for me and instructed me to go and plead my case at the financial aid office. Upon checking my balance, I was told I only have $900 to pay. Thank God for this miraculous debt cancellation. Second Kings 4:6 declares, "And it came to pass, when the vessels were full, that she said unto her son, Bring me yet a vessel. And he said unto her, there is not a vessel more. And the oil stayed. Then she came and told the man of God. And he said, Go, sell the oil, and pay thy debt, and live thou and thy children of the rest."

—Sis. A.

Recently, our Father in the Lord decreed over my wife and I that it is our season of harvest and said that we need to learn how to harvest. God blessed my wife and I in a supernatural way. Someone blessed us with over $1,000. Afterwards, God told me to call the debt collectors. Before I called, we decreed what we wanted our debt to be reduced. After being told it was impossible, and being directed to many people, God lowered a $20,000 debt to $1,400. Two days later, I got paid from my job with excess money. I was dumbfounded and started tracing where the deposit came from. Last Sunday our Father in the Lord also said that someone will send a text of good news before 3:30PM. My wife received a text of good news at 3:20 p.m. that same day. I give God all the glory and praise. Luke 1:45 declares, "And blessed is she that believed: for there shall be a performance of those things which were told her from the Lord."

—Bro. K.

Glory be to God. I thank God for His favor. I want to thank God for reducing a credit card debt I owed. I owed a credit card company around $3,100 and I was not able to get a loan for school for the upcoming semester because of the debt and the "charged off account." I had previously used this card to make payments for my school and the credit card company had charged me extra fees, sent the amount to collections and was also trying to take me to court. I spoke to the law firm that they sent the debt collection to on after anointing the letter by faith the previous week and informed them, that I would not be paying the full $3,000. The representative told me to write a letter to settle the credit card in the amount I could pay. Immediately, I wrote a letter that I wanted to make a settlement for $1,500 and to the glory of God, I got a call back that instead of paying over $3,000 to settle the credit card debt, all I have to pay is $1,600. I was able to pay the balance and I no longer have any credit card debt to the glory of God. Proverbs 3:5–6 declares, "Trust in the Lord with all thine heart; and lean not unto thine own understanding. In all thy ways acknowledge him, and he shall direct thy paths."

—Sis. A.

I want to give God all the glory and the praise because for a while, I have not been able to go back to school due to a debt of about $10,000. My Mother in the Lord has helped to call my school and send letters requesting for the cancellation of the debt. A sister in the Lord shared a testimony about how her debt was reduced and totally paid off and that triggered my step of faith. I then call the school by faith and I was told I now owe $2,000 instead of over $10,000. The reinstatement process has begun for the fall session and I believe that the remaining $2,000 is already canceled in Jesus name. Joel 2:26–27 declares, "And ye shall eat in plenty, and be satisfied, and praise the name of the Lord your God, that hath dealt wondrously with you: and my people shall never be ashamed. And ye shall know that I am in the midst of Israel, and that I am the Lord your God, and none else: and my people shall never be ashamed."

—Sis. O.

Before my Father in the Lord made a decree over me, I had serious chest pain. The pain was so excruciating that I cannot even sleep. After my Father in the Lord prayed for me and I partaking of the communion the chest pain stopped instantly and I was able to sleep like a baby. I give God all the praise. This is nothing but a miracle of God, I cannot explain it. Matthew 8:17 states, "That it might be fulfilled which was spoken by Esaias the prophet, saying, Himself took our infirmities, and bare our sicknesses."

—Sis. N.

I want to give God all the glory for preserving me from an accident on the highway while I was heading home. I was driving on the far-right lane on I-95 in the DC Metro and decided to stay in that lane until I reached my exit. In the middle lane of that highway, a car started spinning uncontrollably and ended up facing the direction of the incoming cars. As a result of this a very big truck ended up swerving into my lane because of the oncoming car but I thank God that I was able to hit the break and did not run into the truck. If I was driving in the middle lane, I would have probably been in that multiple accidents that hit the car that was spinning. Additionally, I thank God because the truck did not hit me while swerving into my lane. I give God all of the glory for preserving me because two days before on the Jeremiah 33:3 Prayer Line, we partook of the Flesh and the Blood of Jesus for mercy, safety and security. The Bible declares in Proverbs 12:21, "There shall no evil happen to the just: but the wicked shall be filled with mischief."

—Sis. O.

I give God all the Glory. The prophetic decree from my Father in the Lord over my family has finally manifested. Our Father in the Lord decree that my family and I will become homeowners. He had instructed us during our breakthrough service at God's Remnant Assembly, Global to possess any land we want by declaring Jeremiah 22:29 (O earth, earth, earth, hear the word of the Lord.) over it. By faith, my family and I obeyed. A week later, to be specific, on October 14 at 3:51 p.m., the property management company emailed us that the owner of the house had asked to inquire from us if we are interested in purchasing the property. We agreed to purchase the property and were approved. All the financial cost was provided supernatural. God was involved in our case and made a way for us. I give God all the praise, we are finally homeowners. The Bible declares in Proverbs 19:21, "There are many devices in a man's heart; nevertheless, the counsel of the Lord, that shall stand."

—Sis. B.

I recently received a certificate in the mail for making the dean's list at Frostburg State University. I don't believe I did a whole lot to deserve the honor myself. My strength alone in the past did not get me to 4.0 GPA level and I know that God was definitely fully involved in my academics for which I give Him all the Glory and Praise. Isaiah 14:26–27 declares, "This is the purpose that is purposed upon the whole earth: and this is the hand that is stretched out upon all the nations. For the Lord of hosts hath purposed, and who shall disannul it? and his hand is stretched out, and who shall turn it back?"

—Bro. J.

I was in a car accident about two years ago and was hospitalized for a week, after being diagnosed with herniated disk, with sever back pain and had since been on a daily pain meds, and physical therapy. I always experience this terrible back pain every day to the point that I cannot bend. I cannot even lift my pocketbook. However, I participated in the last Holy communion on June 6, 2020, on the Jeremiah 33:3 prayer line, I witnessed immediate healing to the praise and glory of God. I have been pain-free since. I have not taken any pain medication since because I am healed. There is no more back pain and I am now bending. I have also started light exercises to the praise and the glory of God. Halleluiah. The Word declares in Acts 10:38, "How God anointed Jesus of Nazareth with the Holy Ghost and with power: who went about doing good and healing all that were oppressed of the devil; for God was with him."

—J. S.

CHAPTER 10

God has Canceled Every Appointment with Death

Only God can protect and preserve us from pandemics, even after following all precautions and CDC guidelines. Understanding the virus and the science of epidemics goes a long way toward explaining the decisions that are being made by public health officials. While we respect our public health officials with the expectation that their recommendations will be healthy and helpful, we must also be praying for them daily. Solomon in 1 Kings 8:15, 24 confirms that only God can fulfil the promises He spoke to his father, David:

> And he said, blessed be the Lord God of Israel, which spake with his mouth unto David my father, and hath with his hand fulfilled it, saying… Who hast kept with thy servant David my father that thou promisedst him: thou spakest also with thy mouth, and hast fulfilled it with thine hand, as it is this day?

God confirms this requirement for long life in Psalm 34:12–13. God wants to help you against your enemies, and the last enemy to be destroyed is death. The way He will do it is by you opening your mouth wide against it. "I will say of the Lord He is my refuge and my fortress: my God; in him will I trust." Saying it is what guarantees it. What you do not say, you will never see. If you must see life triumph over death, then say it and say it continually. Never mind whether the people hearing you believe it or not. God will watch over His Word in your mouth to perform it.

Psalms 57:2 declares, "I will cry unto God most high; unto God that performeth all things for me." Elizabeth concurred with Mary in Luke 1:45 regarding the performance of the Word that is believed and spoken, "And blessed is she that believed: for there shall be a performance of those things which were told her from the Lord."

Partakers of Jesus's Divine Life

Second Peter 1:3–4 declares:

> According as his divine power hath given unto us all things that pertain unto life and godliness, through the knowledge of him that hath called us to glory and virtue. Whereby are given unto us exceeding great and precious promises: that by these ye might be partakers of the divine nature, having escaped the corruption that is in the world through lust.

We must look unto Abraham, our father, and Sarah that God called blessed and increased (Isa. 51:1–2). The Lord wants to do the same—even much more—for us.

Jesus died primarily to connect us to the Abrahamic covenant and blessings, one of which is the blessing of long life. Not just any kind of life, but a good one, a good old age. The Bible accounted that Abraham was old and well-stricken in age, and the Lord had blessed him in everything (Gen. 24:1). God gave him long life coupled with incontestable fortune, enviable, enemy-provoking opulence. He was never a liability to his children. He bought the place where Isaac and Jacob were buried. He was an emperor who had an empire that consisted of three hundred and eighteen trained servants. It's a great privilege that Christ had connected us to Abraham through his death, burial, and resurrection. He did not only die to connect us to the Abrahamic covenant heritage of long life and prosperity; He also died to redeem our souls from death.

God's children do not die. They only sleep. Jesus said, "Lazarus is sleeping," and He is going to Bethany to wake Him out of sleep (John 11:11). First Thessalonians 4:13 states, "But I would not have you to be ignorant, brethren, concerning them which are asleep, that ye sorrow not, even as others which have no hope."

Christians are not born to die. At the end of their days here on earth, Christians sleep. The departure of a Christian from the earth is supposed to be a thing of joy. Men are to congratulate their children and children's children to the fourth generation for a life well spent. God's children are created for life. Jesus declares in John 10:10, "The thief cometh not, but for to steal, and to kill, and to destroy: I am come that they might have life, and that they might have it more abundantly."

Christians are to sleep at a full old age. Everybody sleeps and goes to bed when night falls and also wakes up again (in resurrection) to a new day.

First Thessalonians 4:13–18 explained:

> But I would not have you to be ignorant, brethren, concerning them which are asleep, that ye sorrow not, even as others which have no hope. For if we believe that Jesus died and rose again, even so them also which sleep in Jesus will God bring with him. For this we say unto you by the word of the Lord, that we which are alive and remain unto the coming of the Lord shall not prevent them which are asleep. For the Lord himself shall descend from heaven with a shout, with the voice of the archangel, and with the trump of God: and the dead in Christ shall rise first. Then we which are alive and remain shall be caught up

together with them in the clouds, to meet the Lord in the air: and so, shall we ever be with the Lord. Wherefore comfort one another with these words.

When night comes, people's greetings will be, "Goodnight" or "Blessed night" or Good evening" or "Blessed evening." You are only permitted to greet people this way at night. Until your night falls, you are not permitted to sleep prematurely. This was one of the reasons why Jesus had to raise the dead, including Lazarus. Until your night comes, your sleep will never come in Jesus Christ's name. You cannot be forced to sleep anymore. Those that are on the edge of sleep when their night of good old age has not come must arise right now. They must wake up in the name of Jesus Christ. You are not permitted to be destroyed by shame, the demon of coronavirus, wicked powers, accidents, terror by night, or destruction that wastes destinies at noonday.

From Minimum Lifetime to Maximum

The minimum covenant number of years for the disobedient children of Israel was seventy years. It was designed for them to perish in the wilderness and never to enter the promised land. It can be extended for them beyond seventy by reason of strength. But this is not so for is, God's children. Isaiah 65:20 states, "There shall be no more thence an infant of days, nor an old man that hath not filled his days: for the child shall die an hundred years old; but the sinner being an hundred years old shall be accursed."

For those who are partaking of God's Word and a lively part of the body of Christ, that is the Church wherein Jesus is the Vine. You have the means to build spiritual strength for powerful spiritual muscles that are needed to enjoy longer years. Psalms 90:10 declares, "The days of our years are threescore years and ten; and if by reason of strength they be fourscore years."

Proverbs 4:7–10 states clearly:

> Wisdom is the principal thing; therefore, get wisdom: and with all thy getting get understanding. Exalt her, and she shall promote thee: she shall bring thee to honour, when thou dost embrace her. She shall give to thine head an ornament of grace: a crown of glory shall she deliver to thee. Hear, O my son, and receive my sayings; and the years of thy life shall be many.

The minimum covenant years for God's redeemed is one hundred and twenty, and you could add to it if you are not satisfied. Genesis 6:3 states, "And the Lord said, my spirit shall not always strive with man, for that he also is flesh, yet his days shall be an hundred and twenty years."

Avoid using your mouth to destroy yourself. Stop allowing anti-God's covenant Words to come out of your mouth. You will have what you say. Hosea 13:9 declares, "O Israel, thou hast destroyed thyself; but in me is thine help." You shall live and not die to declare the works of the Lord" (Ps. 118:17).

There is nothing wrong about good old age where you return to the days of your youth. Actually, we don't grow old; we grow young as we return to the days of our youth. Job 33:25 declares, "His flesh (skin) shall be fresher than a child's: he shall return to the days of his youth."

If God rejuvenated the skin of Namaan, the Syrian leprous general who had no covenant relationship with God only because he obeyed the words of Elisha, the prophet, how much more will God do for His own children that are in covenant relationship with Him. Second Kings 5:14 illuminates, "Then went he down, and dipped himself seven times in Jordan, according to the saying of the man of God: and his flesh came again like unto the flesh of a little child, and he was clean."

You do not have to die like a fool in the order of Abner. You have decreed in your heart that there is God, and Great Jehovah must show up in your situation and grant your life to the fullest.

Moses pronounced these blessings upon God's children who are from the tribe of Asher in Deuteronomy 33:24–25, and we are, by covenant, the Israel of God: "And of Asher he said, Let Asher be blessed with children; let him be acceptable to his brethren, and let him dip his foot in oil. Thy shoes shall be iron and brass; and as thy days, so shall thy strength be."

As you grow old, so must you return to the days of your youth, and rather than confess that you are growing old, you should say you are growing younger, and as your age is, so shall your strength be renewed with vigor.

Caleb testifies in Joshua 14:10–12:

> And now, behold, the Lord hath kept me alive, as he said, these forty and five years, even since the Lord spake this word unto Moses, while the children of Israel wandered in the wilderness: and now, lo, I am this day fourscore and five years old. As yet I am as strong this day as I was in the day that Moses sent me: as my strength was then, even so is my strength now, for war, both to go out, and to come in. Now therefore give me this mountain, whereof the Lord spake in that day.

Zechariah 8:4 states, "Thus saith the Lord of hosts; There shall yet old men and old women dwelt in the streets of Jerusalem, and every man with his staff in his hand for very age."

It was said of Sarah who was already stricken in age in Genesis 18:11 that Abimelech, the king of Gerar, took her into the king's residence to marry her. This was recorded after Genesis 18. There was a type of resurrection transformation or transfiguration that had taken place in the body of Sarah between Genesis 18 and 20. While she was stricken in age in chapter 18, she was now very beautiful to the point of catching the king's attention in chapter 20.

Genesis 20:1–7 declares:

> And Abraham journeyed from thence toward the south country, and dwelled between Kadesh and Shur, and sojourned in Gerar. And Abraham said of Sarah his wife, she is my sister: and Abimelech king of Gerar sent and took Sarah. But God came to Abimelech in a dream by night, and said to him, Behold, thou art but a dead man, for the woman which thou hast taken; for she is a man's wife. But Abimelech had not come near her: and he said, Lord, wilt thou slay also a righteous nation? Said he not unto me, she is my sister? and she, even she herself said, He is my brother: in the integrity of my heart and innocence of my hands have I done this. And God said unto him in a dream, Yea, I know that thou didst this in the integrity of thy heart; for I also withheld thee from sinning against me: therefore, suffered I thee not to touch her. Now therefore restore the man his wife; for he is a prophet, and he shall pray for thee, and thou shalt live and if thou restore her not, know thou that thou shalt surely die, thou, and all that are thine.

Choose Eternal Life by Speaking God's Word

Deuteronomy 30:19 declares, "I call heaven and earth to record this day against you, that I have set before you life and death, blessing and cursing: therefore choose life, that both thou and thy seed may live." You live long by choosing to. Even though the provision for it has been made available from God's Word, it is only your choice that will deliver it to you.

Stephen chose to die by surrendering his spirit to death (Acts 7:59–60). Contrarily, Paul chose to live. Acts 14:19–20 declares:

> And there came thither certain Jews from Antioch and Iconium, who persuaded the people, and having stoned Paul, drew him out of the city, supposing he had been dead. Howbeit, as the disciples stood round about him, he rose up, and came into the city: and the next day, he departed with Barnabas to Derbe.

On another occasion, he spent a night and a day in the deep, but he came out alive and well (2 Cor. 11:25)! He refused to commit his spirit to death by calling unto God to keep him alive, and God answered him. He committed his life unto God.

First Timothy 1:12 states, "For the which cause I also suffer these things: nevertheless I am not ashamed: for I know whom I have believed, and am persuaded that he is able to keep that which I have committed unto him against that day."

Paul's advice to young Timothy, his son in the Gospel, in this regard is in 2 Timothy 1:14, 2:2, "That good thing which was committed unto thee keep by the Holy Ghost which dwelleth in us… And the things that thou hast heard of me among many witnesses, the same commit thou to faithful men, who shall be able to teach others also."

God's Word Energizes God's Angels to Perform

Isaiah 44:24–26 declares:

> Thus saith the Lord, thy redeemer, and he that formed thee from the womb, I am the Lord that maketh all things; that stretcheth forth the heavens alone; that spreadeth abroad the earth by myself. That frustrateth the tokens of the liars,

and maketh diviners mad; that turneth wise men backward, and maketh their knowledge foolish. That confirmeth the word of his servant, and performeth the counsel of his messengers; that saith to Jerusalem, thou shalt be inhabited; and to the cities of Judah, Ye shall be built, and I will raise up the decayed places thereof.

When you declare the exceeding, great, and precious promises of God that promise eternal life over yourself (2 Pet. 1:3–4), the angels of God will then be activated at God's command to enforce that which you have declared. The angels are ministering spirits sent forth as your messengers. They hearken to the voice of His Word (Ps. 103:20), and as the Father has sent Him (Jesus), so He has sent us. So they are compelled to carry out whatever command we give them.

God has given His angels charge over you to keep you in all of your ways (Ps. 91:11). The Amplified version of Psalms 91:11 states, "For He will command His angels in regard to you, to protect and defend and guard you in all your ways [of obedience and service]."

God's angels are His agents for our preservation, defense, and security. They are there to ward off all evil and devour all plagues. Angels are messengers of destiny. They are God's Salvage Forces. Their job is to bring you out of every danger. Angelic provision is your covenant heritage. Instruct them directly and exactly what you want them to do. This is because God's angels hearken unto the voice of your word (Ps. 103:20). One of the angels came down to deliver Shadrach, Meshach, and Abednego who they trusted in inside the fiery furnace of death and destruction, and another angel of God shut the mouth of devouring lions, even before Daniel was wrongfully placed into their den (Dan. 3:28, 6:22).

The angels of God have a deliverance ministry to you. They are keepers of covenant people and preservers of covenant destinies. They are heaven's firefighters, commissioned to quench the fire and swallow up death in victory. They come as God's rescue agents, and they're always there for you. That is why God said in Psalm 81:10, "Open your mouth wide, and I will fill it." Therefore, say these confessions out loud continuously, receive and believe it, and trust in the faithfulness of God who can never lie (Num. 23:19; 1 Sam. 15:29; Heb. 6:18, Titus 1:2).

No matter how accurate and loud your declarations of long life are, if you doubt, they are rendered ineffective. But when you sincerely trust God for anything you utter, you have committed Him to performing it. While Jacob was blessing Joseph in Genesis 48:15–16, he professed, "God, before whom my fathers, Abraham and Isaac did walk, the God which fed me all my life long unto this day, the Angel which redeemed me from all evil, bless the lads." Remember, Jacob lived up to 147 years because his angels were at work on His behalf.

The angels of many Christians have been redundant since they turned their lives to the Lord because they have never issued a command to those angels that are at their service. God's angels can only be activated in you by your bold and not beggarly command. The Word of God declares, "Concerning the work of my hands command ye me" (Isa. 45:11). We give orders to the angels of God to take action, according to God's Word. Elisha prayed that his enemies should be struck with blindness, and the angels of God assigned to him went into action immediately. Elisha issued the command (2 Kings 6:19–22).

Jesus described the angels as harvesters in Matthew 13:39, "The enemy that sowed them is the devil; the harvest is the end of the world; and the reapers are the angels;" and if the words we speak are seeds, it means the angels harvest our words by bringing them to pass. Your tongue is the key that turns them on. Anything you say is what they do. That is why God warned Moses to "beware of him" (Ex. 23:21). We are also warned in Ecclesiastes 5:6, "Suffer not thy mouth to cause thy flesh to sin; neither say thou before the angel, that it was an error: wherefore should God be angry at thy voice, and destroy the work of thine hands?"

This is a very potent clause in the ministry of angels, and in giving orders to the angels, you must speak life all the time. Say only what God has said. Start putting the angels to work effectively. The supernatural security arranged around you (God's angels) is so impenetrable that even Satan can never access you.

God's Word Cast out Fear

When you live in fear, even God's hands are folded. That does not mean fear won't come, but you have to resist fear by submitting, believing, and confessing God's Word (James 4:7). God couldn't stop the devastation that came upon Job because his fear opened the door to it. Jesus died so "that through death he might destroy him that had the power of death, that is, the devil; And deliver them who through fear of death were all their lifetime subject to bondage" (Heb. 2:14, 15). The fear of death is the weapon Satan uses in afflicting people with death. That is why you must receive, believe, confess, and begin to act on God's Word.

Len Strazewski asked whether sunshine and warm weather will bring an end to face masks, physical distancing, and other pandemic mitigation tactics. He asked because several states in the United States were already easing the stay-at-home orders by the end of May 2020, but according to him, the joy of the release of COVID-19 restrictions would be short-lived. He cited Marc Lipsitch, a professor of epidemiology at the Harvard T. H. Chan School of Public Health and director of the Center for Communicable Disease Dynamics who said that summer may slow the spread of the coronavirus a bit, but it would be back by fall with a second wave that looked a lot like the first wave. Lipsitch said, "Almost every government is talking about lifting control measures. Not every government, but many, because of the economic burdens. Given the fairly high caseloads that we have in the United States, that's a really risky thing to do right now."

Lipsitch added that testing will be important and medical researchers need to learn more about infection rates. He explained that preliminary research indicates that rates may vary widely around the country, and a real understanding may have to wait until comprehensive serological testing. He reiterated that local leaders will need to understand more about who gets infected before they can make good decisions about openings and staying open.

Sociological factors, such as poverty and transportation, may be important determinants in understanding infection, and serological surveys may help in understanding who gets infected and which intervention and mitigation tactics are most valuable. Controlling the virus may call for a return to the tactics that had worked in spring and a continued focus on maintaining resources such as personal protective equipment and increasing viral testing.

Furthermore, Strazewski cited Lipsitch who addressed the social stresses of COVID-19 mitigation and said he would put more resources to mitigating the social effects of these countermeasures, and in addition to improving testing and medical surveillance, he would provide additional resources to "making sure people have enough to eat, making sure education can continue" and mitigating the mental health issues created by the strain of changing lifestyles to fight COVID-19.[156]

Quentin Fottrell reported that Coronavirus cases in the US had surpassed two million and had risen by double-digit percentages in sixteen US states that had loosened restrictions since Memorial Day of the year 2020. She cited the Organization for Economic Cooperation and Development who released its twice-a-year economic outlook on Wednesday and presented two scenarios in which the coronavirus continued to recede and another where a second wave of rapid contagion erupted later in the year 2020. Fottrell stressed that many epidemiologists had advised on exercising more caution when talking about the reduced prospect of a second wave. He also cited Gregory Poland who substantiated this fact with the great influenza pandemic of 1918 where the second wave was worse than the first, partly due to a more virulent strain of the virus. And another complication is that flu and SARS-CoV-2 have almost identical symptoms: fever, coughing, night sweats, aching, tiredness, nausea, and diarrhea in severe cases.

Like all viruses, neither are treatable with antibiotics. They can both be spread through respiratory droplets via coughing and sneez-

---

[156] Len Strazewski, "Harvard Epidemiologist: Beware COVID-19's Second Wave this Fall," AMA Public health, 2020, Accessed June 13, 2020, https://www.ama-assn.org/delivering-care/public-health/harvard-epidemiologist-beware-covid-19-s-second-wave-fall.

ing yet hail from different virus families. There is still no universal flu vaccine, even though scientists have been researching the flu since the 1940s.

According to Fottrell, Poland likens our desire to get back to normal life to the fable of the tortoise and the hare and advocates' clear consistent messaging.

> The race doesn't always belong to the swiftest. The public and political pressure is for a vaccine as soon as possible. Public pressure is not data. Poland explained that approximately 10% to 20% at the very most of the US population will be immune to the new coronavirus next time around. He said, about 70% to 80% of us are immunologically naïve though people think because we hit Memorial Day and we have nice weather that it's over however when coronavirus hit earlier this year, 99% of the seasonal influenza was actually over but this won't happen next time in addition to the fact that they have similar symptoms.

Furthermore, Fottrell cited Mike Ryan who had warned of complacency surrounding relaxation of social distancing measures. Ryan said, "Continue to put in place the public-health and social measures, the surveillance measures, the testing measures and a comprehensive strategy to ensure that we continue on a downwards trajectory, and we don't have an immediate second peak." Additionally, according to health professionals, flattening the curve of new cases through social distancing, testing, and contact tracing will help to avoid overwhelming the health care system during any possible second wave.[157]

---

[157] Quentin Fottrell, "Yes, America Needs to Brace Itself for a Second Wave of Coronavirus," *MarketWatch*, 2020, Accessed June 13, 2020, https://www.marketwatch.com/story/the-coronavirus-only-knows-one-thing-and-that-is-to-infect-another-host-why-america-should-brace-for-a-second-wave-2020-06-10.

While it is good to put up with all the measures outlined by health professionals and to try as much as possible to nullify the fatigue experienced by the lockdown, we must be sure that we do not give room for fear. It's a covenant requirement for long life needed to cancel appointments with death. Psalms 91:5 declares, "Thou shalt not be afraid for the terror by night; nor for the arrow that flieth by day." The trick of the enemy is to capture his God's children with fear. The Scriptures alluded in Proverbs 29:25, "The fear of man bringeth a snare: but whoso putteth his trust in the Lord shall be safe." Fear gave the devil an in-road into Job's life to afflict him. Job confessed, "For the thing which I greatly feared is come upon me, and that which I was afraid of is come unto me" (Job 3:25).

Nicole Brown cited Ron Elfenbein's observation that doctors "don't understand" why some formerly healthy people can have coronavirus symptoms that linger for many weeks or even months. He noted that while most people with mild cases of COVID-19 recover in about two weeks, according to the World Health Organization, some who refer to themselves as "long haulers" suffer debilitating symptoms for much longer, even after initially improving. Brown also cited a recent Dutch study which looked at about 1,600 people who reported coronavirus symptoms, 91 percent of whom were never hospitalized, and found that a vast majority said they continued to suffer health problems like extreme fatigue or shortness of breath nearly three months later.

The average age of the people surveyed was fifty-three. Elfenbein states, "These people reported that they still had symptoms shortness of breath, cough, headache, intermittent fevers, brain fog, trouble concentrating, chest pain, palpitations, things like that that continued for months and months and months."

In explaining the scary part of the findings, Elfenbein noted that when we observe these people, 85 percent of them considered themselves healthy before this happened, and afterward, only 6 percent reported they were healthy, making up everyday people that had no medical problems. Almost half of the people in the study said they could no longer exercise, and about 60 percent said they had difficulty walking, according to the group that commissioned the research.

Elfenbein said, "We really don't understand the science behind this, and we don't really understand the pathophysiology why this is continuing to go on." He also asked, "Could it be that it's your immune response that's causing that? Or could it be that you have some late reactivation of the virus still inside your body, meaning that it's still in there and reactivating from time to time to cause these symptoms?" He added that doctors don't know the answers to those questions yet, and "the big problem" is they don't know how to treat the ongoing symptoms.[158]

Annie Vainshtein observed that if someone is tested too early one day after potential exposure, their viral load may be below the threshold of detection, rendering a negative result, and alternatively, if someone is tested too late when they're at the tail end of their infection; or if they're only shedding a little bit of the virus, the viral load may also be too low to be detected. However, knowing what's early or late for each person depends on the course of that person's symptoms and sickness because this virus is not a typical virus.

Vainshtein documented a nature study which showed peak viral load to be around two days before symptoms onset and that there have also been widely varied timelines given on how long it takes for symptoms to show up after exposure. She stated that on average, people start to get symptoms about five days after they've been infected, but some people are getting sick shortly after exposure while others have seen two weeks pass before experiencing symptoms.

She explained that the outward appearance of the virus neurological issues, blood clots, blue toes, and pneumonia can be as perplexing as its path inside the body as the virus tends to first begin in the nose and the throat but can quickly spread into the lungs. It can also lodge itself along the lining of blood vessels and push even further, damaging and attacking different organs.

---

[158] Nicole Brown, "Doctors 'Don't' Understand Why Some Coronavirus 'Long Haulers' Have Symptoms for Months," *CBS News*, 2020, Accessed June 17, 2020, https://www.cbsnews.com/news/coronavirus-symptoms-long-haulers/.

Vainshtein added that it all depends on when a test is taken as it is possible the virus may have already traveled beyond the original sites of entry, one's nose or throat, and that scientists are beginning to consider whether saliva tests where a patient spits into a cup may be better equipped to detect the virus across the board both in mild cases and reliably over a longer period of time.[159]

Achenbach, et al., observed that the novel coronavirus can be a killer or no big deal, and in some other cases, it can put a person in the intensive care unit on a ventilator, isolated from family, facing a lonely death, or it can come and go without leaving a mark, a ghost pathogen, more rumor than reality. As of June 15, 2020, COVID-19 has killed more than 400,000 people globally, and scientists are still trying to understand the wildly variable nature of COVID-19, the disease caused by the virus.

Achenbach, et al., explained that among scientists' lines of inquiry are whether distinct strains of the coronavirus are more dangerous. Does a patient's blood type affect the severity of the illness? Do other genetic factors play a role? Are some people partially protected from COVID-19 because they've had recent exposure to other coronaviruses? They noted that much of the research remains provisional or ambiguous, and for now, scientists can't do much better than say that COVID-19 is more likely to be worse for older people, often described as over the age of sixty, and for those with chronic conditions such as hypertension, diabetes, lung disease, and heart disease. They also noted that social and demographic factors, including sex, race, ethnicity, income, and access to quality health care play major roles in how this pandemic affects people and who suffers the most. Therefore, the ultimate goal of many researchers is to develop a personalized risk score so that a person who has COVID-19 or remains vulnerable to catching the disease would have some idea of how to navigate the pandemic.

---

[159] Anne Vainshtein, "Why Some People Get Coronavirus Symptoms but Still Test Negative," *San Francisco Chronicle*, 2020, Accessed June 17, 2020, https://www.sfchronicle.com/bayarea/article/Why-some-people-get-coronavirus-symptoms-but-15342542.php.

They added that some children infected with the coronavirus have severe, sometimes fatal Kawasaki-like symptoms which affect multiple organs—"the gut, the heart, the skin, the eyes." They cited health officials in the United Kingdom who had released two different measures of risk. One developed by the National Health Service looks at age, gender, and very granular medical factors such as whether you have preexisting conditions such as high blood pressure or diabetes and those at low risk are asked to social distance as the economy reopens. Those at higher risk are asked to "shield," which means staying inside as much as possible and avoiding contact with others.[160]

Beezy Marsh reported in the Daily Mail that tens of thousands more COVID-19 victims may be identified due to the innovation of a "game-changing" blood test which will offer a potentially massive boost to the battered economy because it can spot 98 percent of cases, even those without symptoms. Marsh noted that scientists fear that existing methods are effective in detecting the virus only in the very sick but that studies show that up to eight in ten cases are so mild that sufferers barely notice they are ill and therefore will not know they have potential immunity.

According to Marsh, Birmingham University's test will put these "hidden" victims on the radar with huge implications for firms, families, and schools and that the test will work by checking for antibodies produced by the immune system when COVID-19 invades cells using its surface "spikes." By doing so, the test picks up many more cases. Marsh cited that the researchers observed that mild victims react to the "spikes," while severe cases seem to react to the virus's main body, and screening for coronavirus has been mired

---

[160] Achenbach, et al., "The Ultimate COVID-19 Mystery: Why Does It Spare Some and Kill Others?" *The Washington Post, Health*, 2020, Accessed June 17, 2020, https://www.washingtonpost.com/health/the-ultimate-covid-19-mystery-why-does-it-spare-some-and-kill-others/2020/06/16/f6acc1a0-ab35-11ea-9063-e69bd6520940_story.html.

in setbacks. There is confusion about general rates of infection and immunity.[161]

Maura Hohman pointed out that medical professionals have been confronting the wide range of symptoms of coronavirus for months and their varying degrees of severity. The World Health Organization estimates that about 16 percent of people with COVID-19 never develop symptoms and can still infect others. According to *Today's* report, those who develop acute respiratory distress syndrome, which is a life-threatening lung injury due to infection, and such had to be hospitalized in the intensive care unit will be more likely to have diminished lung function afterward. She cited another study out of China that discovered from about 20 percent of patients had heart damage during hospitalization, and International Society of Nephrology disclosed that up to 50 percent of people with severe disease develop kidney abnormalities; likewise, other research suggests that more than one-third of patients may experience dizziness, headache, and taste and smell impairment for an indefinite period of time.[162]

God's Word declares in Matthew 12:36, "But I say unto you, that every idle word that men shall speak, they shall give account thereof in the day of judgment." The devil specializes on making men and women use their tongues against themselves. The issue is whether we will choose to experience His blessings and enjoy His presence by trusting in His spoken Word.

God's Word is a living seed. Likewise, so is every word that comes out of your mouth. "The seed is the word of God" (Luke 8:11). And the Bible declares, "While the earth remaineth...seed

---

[161] Beezy Marsh, "The 'Game-Changer' Blood Test: Tens of Thousands More COVID-19 Victims May be Identified Thanks to New Check that Can Spot 98 Percent of Cases, Even in People with No Symptoms," dailymail.com, 2020, Accessed June 17, 2020, https://www.dailymail.co.uk/news/article-8428961/New-blood-test-spot-coronavirus-victims-without-symptoms.html.

[162] Maura Hohman, "90 Days After Coronavirus Diagnosis, 32-year-old Still Has Symptoms: 'So Frustrating,'" *Today*, 2020, Accessed June 17, 2020, https://www.today.com/health/symptoms-covid-woman-has-coronavirus-symptoms-over-90-days-t184406.

time and harvest shall not cease" (Gen. 8:22). Galatians 6:7–8 buttressed, "Be not deceived; God is not mocked: for whatsoever a man soweth, that shall he also reap. For he that soweth to his flesh shall of the flesh reap corruption; but he that soweth to the Spirit shall of the Spirit reap life everlasting."

People who talk problems, sickness, and death always have them, which is why we must be extra careful regarding the use of our tongues. You are not only expected to say it but to also shout it loud. The Bible says, "Let them shout for joy, and be glad" (Ps.35:27). You need to continually say and shout your covenant heritage of long life to terminate every appointment with death either by sickness, disease, or any form of tragedy, and all your enemies will hear and submit themselves to that Word, and this will make them to subsequently fade out of their hiding places in your life and destinies (Ps. 18:44–45).

No power in heaven, on earth, or under the earth should contend for your glorious body which is the temple of the Holy Spirit (1 Cor. 6:16–20). Your body has been prepared for the habitation of the Spirit of God (Heb. 10:5). Jude 1:9 declares, "Yet Michael the archangel, when contending with the devil he disputed about the body of Moses, durst not bring against him a railing accusation, but said, The Lord rebuke thee." The church in the wilderness might be a type of the body of Moses, but we, the New Testament church, are the body of Christ (Rom. 12:5, 1 Cor. 12:27, Eph. 4:12).

As someone who has witnessed God's mighty miracles in my own life and whom God raised from a ghastly car accident back to life by the power of His resurrection life to serve this generation and generations to come, that same God of miracles will deliver you from COVID-19 and any other pandemic in Jesus Christ name. Now is the time to hold on to the Words of Jesus Christ spoken in Revelation 22:20, "He which testifieth these things saith, Surely I come quickly. Amen. Even so, come, Lord Jesus."

Therefore, this book of God's law must not depart from our mouths, but we must meditate on it day and night so as to do all that it requires. This will deliver to us prosperity of the spirit, soul (mind), and body (3 John 2), and we will have good success (Josh. 1:8).

Begin to confess this Word of eternal life for a prosperous long life and a fulfilled life for those who will be caught up to meet the Lord in the air when He returns once a week as you pray unto God.

Receiving Eternal Life in an Abundant Measure: You Will Have What You Say

> And God said, Let us make man in our image, after our likeness: and let them have dominion over the fish of the sea, and over the fowl of the air, and over the cattle, and over all the earth, and over every creeping thing that creepeth upon the earth.
>
> Who is she that looketh forth as the morning, fair as the moon, clear as the sun, and terrible as an army with banners? (Genesis 1:26; Song of Solomon 6:10)

Confess and say, "Father, we are made in your image, and we look exactly like you and through Jesus Christ we have dominion over the sea, earth, and the air. We have dominion over everything, including Satan, sin, death, hell, shame, poverty, sickness, disease, and all the powers of darkness. We are as the morning, fair as the moon, clear as the sun, and terrible as an army with banners of victory and triumph in Jesus Christ name."

> And ye shall serve the Lord your God, and he shall bless thy bread, and thy water; and I will take sickness away from the midst of thee. There shall nothing cast their young, nor be barren, in thy land: the number of thy days I will fulfil. I will send my fear before thee and will destroy all the people to whom thou shalt come, and I will make all thine enemies turn their backs unto thee. And I will send hornets before thee, which

shall drive out the Hivite, the Canaanite, and the Hittite, from before thee. (Exodus 23:25–28)

Confess and say, "Father, we are serving you wholeheartedly, and you have blessed our bread and water. You have taken all sicknesses and diseases from our midst. Nothing will cast her young, nor be barren in our lives, and the number of our days you will fulfil. You have sent your fear before us, and you are destroying all opposition on our path as you make all our enemies to turn their back on us. You have sent hornets before us and you have driven away all the giants that are in our promised land, in Jesus Christ's name."

And I will give peace in the land, and ye shall lie down, and none shall make you afraid: and I will rid evil beasts out of the land, neither shall the sword go through your land. (Leviticus 26:6)

Confess and say, "Father, you have given us peace in this land, and whenever we lie down to sleep, none shall ever make us afraid. You have rid all evil beasts out of our land, and no sword of destruction shall go through our dwelling place, in Jesus Christ's name."

And the cloud of the Lord was upon them by day, when they went out of the camp. And it came to pass, when the ark set forward, that Moses said, Rise up, Lord, and let thine enemies be scattered; and let them that hate thee flee before thee. And when it rested, he said, Return, O Lord, unto the many thousands of Israel.

Surely goodness and mercy shall follow me all the days of my life: and I will dwell in the house of the Lord forever.

A fire goeth before him, and burneth up his enemies round about. His lightnings enlightened the world: the earth saw, and trembled.

Behold, I stand at the door, and knock: if any man hear my voice, and open the door, I will come in to him, and will sup with him, and he with me. (Numbers 10:34–36; Psalm 23:6, 97:3–4)

Confess and say, "Father, as we go out today as your habitation and as the ark of your glory, rise up, and let all our enemies be scattered. Let those who hate us flee before us, and as we return, return with us in your goodness and mercy. The spirit of sin, death, the grave, and hell will not return with us, but only goodness and mercy will always return with us. Let your fire go ahead of us to burn up all enemies, including the last enemy, which is death, and let the light of your Word enlighten us. We open the door of our hearts and life to Jesus Christ, and He is even dining with us right now as we declare His Word, in Jesus Christ's name."

And he stood between the dead and the living; and the plague was stayed.

I am the God of Abraham, and the God of Isaac, and the God of Jacob? God is not the God of the dead, but of the living.

And beside all this, between us and you there is a great gulf fixed: so that they which would pass from hence to you cannot; neither can they pass to us, that would come from thence.

And to Jesus the mediator of the new covenant, and to the blood of sprinkling, that speaketh better things than that of Abel.

We know that we have passed from death unto life, because we love the brethren. He that loveth not his brother abideth in death. (Numbers 16:48; Matthew 22:32; Luke 16:26; Hebrews 12:24; 1 John 3:14)

Confess and say, "Father, you are the God of Abraham, the God of Isaac, and the God of Jacob. You are not the God of the dead. Therefore, we, your people in the land of the living, cannot crossover to the region of the dead because of the great gulf of the cross of Jesus Christ and His blood that is between the living and the dead. His Passover blood is speaking eternal life over us. Jesus Christ, our heavenly high priest after the order of Melchizedek, is standing between the living and the dead, and we know we have eternally passed from the dead to the land of the living through the death, burial, resurrection, ascension, and glorification of Jesus Christ. In Jesus Christ's name."

And it came to pass, that on the morrow Moses went into the tabernacle of witness; and, behold, the rod of Aaron for the house of Levi was budded, and brought forth buds, and bloomed blossoms, and yielded almonds.

I will make an everlasting covenant with you, even the sure mercies of David.

Instead of the thorn shall come up the fir tree, and instead of the brier shall come up the myrtle tree: and it shall be to the Lord for a name, for an everlasting sign that shall not be cut off.

Even unto them will I give in mine house and within my walls a place and a name better than of sons and of daughters: I will give them an everlasting name, that shall not be cut off. (Numbers 17:8; Isaiah 55:3, 13, 56:5)

Confess and say, "Father, thank you for exchanging every thorn in our lives for fir trees and every brier for myrtle trees. This is an everlasting sign to us that cannot be cut off. Thank you for making an everlasting covenant with us, even the sure mercies of David, and for giving us an everlasting name that cannot be cut off. Thank you, Father, for causing our rod to blossom and bud, bringing forth fruits of the spirit, even the fruits of eternal life. In Jesus Christ's name."

Now these are the commandments, the statutes, and the judgments, which the Lord your God commanded to teach you, that ye might do them in the land whither ye go to possess it. That thou mightest fear the Lord thy God, to keep all his statutes and his commandments, which I command thee, thou, and thy son, and thy son's son, all the days of thy life; and that thy days may be prolonged. Hear therefore, O Israel, and observe to do it; that it may be well with thee, and that ye may increase mightily, as the Lord God of thy fathers hath promised thee, in the land that floweth with milk and honey. Hear, O Israel: The Lord our God is one Lord. And thou shalt love the Lord thy God with all thine heart, and with all thy soul, and with all thy might. And these words, which I command thee this day, shall be in thine heart: And thou shalt teach them diligently unto thy children, and shalt talk of them when thou sittest in thine house, and when thou walkest by the way, and when thou liest down, and when thou risest up. And thou shalt bind them for a sign upon thine hand, and they shall be as frontlets between thine eyes. And thou shalt write them upon the posts of thy house, and on thy gates. And it shall be, when the Lord thy God shall have brought thee into the land which he sware unto thy fathers, to Abraham, to Isaac, and to Jacob, to give thee great and goodly cities, which thou buildedst not. And houses full of all good things, which thou filledst not, and wells digged, which thou diggedst not, vineyards and olive trees, which thou plantedst not; when thou shalt have eaten and be full. (Deuteronomy 6:1–11)

Confess and say, "Father, we are keepers of God's Word. Therefore, our years and that of our children and children's children are prolonged. We have received grace to observe to do God's Word. Therefore, we are increasing mightily in the land that flows with milk and honey. By doing God's Word, we have been blessed with great and goodly cities, which we have not built, and houses filled with riches, wealth, and prosperous businesses, which we did not labor for. In Jesus Christ's name."

> And of Asher he said, Let Asher be blessed with children; let him be acceptable to his brethren, and let him dip his foot in oil. Thy shoes shall be iron and brass; and as thy days, so shall thy strength be. (Deuteronomy 33:24–25)

Confess and say, "Father, the blessing of Asher is on our head as the spiritual Israel of God, and so we are acceptable to all our brethren. We have dipped our feet in the oil of God's favor, and our shoes are as iron and brass. As our days are, so is our strength. We are getting stronger more and more by the Word of the Lord. In Jesus Christ's name."

> And now, behold, the Lord hath kept me alive, as he said, these forty and five years, even since the Lord spake this word unto Moses, while the children of Israel wandered in the wilderness: and now, lo, I am this day fourscore and five years old. As yet I am as strong this day as I was in the day that Moses sent me: as my strength was then, even so is my strength now, for war, both to go out, and to come in. Now therefore give me this mountain, whereof the Lord spake in that day; for thou heardest in that day how the Anakims were there, and that the cities were great and fenced: if so be the Lord will be with

me, then I shall be able to drive them out, as the Lord said.

Neither give place to the devil. (Joshua 14:10–12; Ephesians 4:27)

Confess and say, "Father, the Lord Jesus Christ has kept us alive, and we are very strong this day. We have returned to the days of our youth, and we are strengthened with all might according to your glorious power for war to go out and to come in. Therefore, we possess every mountain of sin, death, debt, sickness, disease, shame, poverty, and distress. We drive them out of our lives, and we give the devil no place in our lives and circumstances. In Jesus Christ's name."

Yet a man is risen to pursue thee, and to seek thy soul: but the soul of my lord shall be bound in the bundle of life with the Lord thy God; and the souls of thine enemies, them shall he sling out, as out of the middle of a sling. (1 Samuel 25:29)

Confess and say, "Father, our souls are bound in the bundle of life with the Lord our God, and the souls of all our enemies are slung out as out of the middle of a sling. In Jesus Christ's name."

And the king lamented over Abner, and said, died Abner as a fool dieth?

The fool hath said in his heart, there is no God.

For there is no remembrance of the wise more than of the fool for ever; seeing that which now is in the days to come shall all be forgotten. And how dieth the wise man as the fool. (2 Samuel 3:33; Psalms 14:1; Ecclesiastes 2:16)

Confess and say, "Father, we will not die as a fool. We shall live and declare the works of God in the land of the living. There is God in our life and circumstances. There is God in our going out and coming in. God is for us, and no one can be against us. In Jesus Christ's name."

> So they hanged Haman on the gallows that he had prepared for Mordecai. Then was the king's wrath pacified.
>
> Whoso diggeth a pit shall fall therein: and he that rolleth a stone, it will return upon him.
>
> He that diggeth a pit shall fall into it; and whoso breaketh an hedge, a serpent shall bite him.
>
> In righteousness shalt thou be established: thou shalt be far from oppression; for thou shalt not fear and from terror; for it shall not come near thee. Behold, they shall surely gather together, but not by me: whosoever shall gather together against thee shall fall for thy sake.
>
> This is the purpose that is purposed upon the whole earth: and this is the hand that is stretched out upon all the nations. For the Lord of hosts hath purposed, and who shall disannul it? and his hand is stretched out, and who shall turn it back? (Esther 7:10; Proverbs 26, 27; Ecclesiastes 10:8; Isaiah 14:26–27, 54:14–15, 17)

Confess and say, "Father, let anyone that has dug or is about to dig a pit for us fall and die in that same pit in the order of Haman who built gallows for Mordecai; and let anyone or anything that will want to break the edge of God's fire around us be consumed by God's fire. We are established in righteousness and we are far from the fear of death and terror. They shall not come near us. Those who will gather or have gathered against us have fallen for our sake, and no weapon formed or fashioned against us shall prosper, and every tongue that rises up or have risen up against us in judgment, we condemn. This is our heritage as God's servants, and our righteousness is of God, says the Lord. This is the purpose that is purposed upon the whole earth, and this is the hand of the Lord that is stretched out upon all the nations to help us. For the Lord of hosts hath purposed to fulfill His Word in our lives and circumstances. Who shall disannul it? His victorious and triumphant hand is stretched out on our behalf. Who shall turn it back? No one, Lord. In Jesus Christ's name."

> He shall deliver thee in six troubles: yea, in seven there shall no evil touch thee. In famine he shall redeem thee from death: and in war from the power of the sword. Thou shalt be hid from the scourge of the tongue: neither shalt thou be afraid of destruction when it cometh. At destruction and famine, thou shalt laugh neither shalt thou be afraid of the beasts of the earth. For thou shalt be in league with the stones of the field: and the beasts of the field shall be at peace with thee. And thou shalt know that thy tabernacle shall be in peace; and thou shalt visit thy habitation, and shalt not sin. Thou shalt know also that thy seed shall be great, and thine offspring as the grass of the earth.
>
> What shall be given unto thee? or what shall be done unto thee, thou false tongue? Sharp arrows of the mighty, with coals of juniper. (Job 5:19–25; Psalm 120:3–4)

Confess and say, "Father, Jesus Christ has delivered us from six troubles and even from the seventh. None shall touch us. The Lord has redeemed us from death as a result of famine and war. Also, He has redeemed us from the power of the sword. We are all hid from the scourge of the tongue. We cut these evil tongues with sharp arrows of the Almighty and coals of juniper. We shall never be afraid of any future destruction, and at the face of destruction, plague, and famine, we shall be filled with laughter of conquest and joy. We shall not be afraid of the beasts of the earth. We are already in league with the stones of the field, and all the beasts of the field are at peace with us. We know by divine revelation that our dwelling places shall be in peace, and we shall go in and out safely into our habitation. Sin shall not be traceable to us. We know that all our seeds are very great. They are flourishing like the grass of the earth. In Jesus Christ's name."

> If iniquity be in thine hand, put it far away, and let not wickedness dwell in thy tabernacles. For then shalt thou lift up thy face without spot; yea, thou shalt be stedfast, and shalt not fear: Because thou shalt forget thy misery and remember it as waters that pass away. And thine age shall be clearer than the noonday: thou shalt shine forth, thou shalt be as the morning. And thou shalt be secure, because there is hope; yea, thou shalt dig about thee, and thou shalt take thy rest in safety. Also thou shalt lie down, and none shall make thee afraid; yea, many shall make suit unto thee. (Job 11:14–19)

Confess and say, "Father, by the blood of Jesus Christ and through the mercy of the Most High, iniquity shall not be found in our life, wickedness shall not dwell in our tabernacles. We shall lift up our faces without spot, shame, and defeat, and we are steadfast and are not afraid. We have forgotten past miseries, which is like the waters that pass away by the blood of the Lamb of God. Our ages are clearer than the noonday, and we are shining forth as the morning. We are fully secured in the Lord because there is hope, and we dig into our life the mercy and grace of God, and so we rest in safety. We shall lie down, and none will make us afraid, and many will look to us for help. In Jesus Christ's name."

> If there be a messenger with him, an interpreter, one among a thousand, to shew unto man his uprightness. Then he is gracious unto him, and saith, deliver him from going down to

the pit: I have found a ransom. His flesh shall be fresher than a child's: he shall return to the days of his youth. He shall pray unto God, and he will be favourable unto him: and he shall see his face with joy: for he will render unto man his righteousness. He looketh upon men, and if any say, I have sinned, and perverted that which was right, and it profited me not. He will deliver his soul from going into the pit, and his life shall see the light. Lo, all these things worketh God oftentimes with man. To bring back his soul from the pit, to be enlightened with the light of the living. (Job 33:23–30)

Confess and say, "Father, we have the Holy Spirit who is your messenger, your interpreter, and one among a thousand in our lives living in us. He has shown us your uprightness, and He has been gracious to us, saying that Jesus Christ has paid the ransom for our souls, and we are eternally delivered from going down into the pit. Our flesh is fresher than a child's flesh, and we have returned to the days of our youth. We have prayed unto God, and He is favorable unto us, and we have seen His face with joy. The Lord has rendered unto us His righteousness. He has not only forgiven our sins, but He has also blotted out our transgressions that can never profit us by the blood of Jesus Christ. He has delivered our souls from going down into the pit, and our lives shall see the light of God. The Almighty God has perfected our lives, and we are enlightened with the light of the living. In Jesus Christ's name."

Have mercy on me, O Lord; consider my trouble which I suffer of them that hate me, thou that liftest me up from the gates of death. That I may shew forth all thy praise in the gates of the daughter of Zion: I will rejoice in thy salvation. (Psalms 9:13–14)

Confess and say, "Father, please have mercy on us and consider our trouble, which we suffer of them that hate us. You have lifted us up from the gates of death that we may show forth your praise in the gates of the daughter of Zion. We will eternally rejoice in your salvation. In Jesus Christ's name."

> Consider and hear me, O Lord my God: lighten mine eyes, lest I sleep the sleep of death.
> But I have trusted in thy mercy; my heart shall rejoice in thy salvation. I will sing unto the Lord, because he hath dealt bountifully with me. (Psalms 13:3, 5–6)

Confess and say, "Father, please consider and hear us, and thank you for enlightening our eyes so we will not sleep the sleep of death. We have trusted in your mercy, and our hearts rejoice in your salvation. We are singing unto the Lord because he has dealt bountifully with us. In Jesus Christ's name."

> For thou wilt not leave my soul in hell; neither wilt thou suffer thine Holy One to see corruption. Thou wilt shew me the path of life: in thy presence is fulness of joy; at thy right hand there are pleasures for evermore. (Psalm 16:10–11)

Confess and say, "Father, you will not leave our souls in hell, and you will never allow us, your holy sons and daughters, to see corruption. You have shown us the path of life because in your presence where we live is the fullness of joy. And at your right hand where we sit, there are pleasures forevermore. In Jesus Christ's name."

> The king shall joy in thy strength, O Lord; and in thy salvation how greatly shall he rejoice. Thou hast given him his heart's desire, and hast not withholden the request of his lips. Selah. For thou preventest him with the blessings of

goodness: thou settest a crown of pure gold on his head. He asked life of thee, and thou gavest it him, even length of days for ever and ever. His glory is great in thy salvation: honour and majesty hast thou laid upon him. For thou hast made him most blessed forever: thou hast made him exceeding glad thy countenance. For the king trusteth in the Lord, and through the mercy of the Most High he shall not be moved. Thine hand shall find out all thine enemies: thy right hand shall find out those that hate thee. Thou shalt make them as a fiery oven in the time of thine anger: the Lord shall swallow them up in his wrath, and the fire shall devour them. (Psalm 21:1–9)

Confess and say, "Father, we that you have made kings (Jesus being the King of kings) shall have joy in your strength, and in your salvation, you have given us our heart's desire. You have never withheld the request of our lips. You have blessed us with the blessings of your goodness and set crowns of pure gold on our heads. We have asked life from you, and you have given us eternal life, even length of days forever and ever. Your glory in our lives is great. You have laid upon us honor and majesty and made us most blessed forever. You have made us exceedingly glad with your countenance. We that you have made kings trust in you, the Most High God, and through your mercy, we shall never be moved. Your hand will locate all our enemies, and your right hand will find out all our haters. You will make them like a fiery oven in the time of your anger. You will swallow them up in your wrath, and the fire of your Holy Spirit shall devour them. In Jesus Christ's name."

My times are in thy hand: deliver me from the hand of mine enemies, and from them that persecute me.

> And when Jesus had cried with a loud voice, he said, Father, into thy hands I commend my spirit. (Psalms 31:15; Luke 23:46)

Confess and say, "Father, our times are in your hands, and you have delivered us from the hands of our enemies and from all that persecute us. Into your powerful, gracious, merciful, holy, righteous, protective, and prosperous hands we commit our spirit, soul, body, and destiny. In Jesus Christ's name."

> Behold, the eye of the Lord is upon them that fear him, upon them that hope in his mercy. To deliver their soul from death, and to keep them alive in famine.
> The fear of the Lord tendeth to life: and he that hath it shall abide satisfied; he shall not be visited with evil. (Psalms 33:18–19; Proverbs 19:23)

Confess and say, "Father, your eyes are upon us because we are walking in the fear of God, and we hope in your mercy. You have delivered our souls from death, and you are keeping us alive in famine. Through the fear of the Lord that tends to life, by which we live, we abide and are satisfied, and we cannot be visited with evil. In Jesus Christ's name."

> The Lord knoweth the days of the upright: and their inheritance shall be forever.
> Lord, make me to know mine end, and the measure of my days, what it is: that I may know how frail I am.
> Mark the perfect man, and behold the upright: for the end of that man is peace.
> Likewise, the Spirit also helpeth our infirmities. (Psalms 37:18, 37, 39:4; Romans 8:26)

Confess and say, "Father, you know our days, and you are our inheritance forever and ever. You have made us to know our end, which is the perfection and peace of God, being like Jesus Christ. The Holy Spirit is helping our infirmities, even as we confess your Word right now. In Jesus Christ's name."

> But God will redeem my soul from the
> power of the grave: for he shall receive me. Selah.
> (Psalm 49:15)

Confess and say, "Father, you have redeemed our souls from the power of the grave, and you have received us in Jesus Christ's name."

> For thou hast delivered my soul from death:
> wilt not thou deliver my feet from falling, that I
> may walk before God in the light of the living?
> (Psalm 56:13)

Confess and say, "Father, because you have delivered our soul from death and you have delivered our feet from falling, we are walking before the Lord for the rest of our lives in the light of the living in Jesus Christ's name."

> Let God arise, let his enemies be scattered:
> let them also that hate him flee before him. As
> smoke is driven away, so drive them away: as wax
> melteth before the fire, so let the wicked perish at
> the presence of God. (Psalms 68:1–2)

Confess and say, "Father, arise and shine in our lives, and let all our enemies including sin, death, shame, fear, depression, oppression, affliction, sorrow, intimidation, disgrace, poverty, sickness, and disease be scattered. Drive them away from our lives as smoke is driven away. Let them melt as wax melt before fire, and let them perish by your consuming fire. In Jesus Christ's name."

They go from strength to strength, every one of them in Zion appeareth before God.

For therein is the righteousness of God revealed from faith to faith: as it is written, The just shall live by faith.

But we all, with open face beholding as in a glass the glory of the Lord, are changed into the same image from glory to glory, even as by the Spirit of the Lord. (Psalms 84:7; Romans 1:17; 2 Corinthians 3:18)

Confess and say, "Father, we go from strength to strength as we appear in Zion. We go from faith to faith because we live by the faith of the Son of God, and we go from glory to glory because we are beholding your face from your Word and as we worship you. This is why we are being transformed into the image of the Son of God by the Spirit of the living God. In Jesus Christs' name."

It is of the Lord's mercies that we are not consumed, because his compassions fail not. They are new every morning: great is thy faithfulness.

For great is thy mercy toward me: and thou hast delivered my soul from the lowest hell. (Psalms 86:13)

Confess and say, "Father, thank you because great is your mercy toward us, and thank you because you have delivered our souls from the lowest hell. It is only by your mercies that we are not consumed, and it's your steadfast love that is upholding us every morning and every day of our lives and throughout eternity. In Jesus Christ's name."

The children of thy servants shall continue, and their seed shall be established before thee.

And immediately I was in the spirit: and, behold, a throne was set in heaven, and one sat on the throne. (Psalms 102:28; Revelation 4:2)

Confess and say, "Father, we your servants and our children shall continue, and our seed shall be eternally established in your throne in Jesus Christ's name."

> For thou hast delivered my soul from death,
> mine eyes from tears, and my feet from falling.
> (Psalm 116:8)

Confess and say, "Father, you have delivered our souls from death, our eyes from tears, and our feet from falling in Jesus Christ's name."

> The right hand of the Lord is exalted: the right hand of the Lord doeth valiantly. I shall not die, but live, and declare the works of the Lord. The Lord hath chastened me sore: but he hath not given me over unto death. Open to me the gates of righteousness: I will go into them, and I will praise the Lord. This gate of the Lord, into which the righteous shall enter. I will praise thee: for thou hast heard me, and art become my salvation. The stone which the builders refused is become the head stone of the corner. This is the Lord's doing; it is marvellous in our eyes. (Psalm 118:16–23)

Confess and say, "Father, your right hand is exalted, and it does valiantly in our lives. We shall live and not die. We shall live to declare the works of the Lord in the land of the living. The Lord hath chastened us sore, but He has not given us over unto death. That is why the gates of righteousness are opened unto us, and we have gone into them and we are praising the Lord. The gate of the Lord into which we the righteous have entered is the gate of heaven here on earth. We live to praise the Lord because He has heard us, and He is our salvation. Jesus Christ, the resurrection and the life, and the stone that the builders refused has become the Chief Cornerstone of our lives. Our lives are the Lord's doing, and it is marvelous in our eyes. "In Jesus Christ's name."

> My help cometh from the Lord, which made heaven and earth. He will not suffer thy foot to be moved: he that keepeth thee will not slumber. Behold, he that keepeth Israel shall neither slumber nor sleep. The Lord is thy keeper: the Lord is thy shade upon thy right hand. The sun shall not smite thee by day, nor the moon by night. The Lord shall preserve thee from all evil: he shall preserve thy soul. The Lord shall preserve thy going out and thy coming in from this time forth, and even for evermore. (Psalm 121:2–8)

Confess and say, "Father, you are the maker of heaven and earth, and you do not slumber nor sleep. Our help comes from you, and you are keeping our feet from being moved. You are our eternal keeper and the shade upon our right hand. The sun shall not smite us by day nor the moon by night. You are preserving our spirit, soul, and body from all evil, just as you preserve our going out and coming in eternally. In Jesus Christ's name."

> Behold, how good and how pleasant it is for brethren to dwell together in unity. It is like the precious ointment upon the head, that ran down upon the beard, even Aaron's beard: that went down to the skirts of his garments.
>
> Wherefore when he cometh into the world, he saith, Sacrifice and offering thou wouldest not, but a body hast thou prepared me.
>
> Yet Michael the archangel, when contending with the devil he disputed about the body of Moses, durst not bring against him a railing accusation, but said, The Lord rebuke thee. (Psalms 133:1–2; Hebrews 10:5; Jude 1:9)

Confess and say, "Father, we are the body prepared for Jesus Christ. Therefore, there could not be any contention over our body because our body is not the Old Testament body of Moses (1 Cor. 10:2) but the body of Christ (1 Cor. 12:27). It is impossible for Satan to raise any dispute over the body of Christ. Therefore, Satan cannot raise any dispute over our body. Our body has been redeemed by the blood of the Lamb of God, and we are flowing in His anointing. We are the body of the anointing of Jesus Christ on the earth, In Jesus Christ's name."

> My son, forget not my law; but let thine heart keep my commandments. For length of days, and long life, and peace, shall they add to thee.
>
> She is more precious than rubies: and all the things thou canst desire are not to be compared unto her. Length of days is in her right hand; and in her left-hand riches and honour.
>
> She is a tree of life to them that lay hold upon her: and happy is everyone that retaineth her.
>
> Hear, O my son, and receive my sayings; and the years of thy life shall be many. I have taught thee in the way of wisdom; I have led thee in right paths. (Proverbs 3:1–2, 15–16, 18, 4:10–11)

Confess and say, "Father, we are your sons and daughters, and we do not forget your law, but our heart is keeping your commandments, and this has added unto us length of days, long life, and peace. Your Word is more precious to us than rubies, and all the things we desire cannot be compared to the wisdom of your Word. We are partakers of the length of days that is in your right hand and the riches and honor that is in your left hand. Your Word is a tree of life to us, and we have laid hold upon your Word. We are eternally joyful and happy because we retain her, and the years of our lives shall be many. In Jesus Christ's name."

> There shall no evil happen to the just: but the wicked shall be filled with mischief.
> Therefore being justified by faith, we have peace with God through our Lord Jesus Christ.
> Moreover whom he did predestinate, them he also called: and whom he called, them he also justified: and whom he justified, them he also glorified. (Proverbs 12:21; Romans 5:1, 8:30)

Confess and say, "Father, there shall no evil happen to us because we are justified by the faith of the son of God through the blood of Jesus Christ, and we have peace with God through our Lord Jesus Christ. There will not be any trace of pity in our lives because we are justified to be glorified in Jesus Christ's name."

> In the way of righteousness is life: and in the pathway thereof there is no death.
> The way of life is above to the wise, that he may depart from hell beneath. (Proverbs 12:28, 15:24)

Confess and say, "Father, in the way of righteousness where we walk is eternal life; in that 'Zoe' pathway thereof, there is no death. The way of life is 'above' to us because we are wise, and we depart from hell beneath in Jesus Christ's name."

> He will swallow up death in victory; and the Lord God will wipe away tears from off all faces; and the rebuke of his people shall he take away from off all the earth: for the Lord hath spoken it. (Isaiah 25:8)

Confess and say, "Father, you swallowed up death in victory, and you have wiped away all tears off our faces. Also, you have rebuked all of our enemies, including death which is the last enemy. Your mouth has spoken this, and it cannot be altered. In Jesus Christ's name."

And your covenant with death shall be disannulled, and your agreement with hell shall not stand.

Can two walks together, except they be agreed?

Verily I say unto you, Whatsoever ye shall bind on earth shall be bound in heaven: and whatsoever ye shall loose on earth shall be loosed in heaven. Again, I say unto you, that if two of you shall agree on earth as touching anything that they shall ask, it shall be done for them of my Father which is in heaven.

For the woman which hath an husband is bound by the law to her husband so long as he liveth; but if the husband be dead, she is loosed from the law of her husband. (Isaiah 28:18; Amos 3:3; Matthew 18:18–19; Romans 7:2)

Confess and say, "Father, thank you for destroying every covenant we have with death, knowingly and unknowingly, and thank you for annulling every agreement we have with hell. We are eternally loosed from the same. By redemption through your blood, we are in complete agreement with Jesus Christ who is the resurrection and life, and we are walking together with Him by His Holy Spirit. Therefore, we bind ourselves to His everlasting life here on earth, and it is bound in heaven. And we lose ourselves from the grip of death, the grave, and hell here on earth, and it is loosed in heaven. In Jesus Christ's name."

But they that wait upon the Lord shall renew their strength; they shall mount up with wings as eagles; they shall run, and not be weary; and they shall walk, and not faint.

Keep silence before me, O islands; and let the people renew their strength: let them come near; then let them speak: let us come near together to judgment. (Isaiah 40:31, 41:1)

Confess and say, "Father, as we wait upon the Lord continually, we renew our strength. We mount up with wings as eagles. We run and we are not never weary; we walk and we do not faint. Every evil inner voice and external voice of death and hell is silenced in our lives by the blood of Jesus Christ. In Jesus Christ's name."

Since thou wast precious in my sight, thou hast been honourable, and I have loved thee: therefore, will I give men for thee, and people for thy life. (Isaiah 43:4)

Confess and say, "Father, we are the remnant of Israel, and you are our only God. You birth us from the belly, and you carried us from the womb even to a very old age that is constantly being renewed like the eagles, making us return to the days of our youth. You have promised to carry us till a glorious hoary hair. You are bearing us on your eagle's wing, and you carry us to deliver us from all troubles of this life. You have restored health unto us, and you have healed us of every emotional and physical wound. We are no more called an outcast, forsaken nor desolate. But we are called Hephzibah, and our lives are called Beulah. The Lord delights in us and we are eternally married to Jesus Christ the resurrection and the life. We have exchanged our death for His life, His righteousness for our sins, His health divine life for our sickness and diseases, His joy for our sorrow, His wealth and riches for our poverty, His strength for our weakness, His wisdom for our foolishness by virtue of our marriage to Him through the blood of Jesus Christ. We are one Spirit with Him, and we have been surnamed Jesus Christ. And because He lives, we shall also live in Jesus Christ's name."

Hearken unto me, O house of Jacob, and all the remnant of the house of Israel, which are borne by me from the belly, which are carried from the womb. And even to your old age I am he; and even to hoar hairs will I carry you: I have made, and I will bear; even I will carry, and will deliver you.

Thou shalt no more be termed Forsaken; neither shall thy land any more be termed Desolate: but thou shalt be called Hephzibah, and thy land Beulah, for the Lord delighteth in thee, and thy land shall be married.

For I will restore health unto thee, and I will heal thee of thy wounds, saith the Lord; because they called thee an Outcast, saying, This is Zion, whom no man seeketh after.

Yet a little while, and the world seeth me no more; but ye see me: because I live, ye shall live also. (Isaiah 46:3–4, 62:4; Jeremiah 30:17; John 14:19)

Confess and say, "Father, you have restored health unto us and you have healed us from every emotional and physical wounds. We are no more called outcasts, forsaken, or desolate, but we are called Hephzibah, and our lives are called Beulah. The Lord delights in us, and we are eternally married to Jesus Christ, the resurrection and the life. We have exchanged death for your life, sin for your righteousness, all sickness and disease for your health and divine life, sorrow for your joy, poverty for your wealth and riches, all debts for your debt-free life, weaknesses for your strength, and foolishness for your divine heavenly wisdom. And by virtue of our union with Jesus Christ through His precious blood, we are one spirit with Him. We have been surnamed Jesus Christ, and because Jesus Christ lives, we too live in Him. In Jesus Christ's name."

Thus saith the Lord, As the new wine is found in the cluster, and one saith, Destroy it not; for a blessing is in it: so will I do for my servants' sakes, that I may not destroy them all.

And I will rejoice in Jerusalem, and joy in my people: and the voice of weeping shall be no more heard in her, nor the voice of crying. There shall be no more thence an infant of days, nor an old man that hath not filled his days: for the child shall die an hundred years old; but the sinner being an hundred years old shall be accursed. And they shall build houses, and inhabit them; and they shall plant vineyards, and eat the fruit of them. They shall not build, and another inhabit; they shall not plant, and another eat for as the days of a tree are the days of my people, and mine elect shall long enjoy the work of their hands. They shall not labour in vain, nor bring forth for trouble; for they are the seed of the blessed of the Lord, and their offspring with them. And it shall come to pass, that before they call, I will answer; and while they are yet speaking, I will hear. (Isaiah 65:8, 19–24)

Confess and say, "Father, just as the new wine is found in cluster, and one declares, destroy it not, for a blessing is in it. That is the reason why we cannot be destroyed because God's blessings are domiciled in our lives. By the unfailing Word of the Lord, God's abundant blessings that are in Christ Jesus are overflowing in and through us. Therefore, we cannot be destroyed. The Lord is rejoicing over us, and the voice of weeping or crying shall not be heard in us.

"In our habitation, there shall not be the death of an infant or youth nor an old man that does not fulfill his days. We build houses and inhabit them. We plant vineyards and eat the fruit of them. We shall not build and another inhabit. We shall not plant and another eat. As the days of a tree are, so shall be the days of we, God's people, and we God's elect shall enjoy the works of our hands for a very long time. We shall not labor in vain nor bring forth trouble. Ourselves and our generation are the seed of the blessed of the Lord, and before we call unto God, He would have answered us. And while we are yet speaking, God is manifesting the answer speedily within the twinkling of an eye. In Jesus Christ's name."

> Behold, I will bring it health and cure, and
> I will cure them, and will reveal unto them the
> abundance of peace and truth. (Jeremiah 33:6)

Confess and say, "Father, you have brought us health and cure, and you have given us the revelation and possession of your abundant peace and truth in Jesus Christ's name."

> I will ransom them from the power of the
> grave; I will redeem them from death: O death, I
> will be thy plagues; O grave, I will be thy destruc-
> tion: repentance shall be hid from mine eyes.
> (Hosea 13:14)

Confess and say, "Father, we have been ransomed by the blood of Jesus Christ from the power of the grave. We have been redeemed from death. O death, Jesus Christ is your plague and grave. Jesus Christ is your destruction. Repentance from this by God shall be hid from God's eyes. In Jesus Christ's name."

> And I will restore to you the years that the
> locust hath eaten, the cankerworm, and the cat-
> erpillar, and the palmerworm, my great army
> which I sent among you. And ye shall eat in
> plenty, and be satisfied, and praise the name of
> the Lord your God, that hath dealt wondrously
> with you: and my people shall never be ashamed.
> And ye shall know that I am in the midst of Israel,
> and that I am the Lord your God, and none else:
> and my people shall never be ashamed. Men do
> not despise a thief, if he steals to satisfy his soul

when he is hungry. But if he be found, he shall restore sevenfold; he shall give all the substance of his house.

For the life of the flesh is in the blood: and I have given it to you upon the altar to make an atonement for your souls: for it is the blood that maketh an atonement for the soul.

The thief cometh not, but for to steal, and to kill, and to destroy: I am come that they might have life, and that they might have it more abundantly.

If any man sees his brother sin a sin which is not unto death, he shall ask, and he shall give him life for them that sin not unto death. There is a sin unto death: I do not say that he shall pray for it. (Joel 2:26–27; Proverbs 6:30–31; John 10:10; Leviticus 17:11; 1 John 5:16)

Confess and say, "Father, the enemy has restored in seven-fold everything stolen from our lives, including the years that the locust, cankerworm, caterpillar, and palmerworm have eaten, and we shall never be ashamed. Jesus Christ has come to give us His life in an abundant measure. We all have His eternal life in us in an abundant measure. We cannot sin unto death. We ask life for one another. We are receiving abundant life of God through the flesh and the blood of Jesus Christ from the communion table of the life of the flesh of Jesus Christ that is in His blood. In Jesus Christ's name."

And after six days Jesus taketh with him Peter, and James, and John, and leadeth them up into an high mountain apart by themselves: and he was transfigured before them. And his raiment became shining, exceeding white as snow; so, as no fuller on earth can white them. (Mark 9:2–3)

Confess and say, Father, the Lord Jesus Christ, the resurrection and the life of God is presently praying in and through us, transfiguring all that pertains to us, including our souls, bodies, character, children, marriage, family, finances, ministry, job, businesses, properties, plans, schedule, going out and coming in as we go from glory to glory. Right now, all of us are appearing in glory because we are already transformed into Christ's image. In Jesus Christ's name."

> And he said to them all, If any man will come after me, let him deny himself, and take up his cross daily, and follow me.
>
> I protest by your rejoicing which I have in Christ Jesus our Lord, I die daily.
>
> That I may know him, and the power of his resurrection, and the fellowship of his sufferings, being made conformable unto his death.
>
> And the very God of peace sanctify you wholly; and I pray God your whole spirit and soul and body be preserved blameless unto the coming of our Lord Jesus Christ. (Luke 9:23; 1 Corinthians 15:31; Philippians 3:10; 1 Thessalonians 5:23)

Confess and say, "Father, thank you for revealing yourself to us as we desire to know you, to experience the power of your resurrection and the fellowship of your sufferings that perfect us. We are conformed to the perfect image of Jesus Christ through the death of His cross that continually mortifies our flesh and its affections thereof. This makes us to resurrect daily because we die daily to overcome the lust of the flesh, the lust of the eyes, and the pride of life. In Jesus Christ's name."

> Behold, I give unto you power to tread on serpents and scorpions, and over all the power of the enemy: and nothing shall by any means hurt you.

Ye are of God, little children, and have overcome them: because greater is he that is in you,
than he that is in the world.

Herein is our love made perfect, that we
may have boldness in the day of judgment:
because as he is, so are we in this world. There is
no fear in love; but perfect love casteth out fear:
because fear hath torment. He that feareth is not
made perfect in love. (Luke 10:19; 1 John 4:4:4,
17–18)

Confess and say, "Father, we are perfected in your love because
God's perfect love in us has expelled all sin and fear of death from
our lives. We can never be tormented by fear again because greater
is the Holy Spirit that is in us than the spirit of the devil, sin, death,
grave, shame, poverty, destruction, and fear that is in the world. We
trample over all scorpions, serpents, and every power of the enemy by
the power of the Holy Spirit that is in us, and nothing shall by any
means hurt us. In Jesus Christ's name."

This is the bread which cometh down from
heaven, that a man may eat thereof, and not die.
I am the living bread which came down from
heaven: if any man eats of this bread, he shall live
forever: and the bread that I will give is my flesh,
which I will give for the life of the world.

Then Jesus said unto them, Verily, verily, I
say unto you, except ye eat the flesh of the Son
of man, and drink his blood, ye have no life in
you. Whoso eateth my flesh, and drinketh my
blood, hath eternal life; and I will raise him up at
the last day. For my flesh is meat indeed, and my
blood is drink indeed. He that eateth my flesh,
and drinketh my blood, dwelleth in me, and I in
him. As the living Father hath sent me, and I live
by the Father: so, he that eateth me, even he shall

live by me. This is that bread which came down
from heaven: not as your fathers did eat manna
and are dead: he that eateth of this bread shall
live forever. (John 6:50–51, 53–58)

Confess and say, "Father, you are the bread that comes down
from heaven. We have eaten the 'bread of life' that you are, and we
shall never die but live forever. We are feeding on your flesh and are
drinking your blood, and so we have eternal life in us. Thank you for
raising us up in the last days, and because we are eating your flesh
and drinking your blood, we are dwelling in you, and you are dwelling in us. We live by the life of the Father of our Lord Jesus Christ.
Therefore, we shall live forever. In Jesus Christ's name."

Jesus said unto her, I am the resurrection,
and the life: he that believeth in me, though he
were dead, yet shall he live. (John 11:25)

Confess and say, "Father, we are called by your name, the resurrection and the life, and we are also known by your name. We
respond to your name because of the blood of Jesus Christ, the blood
of the everlasting covenant, and we can never respond to the name
of sin, death, hell, poverty, sickness, disease, and the grave. In Jesus
Christ's name."

I am the true vine, and my Father is the
husbandman.
I am the vine, ye are the branches: He that
abideth in me, and I in him, the same bringeth
forth much fruit: for without me ye can do
nothing.
I can do all things through Christ which
strengtheneth me. (John 15:1, 5, Philippians
4:13)

Confess and say, "Father, you are the Vine, and we are your fruitful branches. The same eternal life flowing in the Vine is flowing in the branches. We abide in you, and your words abide in us. Therefore, we ask for eternal life in an abundant measure, and it is given to us. We can do all things through Jesus Christ who strengthens us. Since death, sickness, disease, poverty, failure, shame, and depression cannot flow inside Jesus Christ, the Vine, they cannot flow in us, the branches as well. As the branches of the Vine, we are firmly attached to the Vine, receiving eternal life from the Vine, and we bring forth much fruit to glorify our Father. In Jesus Christ's name."

> Whom God hath raised up, having loosed the pains of death: because it was not possible that he should be holden of it. (Acts 2:24)

Confess and say, "Father, we have been raised together with Jesus Christ from the dead because God has loosed the pains of death from us, and it is impossible for the spirit of death and the grave to hold us back eternally. In Jesus Christ's name."

> And Peter said unto him, Aeneas, Jesus Christ maketh thee whole.
> Who hath saved us, and called us with an holy calling, not according to our works, but according to his own purpose and grace, which was given us in Christ Jesus before the world began. But is now made manifest by the appearing of our Saviour Jesus Christ, who hath abolished death, and hath brought life and immortality to light through the gospel. (Acts 9:34; 2 Timothy 1:9–10)

Confess and say, "Father, Jesus Christ has made us whole and He has saved us and called us with a holy calling, not according to our works but according to his own purpose and grace, which was given to us in Christ Jesus before the world began. But it's now made manifest by the appearing of our Savior, Jesus Christ, who has abolished death on the cross of Calvary and has brought life and immortality to light through the Gospel. In Jesus Christ's name."

> For in him we live, and move, and have our being; as certain also of your own poets have said, For we are also his offspring.
> To them who by patient continuance in well doing seek for glory and honor and immortality, eternal life. (Acts 17:28: Romans 2:7)

Confess and say, "Father, in Jesus Christ, we live, move, and have our being, and our Redeemer receives all the glory, honor, immortality, and eternal life forever. In Jesus Christ's name."

> For sin shall not have dominion over you: for ye are not under the law, but under grace.
> But if the Spirit of him that raised up Jesus from the dead dwell in you, he that raised up Christ from the dead shall also quicken your mortal bodies by his Spirit that dwelleth in you.
> The eyes of your understanding being enlightened; that ye may know what is the hope of his calling, and what the riches of the glory of his inheritance in the saints. And what is the exceeding greatness of his power to us-ward who believe, according to the working of his mighty power which he wrought in Christ, when he raised him from the dead, and set him at his own right hand in the heavenly places far above all principality, and power, and might, and dominion, and every name that is named, not only in this world, but also in that which is to come. And hath put all things under his feet and gave him to be the head over all things to the church,

which is his body, the fulness of him that filleth all in all. And hath raised us up together and made us sit together in heavenly places in Christ Jesus.

Remember that Jesus Christ of the seed of David was raised from the dead according to my gospel. (Romans 6:14, 8:11; Ephesians 1:18–23, 2:6; 2 Timothy 2:8)

Confess and say, "Father, your Holy Spirit that raised Jesus Christ from the dead dwells in us, and it is giving life to our mortal bodies right now the same way Jesus Christ was raised from the dead by the Holy Spirit according to the Gospel. Therefore, sin, death, sickness, disease, sorrow, poverty, shame, fear, depression, failure, and powers of darkness cannot have dominion over us. We have been made to sit with Jesus Christ in the heavenly places, far above all principalities and powers and might, and every name that is named, and Jesus has placed everything under our feet, including death, the last enemy, by the exceeding greatness of His mighty power which He wrought in Christ Jesus when He raised Him from the dead. In Jesus Christ's name."

For the law of the Spirit of life in Christ Jesus hath made me free from the law of sin and death.

There hath no temptation taken you but such as is common to man: but God is faithful, who will not suffer you to be tempted above that ye are able; but will with the temptation also make a way to escape, that ye may be able to bear it.

[A]gainst such there is no law. (Romans 8:2; 1 Corinthians 10:13; Galatians 5:23)

Confess and say, "Father, you have delivered us from every temptation that is common to man by your faithfulness, and you will not allow us to be tempted above what we can handle. But we trust that you have made a way of escape for us out of every temptation, and this way of escape is Jesus Christ who is the Way. We are operating the law of the spirit of life in Christ Jesus. Therefore, we are free from the law of the sin and death. The fruit of spirit manifesting in our lives has annulled the law of sin and death, and against such, there is no law. In Jesus Christ's name."

> For to be carnally minded is death; but to be spiritually minded is life and peace.
>
> Because the creature itself also shall be delivered from the bondage of corruption into the glorious liberty of the children of God. (Romans 8:6, 21)

Confess and say, "Father, we are not carnally minded but are spiritually minded, and you have delivered us from the bondage of corruption into the glorious liberty of the children of God. In Jesus Christ's name."

> He that spared not his own Son, but delivered him up for us all, how shall he not with him also freely give us all things?
>
> Now unto him that is able to do exceeding abundantly above all that we ask or think, according to the power that worketh in us.
>
> According as his divine power hath given unto us all things that pertain unto life and godliness, through the knowledge of him that hath called us to glory and virtue. (Romans 8:32; Ephesians 3:20; 2 Peter 1:3)

Confess and say, "Father, because you have given us Jesus Christ, you have also given us freely all things that pertain unto life and godliness through your exceeding great and precious promises, and you are working in our lives exceedingly and abundantly above what we ask or think according to the power of your Holy Spirit that is at work in us. In Jesus Christ's name."

> He that spared not his own Son, but delivered him up for us all, how shall he not with him also freely give us all things? Who shall lay anything to the charge of God's elect? It is God that justifieth. Who is he that condemneth? It is Christ that died, yea rather, that is risen again, who is even at the right hand of God, who also maketh intercession for us. Who shall separate us from the love of Christ? shall tribulation, or distress, or persecution, or famine, or nakedness, or peril, or sword?
>
> Nay, in all these things we are more than conquerors through him that loved us. For I am persuaded, that neither death, nor life, nor angels, nor principalities, nor powers, nor things present, nor things to come. Nor height, nor depth, nor any other creature, shall be able to separate us from the love of God, which is in Christ Jesus our Lord.
>
> For if we would judge ourselves, we should not be judged.
>
> [A]nd mercy rejoiceth against judgment. (Romans 8:32–35, 37–39; 1 Corinthians 11:31; James 2:13)

Confess and say, "Father, No one can place any judgment on us, for your mercy upon us rejoices over every evil judgment. We judge ourselves of all sin, iniquity, disobedience, transgression, and wickedness. Son of David, please have mercy on us as you grant us grace, not only to confess our sins but to forsake them all. Because we have judged ourselves, we shall not be judged. Therefore, nothing can separate us from the love of God, which is in Christ Jesus.

"Tribulation, distress, persecution, famine, nakedness, peril, sword, death, life, angels, principalities, powers, things present, things to come, height, depth, or any other creature cannot separate us from the love of God which is Christ Jesus our Lord and Savior. In and through all these things, we are more than conquerors through Him that loved us. In Jesus Christ's name."

> And God hath both raised up the Lord, and will also raise up us by his own power.
> What? know ye not that your body is the temple of the Holy Ghost, which is in you, which ye have of God, and ye are not your own? For ye are bought with a price: therefore, glorify God in your body, and in your spirit, which are God's.
> Christ is the head of the church: and he is the saviour of the body. (1 Corinthians 6:14, 19–20; Ephesians 5:23)

Confess and say, "Father, we have been raised up by your resurrection power that raised up the Lord Jesus Christ from the dead, and through that same power, we are living in your sight (Hosea 6:1–2). Our body is the temple of the Holy Ghost. We are not ours, but we are born of God. We have been bought with the price of the blood of Jesus Christ. Therefore, we glorify God in our spirit, soul, and body, which belong to Jesus Christ who is the head of the church and the Savior of our body. No sickness, disease, or death is permitted to dwell in our body because they cannot dwell together with the Holy Spirit that lives in us. In Jesus Christ's name."

> Who delivered us from so great a death, and doth deliver: in whom we trust that he will yet deliver us.
> Now thanks be unto God, which always causeth us to triumph in Christ, and maketh manifest the saviour of his knowledge by us in every place.

Who hath delivered us from the power of darkness, and hath translated us into the kingdom of his dear Son. In whom we have redemption through his blood, even the forgiveness of sins. And having spoiled principalities and powers, he made a shew of them openly, triumphing over them in it. (2 Corinthians 1:10, 2:14; Colossians 1:13–14, 2:15)

Confess and say, "Father, you have delivered us from so great a death, even from the powers of darkness, and you are presently delivering us. We also trust that you will yet deliver us from every death trap set for us by the enemy. You have translated us into the kingdom of Jesus Christ where there is no sin, death, nor grave, for it is only in you that we have redemption through the blood of Jesus Christ, even the forgiveness of sins. Thank you for spoiling principalities and powers and publicly disgracing them on our behalf. Thank you for causing us to always triumph in Jesus Christ over all enemies, including death, the last enemy. In Jesus Christ's name."

For thou hast been a shelter for me, and a strong tower from the enemy. I will abide in thy tabernacle forever: I will trust in the covert of thy wings. Selah. For thou, O God, hast heard my vows: thou hast given me the heritage of those that fear thy name. Thou wilt prolong the king's life: and his years as many generations. He shall abide before God for ever: O prepare mercy and truth, which may preserve him. So, will I sing praise unto thy name for ever, that I may daily perform my vows.

Honor thy father and mother; which is the first commandment with promise. That it may be well with thee, and thou mayest live long on the earth. (Ephesians 6:2–3, Psalms 61:3–8)

Confess and say, "Father, you are our shelter and a strong tower from the enemy. We are safe in your name, which is a strong tower where we eternally dwell (Prov. 18:10). We abide in your tabernacle forever, and we are dwelling under the shadow of your wings. Thank you, Father, for giving us the heritage of those that fear your name, and because we are firmly joined to you, our life is prolonged by your eternal life. We are your kings, and our years shall be as many generations.

"We are abiding before God forever. We are walking in the prepared mercy and truth of God that preserves our life, and we are singing praise unto the name of the Lord forever as we perform our daily commitment to dwell in God's presence. We honor our spiritual and physical fathers and mothers, and it is well with us. It is well with our soul, and we live a long, prosperous, and Christ-centered life with God's goodness here on earth. In Jesus Christ's name."

But as it is written, Eye hath not seen, nor ear heard, neither have entered into the heart of man, the things which God hath prepared for them that love him. But God hath revealed them unto us by his Spirit: for the Spirit searcheth all things, yea, the deep things of God.

Who hath delivered us from the power of darkness, and hath translated us into the kingdom of his dear Son? In whom we have redemption through his blood, even the forgiveness of sins. Who is the image of the invisible God, the firstborn of every creature? For by him were all things created, that are in heaven, and that are in earth, visible and invisible, whether they be thrones, or dominions, or principalities, or powers: all things were created by him, and for him. And he is before all things, and by him all things consist. And he is the head of the body, the church: who is the beginning, the firstborn from the dead; that in all things he might have the preeminence. For it pleased the Father that in him should all fulness dwell. And, having made peace through the blood of his cross, by him to reconcile all things unto himself; by him, I say, whether they be things in earth, or things in heaven. (1 Corinthians 2:9–10; Colossians 1:13–20)

Confess and say, "Father, you have delivered us from the powers of darkness, and you have translated us into the kingdom of your dear Son, Jesus Christ, and it is in Him we have redemption through His blood, even the forgiveness of sins. He is the image of the invisible God, the firstborn of every creature, and by Him were all things created, including the things that are in heaven, in earth, visible and invisible, whether they be thrones or dominions or principalities or powers. All things were created by Him and for Him.

"Jesus Christ is before all things, and by Him, all things consist. He is the head of the body, the church that we are. He is the beginning and the firstborn from the dead that in all things, He might have preeminence, for it pleases the Father that in Him should all fullness dwell, and having made peace through the blood of His cross, by Him to reconcile all things unto Himself, including our precious life by Him, I say, whether they be things in earth or things in heaven or under the earth. Eyes have not seen, ears have not heard, and it has not entered the heart of man the great things God has prepared for us because we love Him, but the Lord has revealed them to us by His Holy Spirit that dwells in us, for the Spirit of God in us is searching all things. Yea, the deep things of God. In Jesus Christ's name."

For this we say unto you by the word of the Lord, that we which are alive and remain unto the coming of the Lord shall not prevent them which are asleep. For the Lord himself shall descend from heaven with a shout, with the voice of the archangel, and with the trump of God:

and the dead in Christ shall rise first. Then we
which are alive and remain shall be caught up
together with them in the clouds, to meet the
Lord in the air: and so shall we ever be with the
Lord. Wherefore comfort one another with these
words. (1 Thessalonians 4:15–18)

Confess and say, "Father, all of us that are alive and remain at
your Second Coming when you descend from heaven with a shout,
with the voice of the archangel, and with the trump of God shall be
caught up together with those who have died in Christ in the clouds
to meet you in the air, and we will be with you forever. We are comforted by the Holy Spirit with these words. In Jesus Christ's name."

For God hath not given us the spirit of fear;
but of power, and of love, and of a sound mind.
(2 Timothy 1:7)

Confess and say, "Father, you have not given us the spirit of sin,
death, grave, hell, fear, shame, sickness, disease, poverty, sorrow,
destruction, or affliction; therefore, we reject these forces from Satan,
that wicked one, and we embrace the spirit of life, power, love, and
sound mind. In Jesus Christ's name."

Forasmuch then as the children are partakers
of flesh and blood, he also himself likewise took
part of the same; that through death he might
destroy him that had the power of death, that is,
the devil. And deliver them who through fear of
death were all their lifetime subject to bondage.
(Hebrews 2:14–15)

Confess and say, "Father, you partake of flesh and blood in order
to destroy Satan that used to have the power of death, and you have
delivered us who were subjected to bondage through fear of death.

We are now walking in the liberty of the Spirit of the Living God. In Jesus Christ's name."

> For the priesthood being changed, there is made of necessity a change also of the law.
> Who is made, not after the law of a carnal commandment, but after the power of an endless life. For he testifieth, Thou art a priest for ever after the order of Melchizedek. (Hebrews 7:12, 16–17)

Confess and say, "Father, we belong to the everlasting priesthood order of Melchizedek that cannot die. Therefore, we are energized by the power of Jesus Christ's endless life. In Jesus Christ's name."

> Being born again, not of corruptible seed, but of incorruptible, by the word of God, which liveth and abideth forever.
> And the world passeth away, and the lust thereof: but he that doeth the will of God abideth forever. (1 Peter 1:23; 1 John 2:17)

Confess and say, "Father, we are born again not of corruptible seed but of incorruptible by the Word of God, which lives and abides forever. This world and its lusts are passing away, but we doers of God's Word abide forever because we have received God's divine life that is in the Word of God. In Jesus Christ's name."

> Who is he that saith, and it cometh to pass, when the Lord commandeth it not?
> He that hath an ear, let him hear what the Spirit saith unto the churches; To him that overcometh will I give to eat of the tree of life, which is in the midst of the paradise of God.

Blessed are they that do his commandments, that they may have right to the tree of
life, and may enter in through the gates into the
city. (Revelation 2:7, 22:14; Lamentation 3:37)

Confess and say, "Father, it is not possible for anyone to decree
any contrary word against your Holy Word, for our lives and destiny,
and it comes to pass. Only the decree of your Word into our lives and
destiny must be fulfilled in our lives according to God's counsel and
purpose for us. As overcomers, we are all ears to hear what the Holy
Spirit is saying unto the churches. As overcomers in God's church, we
are feeding on Jesus Christ, the Word of God, who is also the tree of
life planted in the midst of God's paradise.

"We bless the name of the Lord for giving us the full right to
the tree of life, Jesus Christ. He has redeemed us by His blood as
kings and priests, and we are reigning with him here on earth. We
have entered the gates and the courts of the new Jerusalem, the city
of God, with thanksgiving, praise, and spiritual worship from our
hearts to the Lord. In Jesus Christ's name."

And God shall wipe away all tears from
their eyes; and there shall be no more death, neither sorrow, nor crying, neither shall there be any
more pain: for the former things are passed away.
And he that sat upon the throne said, Behold, I
make all things new. And he said unto me, write:
for these words are true and faithful. (Revelation
21:4–5)

Confess and say, "Father, you have wiped away all tears from our
eyes, and there is no more death, sorrow, nor crying—neither pain or
shame. For the former things have passed away from our lives, and
right now, you have made all things new. Since this has been written
down with our tongues, which are the pen of the ready writer (Ps.
45:1), our lives are now being read by everyone as a brand-new letter

of the life of Jesus Christ, and your powerful Words in our lives are true and faithful. In Jesus's Christ name."

He that dwelleth in the secret place of the Most High shall abide under the shadow of the Almighty. I will say of the Lord, He is my refuge and my fortress: my God; in him will I trust. Surely, he shall deliver thee from the snare of the fowler, and from the noisome pestilence. He shall cover thee with his feathers, and under his wings shalt thou trust: his truth shall be thy shield and buckler. Thou shalt not be afraid for the terror by night; nor for the arrow that flieth by day. Nor for the pestilence that walketh in darkness; nor for the destruction that wasteth at noonday. A thousand shall fall at thy side, and ten thousand at thy right hand; but it shall not come nigh thee. Only with thine eyes shalt thou behold and see the reward of the wicked. Because thou hast made the Lord, which is my refuge, even the Most High, thy habitation. There shall no evil befall thee, neither shall any plague come nigh thy dwelling. For he shall give his angels charge over thee, to keep thee in all thy ways. They shall bear thee up in their hands, lest thou dash thy foot against a stone. Thou shalt tread upon the lion and adder: the young lion and the dragon shalt thou trample under feet. Because he hath set his love upon me, therefore will I deliver him: I will set him on high, because he hath known my name. He shall call upon me, and I will answer him: I will be with him in trouble; I will deliver him and honor him. With long life will I satisfy him and shew him my salvation. (Psalm 91)

Finally, I strongly believe the reason why you are able to read this book is because it was endorsed by the Lord. He desires to reveal His will regarding victory and an ultimate triumph over the last enemy, which is death unto you. Jesus Christ destroyed death by death on the cross of Calvary, and we must enforce that triumph in our lives. Every encounter with the secret of God brings an added security to the one that has the encounter because every discovery culminates in a delivery. When you discover divine healing, it becomes your natural possession. It is the same thing for protection and access to eternal life to cancel every appointment with death.

COVID-19 reminds us that lasting contentment, security, and happiness is not to be found in this present world system but only in Jesus Christ. Hebrews 11:10 declares concerning Abraham, "For he looked for a city which hath foundations, whose builder and maker is God." As Christians, we must live with the hope of a better world yet to come. However, the essential practice at the moment is to keep our "healthy distance" from others, which does not necessarily mean taking care of ourselves but of others. Our viewpoint and mission must be the common good, and we need to do that which is needful to protect the well-being of others.

The three Christian "must have" virtues are faith, love, and hope. The faith we have in Christ will sustain us because we live by His faith (Hab. 2:4; Rom. 1:17; Gal. 2:20, 3:11; Heb. 10:38). The love for God in our hearts and the love of God we have for others— loving men as Christ loves us—will define who we are because by love, we serve one another, and the world will know us by our love for one another (Gal. 5:6; John 13:34–35). Also, because our hope is in God, we are to move forward in the midst of difficulties (Ex. 14:15; Rom. 4:18, 5:4–5, 8:24–25, 12:12, 15:13).

The COVID-19 pandemic crisis has revealed the enormous social and economic inequality in all nations, but one that is most clearly evident is in the developing nations where people are experiencing the greatest impact of the global pandemic. As God's children, we have a responsibility to help those who are in need now and, as at all times, to build a world where there is justice and equity. Galatians 5:13 declares, "For, brethren, ye have been called unto liberty; only use not liberty for an occasion to the flesh, but by love serve one another."

Friend, you still have a long way to go, so make the most of living for God and to fulfill His purpose for your life. You are not created to die like a beast. You have a heritage of long life in Christ Jesus. Because Jesus lives, we shall live also. No one is permitted to welcome or greet you with a "Goodnight" in the morning, afternoon, or evening. We are sons and daughters of light. This is the day the Lord has made.

We are a "Good morning" people of God and not a "Goodnight" or "Good evening" defeated people. The world had experienced the night season of weeping and sorrow from COVID-19 and previous pandemics, but this is the morning season of the church, and our joy has come in the morning. Therefore, it is imperative for the church of God to awake out of sleep because we are of the day (Ps. 30:5; Rom. 13:11).

First Thessalonians 5:4–8 declares:

> But ye, brethren, are not in darkness, that that day should overtake you as a thief. Ye are all the children of light, and the children of the day: we are not of the night, nor of darkness. Therefore, let us not sleep, as do others; but let us watch and be sober. For they that sleep, sleeps in the night; and they that be drunken are drunken in the night. But let us, who are of the day, be sober, putting on the breastplate of faith and love; and for an helmet, the hope of salvation.

The Lord has declared in Isaiah 34:16, "Seek ye out of the book of the Lord, and read: no one of these shall fail, none shall want her mate: for my mouth it hath commanded, and his spirit it hath gathered them."

You are a child of a glorious destiny and not destitute. You are not created to be unfulfilled. You are not to be terminated until you can say like Simeon, Jesus, Paul, and Peter, "It is finished" (Luke

2:29; John 19:30; 2 Tim. 4:7, 2; Pet. 1:13–14). We are privileged to be a partaker of the divine life of God. Cancelling appointments with death come with covenant responsibilities. Wisdom dictates that we put God's Word to work. Jesus described whosoever hears His sayings and does them is likened to a wise man (Matt. 7:24).

One of the things I have done in this book is to introduce you to the Holy Ghost power that is domiciled inside God's Word. God upholds all things by the Word of His power (Heb. 1:3) because all things are made by the Word, and without the Word was anything made that was made (John 1:1–5). Thank God for science, psychology, governments, and all efforts of men, but if all things were made by the Word and they are made by the Word, then we must reasonably conclude that all things must be and remain under the control of God's Word.

If we are made by the Word, then we must be ruled by God's Word and nothing else. Every other thing must comply, including pandemics, when the Word of God is at work. If our lives and destinies are created by God's Word, then they must be navigated, controlled, and move at the trajectory of God's Word. Every child of God is a tree of righteousness (Isa. 61:3), and every tree needs adequate sunlight for survival, which is simply the process of photosynthesis. Jesus Christ is our Sun of righteousness (Mal. 4:2), and as trees of righteousness, we must adequately expose ourselves (the trees of righteousness) to God's Word (the sun of righteousness with healing in His wings).

Cancelling appointments with death by experiencing long lives that are full of health and vitality or by being caught up to meet Jesus Christ in the air is absolutely dependent on the quality of light we access, believe, and experience from God's Word. Jesus said in Matthew 16:28, "Verily I say unto you, there be some standing here, which shall not taste of death, till they see the Son of man coming in his kingdom." This has been fulfilled and will still be fulfilled in the lives of God's people.

Remember, Isaiah 30:26 declared regarding the days we are living in, "Moreover the light of the moon shall be as the light of the sun, and the light of the sun shall be sevenfold, as the light of seven days, in the day that the Lord bindeth up the breach of his people, and healeth the stroke of their wound." It is time for us to rise and shine with an exponential level of gross light in gross darkness (Isa. 60:1–2).

However, we must never forget that God is greater than the enemy because greater is the Spirit of Jesus Christ that lives in us than all of the devil's evil forces, including COVID-19 and future pandemics that are in the world (1 John 4:4). Our God must be magnified (Psa. 35:27, 40:16), and we must believe, confess, and obey His Word during COVID-19 and a post-COVID-19 world. God's wisdom from His Word dictates to us that nothing must catch God's people by surprise. We must always come to the throne of grace, which is that inner private closet, to obtain mercy and find grace to help us in times of need (Heb. 4:16). We must arm ourselves with God's Word, which is the sword of the Spirit (Eph. 6:17). To walk triumphantly for the Lord will always cause us to triumph in Christ Jesus (2 Cor. 2:14).

I pray that every reader will be ruled and guided by the Word of God so as to fulfill destiny to the fullest and not be terminated by the powers of darkness that have covered the earth. Again, it is time to arise and shine, for our light has come, and the glory of God is risen upon us that we may boldly declare, "The last enemy that shall be destroyed is death... O death, where is thy sting? O grave, where is thy victory? And (Jesus) hath put all things (including death) under his feet (we the body of Christ) and gave him to be the head over all things to the church" (1 Cor. 15:26, 55; Eph. 1:22). Hallelujah!

ABOUT THE AUTHOR

Akintayo Emmanuel is a seasonal global speaker and breaker of the Word of God. He is a geneticist by profession, and a missionary by calling according to the election of grace.